"*Nature-Based Allied Health Practice* is a wonderful and insightful book that explores the transformative power of nature as a t... who has experienced the benefits of outdoor ther... therapist, behavior analyst, and educator, I found ... resource that offers a fresh perspective on the hea... authors expertly weave together personal anecdotes, scientific research, and practical tips to illustrate how being in nature can have a profound impact on our physical, mental, and emotional wellbeing. In addition, the authors highlight the ways in which nature can complement therapeutic interventions in all fields. Who knew that there was such a powerful therapeutic tool waiting for you right outside your door to incorporate into your therapeutic practice."

—Marlene Sotelo, EdD, BCBA-D, MT-BC

"*Nature-Based Allied Health Practice* will transform your perception of the power of nature and its infinite possibilities as a therapeutic tool. Utilizing their extensive knowledge, authors Amy Wagenfeld and Shannon Marder inspire readers to take therapy outdoors (or bring it inside) to increase cognitive function, regulate the sensory systems, and strengthen family ties. This evidence-based and accessible guide is a must-read for those interested in interacting with nature for social, cognitive, and physical wellbeing. Teeming with anecdotes, scientific research, and practical tips, *Nature-Based Allied Health Practice* educates and inspires while providing a fresh approach."

—Amy KD Tobik, Editor-in-Chief, *Exceptional Needs Today*

"Amy and Shannon's inspiring resource beautifully combines theory, evidence, and real-life examples of nature based therapy. It uniquely positions nature-based therapy as an evidence-based intervention across the life span, empowering allied health professionals to confidently partner with nature for the wellbeing of our clients, communities, and ourselves."

—Bronwyn Panter, Nature OT

"In a time of profound mental health needs, *Nature-Based Allied Health Practice* is just what the doctor ordered to help all our patients heal and thrive."

—Mona Hanna-Attisha, Flint pediatrician, author of
*What the Eyes Don't See: A Story of Crisis, Resistance,
and Hope in an American City*

NATURE-BASED
ALLIED HEALTH PRACTICE

of related interest

With Nature in Mind
The Ecotherapy Manual for Mental Health Professionals
Andy McGeeney
Foreword by Lindsay Royan
ISBN 978 1 78592 024 0
eISBN 978 1 78450 270 6

How to Get Kids Offline, Outdoors, and Connecting with Nature
200+ Creative Activities to Encourage Self-Esteem, Mindfulness, and Wellbeing
Bonnie Thomas
ISBN 978 1 84905 968 8
eISBN 978 0 85700 853 4

NATURE-BASED ALLIED HEALTH PRACTICE

Creative and Evidence-Based Strategies

Amy Wagenfeld
and Shannon Marder

Jessica Kingsley Publishers
London and Philadelphia

First published in Great Britain in 2024 by Jessica Kingsley Publishers
An imprint of John Murray Press

1

Copyright © Amy Wagenfeld and Shannon Marder 2024

The right of Amy Wagenfeld and Shannon Marder to be identified as the Authors of the Work
has been asserted by them in accordance with the Copyright, Designs and Patents Act 1988.

A CIP catalogue record for this title is available from the British Library and the Library of Congress

ISBN 978 1 80501 008 1
eISBN 978 1 80501 009 8

Printed and bound in the United States by Integrated Books International

Jessica Kingsley Publishers' policy is to use papers that are natural, renewable and recyclable
products and made from wood grown in sustainable forests. The logging and manufacturing
processes are expected to conform to the environmental regulations of the country of origin.

Jessica Kingsley Publishers
Carmelite House
50 Victoria Embankment
London EC4Y 0DZ

www.jkp.com

John Murray Press
Part of Hodder & Stoughton Limited
An Hachette UK Company

For all the practitioners who have dared to take it outside with their clients, those who have benefitted from receiving therapy outside, and all who, by reading this book, will be inspired to do so in the future. Go outside and reap the benefits that nature offers. It will change your life, for the better.

Contents

Abstracts

Chapter 1: Introduction

This book introduces healthcare professionals, including mental health providers to the value of therapy outdoors and provides straightforward, practical, and doable strategies to consider when facilitating the option of offering therapy services outdoors. The book begins with a chapter discussing important ethical considerations, such as ensuring the client privacy and safety, that are associated with providing therapy outdoors. What follows is an overview of the seminal and current evidence-based research that supports the global benefits of being outdoors and the theories that align with nature and health. The remainder of the book is organized in a developmental, lifespan fashion, beginning with chapters on children and youth and families followed by adolescence, young adulthood, adulthood, and older adulthood. Each of these age spans focuses on the developmental tasks associated with them and specific evidence that supports the applicable client population's connections with being outdoors, in nature. Also featured are personal stories shared by those who love nature and exemplar case narratives with photographs of current therapy programs offered outside and any evidence research that supports these incredible programs that are facilitated outdoors. A concluding chapter provides resources and suggested ways to measure program outcomes, and the Appendix includes program readiness guides.

Chapter 2: Above All, Do No Harm

Ethical philosophy was introduced in the fifth century BCE by the philosopher Socrates. A contemporary definition of ethics is that they are a way to actualize values and to serve as a system of beliefs held by a group that operationalizes what is good and bad or right and wrong. In practice, ethics are used to guide decision making, including how to protect client privacy and confidentiality and facilitate therapy in a safe environment. Protecting client privacy and confidentiality is a high priority in the therapeutic relationship. Practitioners need to be vigilant about providing a safe environment for clients as well as themselves. In short, and above all, practitioners must do no harm. In this chapter, these issues as they relate to ethical practice are explored and contextualized to bringing therapy services outdoors so that both client and therapist can reap the benefits of being in nature.

Chapter 3: Being in Nature Is Good for Your Health

This chapter explores the expansive evidence base that supports the benefits of interaction with nature. While nature is good for health and wellbeing, the intention of this chapter is to expand this perspective of nature being good for health and wellbeing, to nature also being an important tool to improve the therapeutic services that practitioners provide. Ideally, all therapy could be "taken outside," but even when circumstances do not allow for taking it outside, there are still health benefits to bringing the outside indoors. The chapter begins with a brief overview of how nature has been used toward health benefits throughout history. It then describes some of the leading theories that explain the mechanisms for how nature heals. What follows is a sharing of some of the evidence-based research that links nature with health and wellbeing. For organizational purposes, here and throughout the book, the research literature related to the therapeutic benefits of nature at all stages of life is organized by type of benefit such as social-emotional, cognitive, and physical. A set of benefits specific to this chapter and relevant to all clients relates to using nature to promote diversity, equity, inclusion, and justice in our communities and with the clients we serve. The chapter concludes with ideas for adapting a nature-based program to a variety of indoor and outdoor environments.

Chapter 4: Children and Families

Childhood begins at birth and ends with the onset of adolescence at about age 12–13 years. This chapter begins with an overview of the social-emotional, cognitive, and physical developmental tasks associated with childhood, which are intertwined and rely on each other to "build" a resilient child, adolescent, and, ultimately, an adult. The chapter continues by exploring the literature that links nature with childhood development and family enrichment. This is important because research supports that children's social-emotional, language/communication, cognitive, and physical and motor development are enriched through meaningful connections with nature. Many of the findings linking nature with childhood development and family enrichment add an extra layer of authenticity and evidence for setting up an outdoor pediatric therapy program. Integrated into the chapter are examples of child- and family-focused outdoor therapy programs and how they have changed the lives of those they serve, and there are also practical ideas for including nature in a pediatric outdoor therapy program.

Chapter 5: Adolescents

Adolescence is a period of tremendous development and change in preparation for adulthood and future health and wellbeing. It begins with the end of childhood, around age 13, and ends when a person enters young adulthood, around age 18. In this chapter, an overview of the typical tasks of adolescence are provided, and this is followed by a discussion of the impacts of nature-based interventions on adolescents, which are focused on social-emotional health, education, and physical health outcomes. The bottom line is that nature can be a positive mediator in adolescent development, yet there is cause for concern because adolescence is a life period often characterized by declines in physical activity and time spent outdoors, in nature. Examples of adolescent-focused outdoor therapy programs and how they have changed the lives of those they serve are integrated into the chapter, as are practical ideas for including nature in an adolescent outdoor therapy program.

Chapter 6: Young Adulthood

Spanning from ages 18 to 25–30 years, young adulthood is also referred to as emerging adulthood. It is the transition period between adolescence and adulthood and, like all other periods of development, has its unique tasks and challenges. This chapter looks at the developmental tasks associated with young adulthood and how research supports that nature-based experiences positively impact this stage of life with regard to social-emotional, cognitive, and physical development, as well as its potential for future positive engagement with nature in adulthood. In this stage, when brain development is reaching its peak, nature can mediate and buffer the challenges of navigating through young adulthood. Examples of young adult focused outdoor therapy programs and how they have changed the lives of those they serve are integrated into the chapter, as are practical ideas for including nature in a young adult outdoor therapy program.

Chapter 7: Adulthood

Adulthood follows young or emerging adulthood and precedes older adulthood. This developmental period extends from age 30 to 65, which is the longest in human development. Adulthood is for most people a period of "good" physical and mental performance, but how people age is multifactorial. The uncontrollable factors that impact aging, such as biological and genetic, are called primary factors. Secondary aging factors refer to elements such as diet, physical activity, and drug and alcohol consumption, which are within our control. In this chapter, some of these factors that are associated with aging are explored. This chapter also provides an exploration of the expansive evidence base of nature-focused research that has been conducted with adults. Much of the research finds that being surrounded by nature and interacting with natural materials have the capacity to improve multiple health outcomes, including mental and physical health, wellbeing, and cognition during adulthood. Examples of adult-focused outdoor therapy programs and how they have changed the lives of those they serve are integrated into the chapter as are practical ideas for including nature in an adult outdoor therapy program.

Chapter 8: Older Adulthood

Older adulthood is understood to begin at age 65. This number is based on the age most commonly found in the research literature. The chapter explores some of the tasks and challenges associated with older adulthood and common misconceptions that can lead to ageism. This chapter looks at the benefits of nature-based interventions for older adults. It also discusses common chronic conditions and potential accommodations; considers the research that supports the benefits of nature connections for older adults; and takes a closer look at a few nature-based programs that have been developed for older adults. In this stage, when older adults are managing chronic conditions and potentially spending more time in leisure, nature can provide both a welcome respite and be an engaging environment. Examples of older adult focused outdoor therapy programs and how they have changed the lives of those they serve are integrated into the chapter as are practical ideas for including nature in an older-adult outdoor therapy program.

Chapter 9: Program Evaluation

Program evaluation can take on many forms and be conducted for various reasons, including seeking funding and outcomes research. Evaluation is a reflective process, and this chapter offers suggestions for how to engage in both quantitative and qualitative study of outdoor therapy programs. Engaging in an evaluation process offers practitioners an opportunity to step back and think about the impact that a program is making on the lives of those we serve and those with whom we work. Research drives innovation, and the reality is that there have been very few published studies that validate why therapy outdoors provided by licensed healthcare professions, such as music therapy, mental health therapies, occupational therapy, physical therapy, recreational therapy, and speech and language therapy, is important. This chapter offers a call to action for all who are interested in facilitating therapy outdoor programs.

Afterword

The authors describe their respective "This Much I Know" experiences that have shaped their love of nature and commitment to incorporating it into practice.

Appendix: Program Readiness Guides

The Appendix provides practitioners with checklists to set up or modify an existing practice to be outdoors or to bring nature inside.

Acknowledgments

I would like to thank the two most important people in my life. To my husband Jeffrey Hsi for his enduring support and encouragement to take my skills and passion as an occupational therapist in different directions that positively changed my life, I am deeply grateful. To our son, David Hsi, who as a wise 13-year-old quietly encouraged his then overwhelmed Mom to "just go out in your garden for a while," you are the true inspiration for the book. That prescient statement transformed my life, for the better. I love you both, very much.

Amy Wagenfeld

I am grateful to Amy Wagenfeld for encouraging me to join this project and mentoring me through years of education and life events. Thank you to Jesse Marder for supporting my interests and being a solid sounding board. Thank you also to Susan and Dan Marder for providing the space and time to work on the project. And lastly, I would like to thank my grandmothers, Ellen, Peggy, Susan, Ethel, Fern, and Dorothy, for inspiring and fueling my enthusiasm and creativity for all things nature, outdoors, and plant related.

Shannon Marder

About the Authors

Amy Wagenfeld, PhD, OTR/L, SCEM, EDAC, FAOTA, is passionate about providing people of all ages, abilities, and cultures equitable, inclusive, and safe access to therapeutic environments in which to regulate their emotional state, engage in physical activity, learn, socialize, and heal. She is on the faculty of the University of Washington's Department of Landscape Architecture and Boston University's Post Professional Occupational Therapy Doctoral Program and is the Principal of Amy Wagenfeld | Design, a therapeutic design consulting organization. Amy is a Fellow of the American Occupational Therapy Association, holds evidence-based design accreditation and certification (EDAC) through the Center for Health Design, specialty certification in environmental modifications (SCEM) through the American Occupational Therapy Association, and certification in Healthcare Garden Design through the Chicago Botanical Garden. Amy was recently awarded both the American Occupational Therapy Association Recognition of Achievement for her unique blending of occupational therapy and therapeutic design, and the American Society of Landscape Architects' Outstanding Service Award.

Shannon Marder, OTD, OTR/L, is most curious about how nature can cultivate community and create a sense of belonging. She is a veteran of the U.S. Navy and graduated from Boston University with a degree in occupational therapy in which her doctoral capstone focused on nature-based interventions to promote socialization among older adults. She has developed curricula for nature-based education programs. Shannon lives in the Pacific Northwest with her husband and sons. Her clinical interests now lie at both ends of the life course: working with young children and older adults.

Contributing Authors

Our book would not be what it is without the generous contributions from the following people and organizations who care and dared to "take it outside" and have flourished. Your work will undoubtedly inspire others to do so. Thank you so much.

Barefoot OT—Marika Austin, MS, OTR/L

Bird Tales—Kathy Lee, PhD, LMSW, and Jessica Cassidy, LMSW, PhD candidate

Cascade Girl Organization's Bee Heroes America—Sharon Schmidt, PMHNP, Psy.D., Certified Master Beekeeper

Central Oregon Veterans Ranch—Alison Perry, MS, LPC

Clinical Specialist in Neurologic Physical Therapy—Kathryn Palano, PT, DPT, MPH, NCS

Destination Rehab—Carol-Ann Nelson, PT, DPT, NCS, MSCS

Empower SCI—Elizabeth Lima Remillard, MS, OTR/L, LSVT BIG, CRS, Carinne Callahan, MS, PT, ATP, and Jessica Goodine, MS, PT, NCS

Hooves 4 Healing—Laura Ryan, OTD, OTR/L

Leg Up Farm—Maura Musselman, Director of Community Engagement

Metro Music Therapy—Chris Monroe, MM, MT-BC, NMT

Monarch School of New England—Kathryn Perry, MA, OTR/L, HTR (lead contributor)

Mood Walks—Canadian Mental Health Association, Ontario Division

Mountain States Hand and Physical Therapy—Pam Bohling, PT, MHS, OCS

Occupational Therapist—Samora Casimir, OTD, OTR/L

Ocean Therapy—Carly Rogers, OTD, OTR/L, and Nancy Miller

Outdoor Kids Occupational Therapy—Laura Park Figueroa, PhD, OTR/L

OT OuTside—Courtney Boitano OTD, OTR/L, BCBA-D

Pacific Quest—Suzanne McKinney, MA

Park Rx America—Robert Zarr, MD

Promise Ranch—Danielle Braman, MSOT, OTR/L, C/NDT

Positive Strides—Jennifer Udler, LCSW-C

P.R.O.D.U.C.E.—Lauren Telesmanic, OTD, OTR/L, and Antonio Fotino, OTD, OTR/L

Rush Oak Park Hospital's Garden Program—Ryan Durkin, OTD, OTR/L, MBA

Serenity Garden (Rocky Mountain College OTD)—Twylla Kirchen, PhD, OTR/L

The Therapeutic Forest—Hannah Broughton, Co-founder and Managing Director, and Caspian Jamie, Co-founder, Speech and Language and Land Lead Therapist

TimberNook—Angela Hanscom, MOTR/L

Triform Camphill Community—Carol Fernandez, JD

Triune Health & Wellness—Judith Sadora, MA, LMFT

Walk with a Doc—Rachael Habash, MA, and David Sabgir, MD, FACC

Willow Family Wellness OT Services—Amanda Hall, MSc.OT, OT Reg. (Ont.), PMH-C, RYT

Yellowstone Boys and Girls Ranch (Rocky Mountain College OT)—Taylor Clark, OTD, OTR/L

We also extend our profound gratitude to those who shared their beautiful drawings, stories, and connections with nature. "This Much *They* Know" is that nature plays a meaningful role in their lives.

CHAPTER 1

Introduction

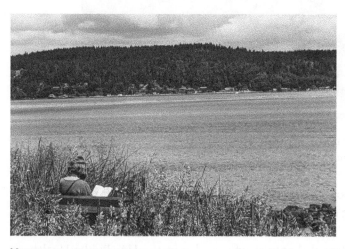

<small>NATURE IS THE GREATEST TEACHER</small>
Photo credit: Rebecca Habtour

Beginning in late 2019, as we faced the challenges of navigating through the mysteries, stresses, and complexities associated with the COVID-19 global pandemic and considered what the new normal may look like, many people turned to nature as a setting in which to exercise, to socialize in responsible ways, to eat, to worship, to learn, and to receive personal services. School administrators began looking at ways to turn school grounds into outdoor classrooms, gyms offered an array of outdoor workouts, outdoor restaurant seating became more common, and even barbers and hairstylists moved salon operations outdoors. What is missing in this lengthy list of "take it outside" innovations? How about therapy services? What if outdoor environments were reconceptualized and reimagined as alternative spaces in which to provide healthcare services? If we look back through archival records, we learn that therapy outdoors is not necessarily a new idea. In their infancy as professions, mental health and occupational therapies were often facilitated in gardens, and going back further, court physicians of ancient times prescribed strolls in the garden to ease stress and angst. We will take a closer look at what the past can tell us about contemporary practice in Chapter 3.

THIS MUCH I KNOW—SAMORA

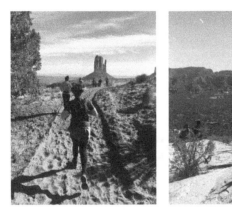

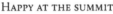

A weekend group hike   Happy at the summit
Photo credits: Samora Casimir

Lieutenant Samora Casimir, OTD, OTR/L, shared, in her own words, how she "takes it outside."

I am an occupational therapist who is also in the U.S. Public Health Service Commissioned Corps, working towards protecting, promoting, and advancing the health and safety of the United States. Pursuing that mission involves providing medical care to various underserved populations, delivering rapid and effective responses to public health needs, and fighting against disease and poor health conditions. During the outbreak of the COVID-19 pandemic, I was working in Red Mesa, Arizona, on a Navajo Native American reservation in a local community outpatient health clinic.

Red Mesa is a stunningly beautiful part of the U.S. It is located within the Four Corners area of the United States (where the borders of Utah, Colorado, Arizona, and New Mexico meet). Red Mesa is approximately three hours northeast of the Grand Canyon and two hours south of Durango, Colorado. Being there was awe-inspiring and humbling, while, at the same time, very isolating. As the clinic's only occupational therapist, I treated clients of all ages by providing individualized one-on-one care and leading small health and wellness groups. While working with the rest of the rehabilitation team, which included physical therapists, we took groups of clients outside for therapy whenever possible. I was working mostly with clients recovering from a stroke or upper-extremity disorders such as carpal tunnel syndrome, trigger finger, shoulder issues, neck and back pain, and various elbow conditions. When addressing the client's holistic health, I found a lot of value in facilitating moderate to vigorous physical activities outside to promote and improve my clients' mental health and physical wellbeing. I discovered that working and just being outside was a positive alternative to the clinical environment; it provided mental relief for the clients, enhanced socialization, and reduced the hospital stigma. The clients enjoyed it much more than being inside, and treatment activities felt more therapeutic and recreational.

In the spring of 2020, I had already been in my position for nearly two years when the COVID-19 restrictions started affecting our lives. The initial fears, ever-changing guidelines, and newly implemented protocols created a situation that felt increasingly isolating. To mediate the loneliness, we went outside. It may seem ironic that initially the large spaces and long distances of the reservation were isolating factors, but that the same vast outdoors became our space to connect. Our therapy staff facilitated 5K walks/runs outside within the community reservation area. We shared the information about the outdoor activities on the local radio stations, posted on the clinic's website and various social media platforms, and shared the details via word of mouth. In addition to walks and runs, I took spin bikes outdoors for small group classes while maintaining six feet between the bikes. Participants reaped the benefits such as safe socializing, stress relief, positive team building, and exercising outside, in addition to physical health benefits such as weight loss and lowered blood pressure.

I believe that part of the reason for the successes I saw in the clinic was due to the connections I fostered outside of the clinic. For example, we invited a client who had "graduated" from all of her occupational and physical therapy sessions to join the rehab team on one of our long weekend hikes. She did not think she could complete the hike, but with some motivation and encouragement, she still joined us. It was great to see her at the end of the hike. She was very grateful that we invited her, that we believed she could do it, and she felt very accomplished. On a larger scale, I participated in numerous outdoor community events and activities such as National Park hikes, health fairs, yard sales on the reservation, and school events. At first, these activities or events may seem trivial, but they were ultimately meaningful and helped me to build relationships with the Navajo community residents. For me it was important to participate in these types of leisure-related activities to learn more about the history and culture of the clients with whom I was working. In addition to my own education, this time outside the clinic also helped me become more grounded in cultural humility, cultural awareness, and cultural sensitivity.

If I were to recommend anything about taking therapy outside, it would be that practitioners can facilitate any type of intervention with just a few needed adaptations. If a client uses a wheelchair, try seated gardening and greenhouse management, host a reading book club outside, lead a meditation or seated yoga hour, or do puzzles and other cognitive activities outside. Why? Because being outside is less stigmatizing than indoor clinical environments and, for many, is much more enjoyable than having an indoor therapy session. And I would also encourage all therapists to practice cultural humility with all clients of diverse ethnic backgrounds and incorporate each client's cultural values into their treatment.

There are good reasons to consider a paradigm shift toward providing therapy outdoors. An ample and ever-increasing body of evidence finds that being in nature improves physical, social-emotional, and mental health. It is also shown to improve cognitive function, regulate the sensory systems, and strengthen family ties. Being in nature is, for many, inspirational, comforting, and restorative.

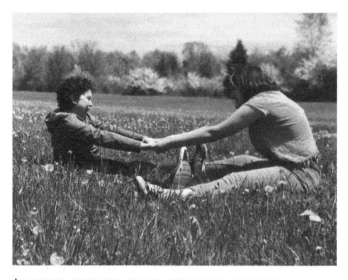

A MOMENT OF SHARED JOY AND INSPIRATION IN NATURE
Photo credit: Nicole Honoré

First Steps

A first step in "taking it outside" is acknowledging that nature matters as it pertains to improved quality of life and health and wellbeing. A next step is to consider that outdoor environments may be an invaluable option for facilitating therapy services. The purpose of this book is to introduce all health professionals, such as social workers, psychologists, occupational, physical, recreational, and speech therapy practitioners, music therapists, athletic trainers, low-vision and blindness practitioners, and other mental health providers to the value of therapy outdoors and to provide straightforward, practical, and doable strategies to consider in facilitating the option of offering therapy services outdoors. Some outdoor programs such as equine, wilderness, or adaptive sports are best facilitated after you have received formal training. Other outdoor therapy programs, such as walking or gardening, do not necessitate any formal training.

In addition to starting a new outdoor or nature-based therapy program, we also advocate for taking your current practice outside. For instance, if you have access to nearby outdoor spaces, when teaching a home exercise program, go outside to practice the repetitions, practice language skills or handwriting activities at a table outside, or practice using adapted utensils to eat during an outdoor picnic. These are small but significant steps to start taking therapy outside in a less formal manner.

While you, the reader, and we, the authors, come to this book identifying as a specific type of health professional, a common umbrella term that we may want to use to describe therapeutic work outdoors is nature therapy. First and foremost, though, it is imperative to acknowledge that you are a licensed provider using the medium of nature therapy within the scope and under the credentials of your practice to improve the health and wellbeing of your clients. It makes such perfect sense! Miyazaki, Song, and Ikei (2015) describe nature therapy as being "a set of practices aimed at achieving 'preventive medical effects' through exposure to natural stimuli that render a state of physiological relaxation and boost the weakened immune functions to prevent diseases" (p.20). This definition bodes well with the overarching goals of therapy and, more so, therapy that involves interaction with nature.

Nature-Based Allied Health Practice is in large part driven by stories. The voices of people of all ages who love nature and the providers who are already "taking it outside" with their clients resonate throughout the book. We want you to feel inspired and empowered to include nature in your respective professional practice. When writing this book, a case narrative provider shared a great quote toward encouraging us to write. Liz Remillard of Empower SCI said, "Be confident and do it; you don't need anyone else's permission. You have the power; give yourself permission to make things happen."

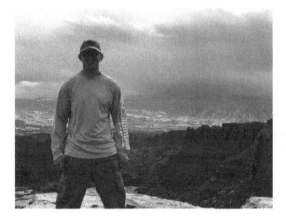

FINDING POWER IN NATURE
Photo credit: David Hsi

Organizing Features

The book begins with a chapter discussing important ethical considerations, such as ensuring client privacy and safety, that are associated with providing therapy outdoors. We review what "do no harm" means and how safety, privacy, and confidentiality take on a whole new level of meaning when therapy is provided outdoors in public spaces. Chapter 3 is an overview of the seminal and current evidence-based research that supports the global benefits of being outdoors and the theories that align with nature and health. The evidence, both self-report studies and physiological biomarker studies, continue to be published at an astonishing rate, and much of it confirms the value of nature as a way to be at our best in body, mind, and spirit. As healthcare practitioners, it is incumbent upon us to constantly be learning in pursuit of providing the best care possible, including learning about innovative practice options such as therapy outside. We continue the chapter by addressing inequities in practice; providing our clients with humble, self-reflective, evidence-based, and client-centered care can be a small step toward righting the inequalities that affect our healthcare and education systems.

The remainder of the book is organized in a developmental, lifespan fashion, beginning with chapters on children, youth, and families followed by adolescence, young adulthood, adulthood, and older adulthood. We focus on the developmental tasks associated with each age range and evidence that supports connections with being outdoors, in nature. A concluding chapter provides resources and suggested ways to measure your program outcomes.

This book also includes several other unique features. They are:

- A series of *Case Narratives*, which are exemplar models of current therapy programs offered outside and the research that supports these programs. The narratives are included in most chapters according to the population that they serve. Each case narrative is accompanied with photographs.
- *Nuggets of Nature*—information linking the positive benefits of nature to health—are included in all chapters. One of these Nuggets of Nature is that exposure to *Mycobacterium vaccae*, a bacterium found in soil, is associated with increased capacity to learn (it is great to get your hands dirty!). Nuggets of Nature are intended to inspire and empower you to take your practice outside. The Nuggets of Nature in the developmental age range chapters also include therapeutic nature-based activities and practical suggestions that, with adaptation, can be applicable to multiple age groups.
- A series of *This Much I Know* testaments are woven into the chapters. These are personal comments and reflections from children, adolescents, young adults, adults, and older adults who are sharing their thoughts about being outside for therapy or simply the joys of experiencing nature and how it is meaningful and purposeful for them. Noteworthy is that we asked children to draw pictures and share a brief explanation of their favorite ways to be in nature. The comments and drawings shared in the developmental-age-range chapters correspond with individuals in that age group.
- An appendix that provides two practical *Readiness Checklists* for two types of outdoor therapy program models. This feature is designed to help you plan, organize, and facilitate the process and ease the transition from indoor to outdoor therapy. The accompanying PDFs can be downloaded from https://library.jkp.com/redeem using the code CCCAPRH.

We invite you to find a cozy place outside or nearby a favorite window and start reading *Nature-Based Allied Health Practice.* And sometime soon, we hope to learn about how you have developed your own unique outdoor or nature-based therapy practice.

CHAPTER 2

Above All, Do No Harm

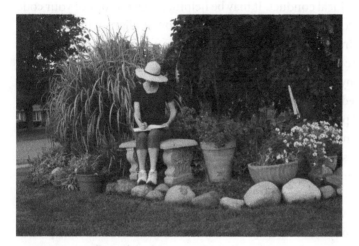

QUIET CONTEMPLATION
Photo credit: Gretchen Ledesma

Introduction

Protecting client privacy and confidentiality is a high priority in the therapeutic relationship. We need to be vigilant about providing a safe environment for clients (the words "client" and "patient" will be used throughout the book) as well as ourselves. In short, above all, we must do no harm. This is a basic but profound ethical principle. Because taking therapy outside adds additional privacy and confidentiality issues that may not arise in traditional practice, as well as the safety realities associated with being outside, it is important to explore ways to minimize these issues so that both client and therapist can reap the benefits of being in nature. Despite any extra strategizing and planning needed to make therapy outside a reality, we want you to be convinced that it is well worth the extra work!

Ethics

If you are a therapist or practitioner reading this book, it is safe to say that your profession has a code of ethics. They often serve as a legal document behooving all of us to practice our respective professions in the most ethical way possible, because ethical practice is a commitment to benefit others, to engage in "genuinely good behaviors," and to "noble acts of courage" (American Occupational Therapy Association [AOTA] 2020, p.i). One side note is that a national professional organization may not enforce the principles in their respective code of ethics. State licensing boards may in fact do so and take legal action if there are proven breaches of ethical conduct. It may be helpful to have a copy of your code of ethics handy as you read this chapter and see how it aligns with the information we are sharing. But first, we need to provide a short historical context of ethics and explore a contemporary vision.

Ethical philosophy was introduced in the fifth century BCE by the philosopher Socrates who believed it to be imperative that everyone receive "rational criticism for their beliefs and practices" (encylopedia.com n.d., para. 1). Some early Greek philosophers also connected the dots between medicine and ethics by describing ethics as "care of the soul" and "art of living" (para. 5). Around this same time, the Hippocratic Oath emerged. Part of the Oath can be summarized as a promise to provide care that "will benefit my patients according to my greatest ability and judgment, and I will do no harm or injustice to them" (History of Medicine Division 2012). To this day, medical professionals often cite the Oath as part of their graduation ceremony. Not only was ethics considered a reflective process guided by feedback from others; it was also a necessary part of medical practice, which we can and do extrapolate to contemporary allied health and mental health practice.

Ethics can be thought of in several ways, including (1) a general pattern or "way of life," (2) a set of rules of conduct or "moral code," and (3) inquiry about ways of life and rules of conduct (encylopedia.com n.d., para. 3). The first concept is more of a spiritual view, the second refers to professional practice, and the third is a more philosophical view of ethics. For our purposes, we are concerned with the view of ethics as a set of rules of conduct. A more contemporary definition of ethics is that they are a means to actualize values and are a system of beliefs held by a group that operationalize what is good and bad or right and wrong, and are used to guide decision making (Gorman 2015).

We look to four principles of ethics described in Tom Beauchamp and James Childress's iconic *Principles of Biomedical Ethics*, first published in 1979. The four principles are respect for autonomy, non-maleficence, beneficence, and justice (Beauchamp and Childress 2019), which are briefly described below.

Respect for autonomy is accepting that the client or patient has the right to make their own choices for treatment if it is within the accepted standards of care. Respect for autonomy also pertains to client confidentiality, privacy, and consent. These are topics that we will come back to shortly as therapy outside could potentially disregard respect for autonomy if it is not facilitated properly.

Non-maleficence is entirely focused on never inflicting harm of any kind on patients or clients. Safety, a reality of outdoor therapy, must take non-maleficence into consideration.

Beneficence requires practitioners to provide therapeutic services that are beneficial to their patients or clients and to do so in a way that avoids or prevents harm. Outdoor therapy has uncontrollable factors such as variations in terrain and weather conditions. When selecting outdoor spaces that meet your client or patient's needs and preparing backup plans for inclement weather, you are taking beneficence into consideration.

Justice pertains to equity and fairness. Every client that we treat, regardless of race, ethnicity, religion, socioeconomic status, sexual orientation, gender identity, age, ability, political view, and/or the insurance policy that they have or do not have, must be afforded the same level of care as everyone else.

Privacy and Confidentiality

In alignment with the ethical principle of respect for autonomy, our clients and patients have the right to privacy and confidentiality as part of the treatment process. This applies to not speaking about them in any identifiable way except when in some type of official treatment meeting. Notes are never to be left out and available for others to read, and never should you photograph them without written permission. These are just a few examples of how we need to apply respect for autonomy. It can become more complex when therapy happens outside rather than in a more self-contained indoor clinic setting where there is more control over who is allowed in the treatment area and who is not. But let's take a step back on this. If you are fortunate enough to have outdoor space as part of the clinic and can install privacy fencing so people cannot peer into the space, then therapy outdoors is an extension of the clinic and there are no additional concerns for maintaining privacy beyond what policies are in place inside the clinic.

If therapy is going to be provided in a public place such as a playground, park, woods, or walking trails, it is a different story because you will have less control to maintain privacy and confidentiality. With that said, many hospitals now have healing gardens on their campuses for family members, patients, and staff to use to rejuvenate, to reflect, and to reduce their stress levels. Spoiler alert: we are going to be spending much more time talking about this in Chapter 3, but for now let's think about these spaces and who uses them. The Legacy Health system in Portland, Oregon, is a superb example of how hospital gardens can be intentionally designed to welcome the public but also serve as a unique place for therapists to take their patients outside for their therapy sessions. It may not be for every patient, but those who elect to have therapy outside do so in the company of the general public. At any given time, you might observe a physical therapist working on ambulation with a patient, a speech therapist and their patient sitting across from each other at a table under a shade canopy having a session, or an occupational therapist working on range of motion and sensory discrimination by having a patient deadhead flowers that are growing on a vertical wall garden. At the same time, staff may be strolling or sitting at tables eating a meal, while community members admire the lush and well-maintained plantings as they move through the garden. While this is a somewhat unusual situation, it works brilliantly, and much kudos is due to the Legacy Health system for their commitment to recognizing the value of nature to promote health and wellbeing.

Let's say that you are electing to use public space for "taking it outside." Jen Udler, the Founder and Director of Positive Strides, shares how she and her team adapt to facilitating their walking therapy in public woodlands in Chapter 7. It involves walking on quieter trails, and if they do encounter someone that they know, there is no acknowledgment or greeting.

Safety

Aligned most closely with the ethical principles of beneficence and non-maleficence is the concept of providing safe therapy. The reality is that being outdoors lacks the predictability that indoor therapy provides. For instance, paving can be rough and bumpy, and the joint spaces between pavers can catch a cane or crutch tip (or high heel!) and lead to a fall. Unpaved paths may be uneven, have divots, rocks, or tree roots that can be a tripping hazard. Playground equipment may be hot to the touch, wood chips may be impossible for wheeled mobility devices to move through, there are insects that may sting and cause adverse reactions, and plants may be toxic. There may not be enough shade for clients to sit underneath and self-regulate. It sounds daunting to try to control for these, but a great deal of forethought and careful consideration of where you are providing therapy and how to prepare your clients to go outside minimizes the safety concerns.

NUGGET OF NATURE: CREATING MEANINGFUL WORKING RELATIONSHIPS

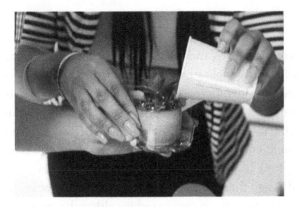

IT TAKES A TEAM TO NURTURE A PLANT
Photo credit: Amy Wagenfeld

When planning a program at an existing facility, some of the first and most important relationships to establish are with the facilities manager or head gardener, and any staff or volunteers who help maintain the facility grounds. Their knowledge base about plants and their care are immeasurable, and a partnership with them can add immense value to your therapy-with-nature program. Your intention should not be to take over their job of maintaining a high level of beauty on the facility grounds. Rather, it is to be respectful and to work together in partnership to have a restorative space in which to facilitate therapy.

Take the time to invite these people to join you for a cup of coffee or tea and share your ongoing vision for a nature-based therapy program. Describe how the foliage, plants, and flowers connect with your intended design to benefit your service users. Explain how you feel a partnership with them will enable clients to reap the benefits of being in nature while receiving their therapies. Just as we strive for interprofessional relationships with other health professions, an equally important interprofessional relationship for any facility-based therapy outdoor program is between therapists and the facilities team.

Shared by Elisabeth Pilgrem, Occupational Therapist, RCOT Merit Award Holder, PDD Social and Therapeutic Horticulture

The bottom line is that you as a therapist need to develop a plan that balances privacy, confidentiality, and safety with the joys of taking it outside, because, above all, we must always do no harm and practice within the ethical guidelines of our professions. To get you started on your journey to taking it outside, we end this chapter with some suggestions for ways to assess risk and facilitate effective, safe, and ethical outdoor therapy.

Risk Assessment

A helpful tool to organize your concerns and manage the challenges associated with providing therapy outdoors is a qualitative risk assessment. Provided below in Table 2.1 is a simplified risk consideration grid, which is based on and adapted from the U.S. Navy's Operational Risk Management system (Naval Postgraduate School n.d.). To use this tool, first spend some time generating a list of potential challenges you could encounter outdoors. Then go through each of the challenges, considering how likely they are to happen and how severe the consequences could be, and assign them a score based on the grid below. Finally, generate a list of mitigating actions you can take to reduce either the probability or the severity of the challenge. It can be helpful to collaborate with a colleague or friend during the process, and it can be rewarding to share your conclusions and plans with supervisors or stakeholders. If you find that the risk cannot be managed, you always have the option to take it outside somewhere else, take it outside another time, or to find a way to bring the outside in.

Table 2.1 Risk consideration grid

			Probability		
			Likelihood of challenge		
			Expected and likely (has occurred many times and may be considered recurrent)	**May occur** (has occurred in the past and can be reasonably expected to occur)	**Not likely** (possible but would be very improbable)
Severity	Consequences of challenge	**Extreme** (death or serious injury)	1	2	3
		Moderate (minor injury)	2	3	4
		Minor (minimal to no injury)	3	4	5

Risk assessment score	Risk assessment level
1–2	High
3	Moderate
4–5	Low

Below are examples of challenges, potential risk assessment scores, and potential mitigating factors.

- **Uneven paving, resulting in a fall—3: moderate risk.** To reduce the likelihood of falling while walking on uneven paving, consider encouraging your clients to wear sturdy shoes, and to use a mobility device if it is medically approved and appropriate. Encourage your client to walk slowly and hold on to a handrail, if available. Before walking, brief your client that there will be uneven paving and that they should watch their step. Ideally, and for safety and communication purposes, whatever path that you choose needs to be wide enough so you and your client can walk side by side.

- **Wood chip paths, resulting in a fall—3: moderate risk.** To reduce the likelihood of falling while walking on a wood chip path, encourage clients to wear sturdy shoes. Consider walking when there is plenty of daylight to improve your client's ability to see the path more clearly. Consider choosing paths that are wide, so that you (the therapist) can always be alongside your client. It is best, though, to avoid wood chip paths entirely. While they are Americans with Disabilities Act (ADA) approved, they can be unnecessarily difficult and frustrating to navigate through.

- **Lack of shade, resulting in sunburn and heat exhaustion—3: moderate risk.** To reduce the consequences of sun exposure, consider carrying an umbrella and using it as a sunshade when needed. Encourage your clients to wear a hat during outdoor activities and to apply sunscreen before meeting. Consider meeting prior to 10 a.m. or after 3 p.m. to avoid the direct overhead sun. To reduce the probability of sunburn or heat exhaustion, reduce the amount of time you spend outside and plan to return to an air-conditioned space. Always carry water bottles for you and your client. The U.S. Centers for Disease Control and Prevention (CDC) website is a resource you can use to help learn more about sun- and heat-related risks: www.cdc.gov/disasters/extremeheat/faq.html.

- **Insect bite, resulting in adverse reaction—4: low risk.** To reduce the risk associated with insect bites, review your client's medical record or ask them if they are allergic to any insect bites and take appropriate precautions as needed, such as carrying and knowing how to use an EpiPen for someone who is allergic to bee stings. Learn about venomous insects in your area. To reduce the probability of a bite, use insect repellent and encourage your client to wear long sleeves and long pants. The U.S. Centers for Disease Control and Prevention (CDC) website is a resource you can use to learn about preventing insect bites: wwwnc.cdc.gov/travel/page/avoid-bug-bites.

- **Lack of available seating, resulting in exhaustion and a fall—3: moderate risk.** To prevent this risk, only choose places where there is seating available, which would require you to preview and screen locations prior to the therapy session. Consider carrying a foldable chair. Ask your clients if they are comfortable sitting on the ground and if they are familiar with fall recovery methods.
- **Seeing familiar people, resulting in a breach of privacy—4: low risk.** Discuss this issue with your clients beforehand and ensure they are comfortable with this risk. Consider choosing a private location, such as the client's backyard, where it is less likely that privacy will be violated.
- **Client has an emotional response, resulting in tears and fatigue—4: low risk.** Guide your client to the nearest seating and allow them the time they need to recompose themselves. Be sure to carry tissues. Consider discussing with them the risk of seeing familiar people, resulting in a breach of privacy beforehand.
- **Client needs to use the restroom—4: low risk.** This is expected, and sites should be selected based on the availability of restrooms and running water. If you are providing wilderness therapy, consult the most relevant literature guiding backcountry etiquette.

With this ethical information in mind, you are now on your way to beginning your journey to taking it outside.

CHAPTER 3

Being in Nature Is Good for Your Health

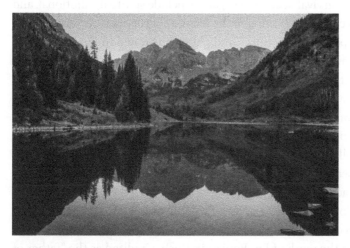

AWE
Photo credit: Chris Monroe

Introduction

You may already have an inkling that experiencing nature can be good for your health—if not, we hope that by the end of this chapter you are convinced. Our intention is also that you see nature as being an important tool to improve the therapeutic services that you provide. Ideally, all therapy could be taken outside, but even when circumstances do not allow for "taking it outside," there are still health benefits to bringing the outside indoors. The chapter begins with a brief overview of how nature has been used toward health benefits throughout history. It then describes some of the leading theories that explain the mechanisms for how nature heals. Then we explore some of the evidence-based research that links nature with health and wellbeing. For organizational purposes, here and throughout the book, the research literature related to the therapeutic benefits of nature is organized by type of benefit such as social-emotional, cognitive, and physical. In this chapter, we address a set of benefits relevant to all clients related to using nature to promote diversity, equity, justice, and inclusion in our communities and with the clients we serve. We close the chapter with ideas for how to adapt a nature-based program to a variety of environments.

Historical Overview

In the earliest days of humanity, nature was essential for survival and subsistence. It was a necessary source for providing food, water, medicine, shelter, and clothing (Beil 2021; Keniger *et al.* 2013). In time, understanding nature's role in our lives grew beyond physical survival needs and began to include spiritual, emotional, and mental health connections. Beginning in the second century BCE, records written by Roman scholars, poets, agronomists, and physicians noted the important relationship between the body and nature, acknowledging it as a pathway to health (Baker 2018). In about 400 BCE, Hippocrates, in his foundational ideals of medical practice, included providing clients with holistic care, which included "drug therapy, diet [recommendations], and physical and mental exercise" (Kleisiaris, Sfakianakis, and Papathanasiou 2014, p.3). Most interesting to us is that Hippocrates' prescribed exercise involved walking outdoors to bring about improved wellbeing. Contemporary evidence-based research fully supports this prescient vision.

Nature-based spaces and gardens have been considered therapeutic since the Middle Ages (Stigsdotter *et al.* 2011). Now, fast-forward about 400 years to the early part of the 19th century, and nature has found its way to the roots of mental health in the U.S. via the work of Dr. Benjamin Rush. Credited as the "father of American psychiatry," Rush deplored the way that individuals with psychiatric conditions were treated, and he lobbied for humane care (Gunderman 2020; Penn Medicine n.d.). Under his tenure at the Pennsylvania Hospital, Rush was instrumental in engaging patients in meaningful tasks such as gardening, and seeing that the hospital grounds included gardens, large swaths of greenery, and paths with walking trails through meadows for patients to experience (Detweiler *et al.* 2012). Likely influenced by Rush's work, "agricultural and gardening activities thus became important elements in both public and private psychiatric hospitals" in the U.S. (p.101).

Using horticulture in a therapeutic capacity to improve the care of veterans took a large step forward during WWI. The enormous number of wounded veterans returning to U.S. hospitals precipitated the start of horticulture use in clinical settings, most notably by occupational therapists, as part of psychiatric and physical rehabilitation.

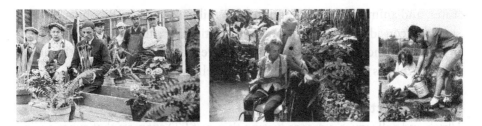

INCORPORATING NATURE INTO OCCUPATIONAL THERAPY
INTERVENTION IS DEEPLY ROOTED IN THE PROFESSION
Photo credit: American Occupational Therapy Association

Moving into the mid-20th century, the Rusk Institute of Rehabilitative Medicine, associated with New York University Medical Center, was the first U.S. medical center to add a greenhouse to its rehabilitation unit in 1959 for interdisciplinary diagnostic and rehabilitative therapy (Detweiler *et al.* 2012, p.101). Unfortunately, after being damaged in 2012 by Hurricane Sandy, the greenhouse was closed. As you will read throughout the book, the practice of infusing nature into therapy, dating back to before the common era (BCE), continues today in many forms and for all people across their lifespan.

Theories Connecting Nature and Health

The ways nature promotes improved health can be described or categorized in many ways; some have sorted the actions into mechanisms such as mitigation, restoration, or instoration—the "perception of restorative potential and outcome without preceding stressors" (Korpela and Ratcliffe 2021, p.2; Pouso *et al.* 2021). Here, we focus on a few powerful restoration theories that have shaped the evidence-based research supporting a relationship between nature and health. The theories include biophilia, stress reduction theory, attention restoration theory, and prospect and refuge theory. All the theories have a bearing on how an outdoor therapy program can be provided, and explanations for why they are important for clients and practitioners alike. As this section provides only a brief overview, interested readers are encouraged to pursue further study of the theories.

Biophilia

E.O. Wilson's theory of biophilia (Wilson 1984) contends that we need nature because it is an essential part of our humanity. People can thrive in nature. Biophilia is also based on the proposition that people have genetically evolved to live in nature, as opposed to living in more modern urban, built environments that limit interaction with nature (Leavell *et al.* 2019). Access to plants, weather, water, and animals all contribute to a biophilic experience. Biophilia can and should be considered when applying therapeutic interventions to promote health or improve function because being in nature and/or interacting with natural materials elicits health benefits simply by their inherent characteristics.

Stress Reduction

Ulrich and colleagues' stress reduction theory (SRT) suggests that experiencing natural environments or viewing nature can reduce a person's experience of stress and may contribute a therapeutic component to recovery from a stressful situation (Ulrich 1984; Ulrich *et al.* 1991). When people are in or view natural environments, they can more quickly recover from the negative health consequences of a stressful experience (Ulrich 1984). In essence, contact with nature may be a buffer or defense to the corrosive psychological and physiological impact of stressful life events (Marselle, Warber, and Irvine 2019). Examples of physiological recovery secondary to nature experiences include reduction in heart rate and blood pressure, reduced sweating, and relaxed muscles (Christiana *et al.* 2021; Corley *et al.* 2021; Leavell *et al.* 2019; Stigsdotter *et al.* 2011; Wolf and Wohlfart 2014). When the SRT is applied to providing care to improve a client's functioning or health, spending time experiencing nature may produce positive health benefits by reducing the client's experience of stress.

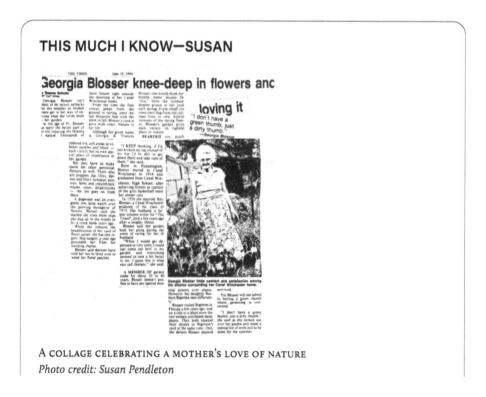

THIS MUCH I KNOW—SUSAN

A COLLAGE CELEBRATING A MOTHER'S LOVE OF NATURE
Photo credit: Susan Pendleton

I grew up in a small village at a time with no computers, internet, smartphones, or social media. Children played outside, all kinds of games, roller skating, etc. I didn't think nature, I lived in it. I gathered wild strawberries growing along a nearby railroad, dug up wildflowers from nearby woods, which my mother planted in her garden, and I spent many summers helping my grandparents in the country. My mother was an amazing gardener; her backyard was full of many varieties of flowers, especially iris. I learned so much from her, not just plants but also birds. Thinking about this, I realize how much these experiences have helped me manage stress. Planting flower beds, having houseplants, watching birds, even the ornery squirrel that tries to dig in my flowerpots—all make life a bit easier.

Attention Restoration

Stephen and Rachel Kaplan's attention restoration theory (ART) suggests that exposure to nature can reduce a person's mental fatigue and restore their ability to attend (Kaplan 1995; Leavell *et al.* 2019). ART proposes that nature can gently fascinate people and that viewing or experiencing nature demands less effort and concentration as compared to a bustling urban, built environment. Thus, when viewing and experiencing nature, a person can more efficaciously recover from mental fatigue (Kaplan 1995; Wolf and Wohlfart 2014). When applied to providing an intervention to reduce dysfunction or promote wellness, spending time viewing and experiencing nature may help clients to softly refocus and thus be better able to engage with their therapy regime.

Prospect and Refuge

Originally proposed by Jay Appleton (1996 [1975]), prospect and refuge theory suggests an evolved survival mechanism in which humans desire and need to have access to spaces that allow them to observe but not to be observed by others. Dosen and Ostwald (2016) describe prospect and refuge as "an allegedly universal, human behavioral and psychological need for places that allow a person to see, but without being seen" (p.9). In the early hunter-gatherer years, occupying these types of spaces was critical for successful hunting. Although we no longer need to subsist on what we hunt, we continue to find comfort in spaces that provide enclosure but also offer opportunities to view the expanse. This preference for enclosure (typically installed on the edge or periphery of an outdoor space, as either permanent or temporary structures) must be considered in outdoor therapy programs, particularly for clients with post-traumatic stress disorder (PTSD) and autism. Time spent in spaces "away" such as tunnels, tents, and other nook spaces allows for self-regulation, composure, and repose.

NUGGET OF NATURE: EQUIGENICS

Equigenics is an important theory that can guide program development. Equigenics refers to places that reduce health inequities. These environments "act to disrupt the usual conversion of socioeconomic adversity to a greater risk of poor health...[and] may include recreational/green areas" (Mitchell *et al.* 2015, p.83). Equigenesis, part of equigenics, also introduced by Dr. Mitchell (2013), is a process of leveling up or down environmental access. An equigenic environment that levels up is understood to benefit those who are disadvantaged more than those who are advantaged, but all people can reap the benefits of the natural space. An equigenic environment that levels down marginalizes those who are advantaged more than those who are disadvantaged. When striving for population health and equity, leveling up is the preferred direction. For example, when conceiving the more desirable leveling-up equigenic effect, access to nature is beneficial to all adults with mental health challenges. Those with mental health challenges who are socially, economically, or otherwise marginalized benefit the most from nature contact; hence, it is critical that they have equitable access to nature, but not at the exclusion of others. This leveling-up effect applies to all groups and populations who experience disadvantage. Many of the clients we serve experience marginalization in some capacity, and therefore the equigenic effect is of great importance, particularly when we consider that interactions between the environment and person are at the heart of how we conceive of health and can impact participation (Dean *et al.* 2018; World Health Organization [WHO] 2001). Dr. Mitchell posed two questions that are worthy of further thought, particularly regarding consideration of the environments in which therapy is facilitated outdoors. He asks, "Can places make us more equally healthy? What features of places might be equigenic?" (Mitchell 2013, para.17).

General Evidence Supporting the Health Benefits of Nature

Until the 1980s there was no evidence-based research to support the value of being in nature, yet there was an intuitive understanding of its value. For instance, Elizabeth Clarke shared in "Gardening as a Therapeutic Experience," published in a 1950 issue of the *American Journal of Occupational Therapy*:

There are many types of activities in which patients may become interested; perhaps one of the most profitable yet relaxing and enjoyable to all those requiring physical exercise is that of gardening. The values derived from gardening, whether the participation is passive or very strenuous, are far reaching and give each person a chance to re-create and express himself. (p.109)

The literature landscape has since changed significantly. Today there is an expansive body of evidence that finds nature contributes to improved health and wellbeing for individuals, groups, and populations (Beil 2021). While there is no clear mechanism to explain why, extensive research shows that nature matters in our lives. What we experience in green or blue spaces can and does recharge and replenish the body and mind (Koh *et al.* 2022; White *et al.* 2013; Yao *et al.* 2022).

Interaction with nature helps reduce stress, increase movement and physical activity, reduce heart rate and blood pressure, and improve a person's capacity to learn, focus, remember, and connect with others (Attwell *et al.* 2019; Christiana *et al.* 2021; Corazon *et al.* 2019; Coventry *et al.* 2021; Howarth *et al.* 2020; Leavell *et al.* 2019; Vella-Brodrick and Gilowska 2022). This line of research got its start from the seminal paper, "View Through a Window May Influence Recovery from Surgery," published in 1984 by Dr. Roger Ulrich. He found that inpatients who were recovering from gallbladder procedures required less pain medication, needed less nursing attention, and were discharged sooner if their hospital room window had a view of green nature as compared to patients whose window looked out onto a brick wall (Ulrich 1984). Since 1984, research has found that every aspect of a person—their mental, physical, and physiological health; their capacity to think, learn, and remember; their sensory wellbeing; their ability to rest and sleep; and their spirituality—is positively impacted by exposure to nature. Where we live or visit also matters as proximity to and/or visiting green and blue natural environments such as parks, forests, gardens, and waterways have been found to be positive factors that influence health and wellbeing (Yeo *et al.* 2020, p.e185). On the other hand, limited access to nature is associated with poorer health and increased stress (Chang and Netzer 2019; Lottrup, Grahn, and Stigsdotter 2013; Pretty, Bragg, and Barton 2006; Shuda, Bougoulias, and Kass 2020).

CASE NARRATIVE: Triune Health & Wellness

Thank you to Ms. Judith Sadora MA, LMFT, for her help in preparing this narrative.

Ms. Judith Sadora MA, LMFT, established Triune Health & Wellness (THW) in 2019 as a systemic psychotherapy clinic to provide psycho-educational workshops, therapy, and experiential ways of healing, for individuals and families. Systemic therapy is an approach that focuses on addressing both intrapersonal issues and relationships between people and groups. Ms. Sadora's clinical practice provides creative ways for clients to heal their trauma and gain a greater sense of self and their communities. Foundational to care is that Ms. Sadora, in her work at THW, understands the implications of generational trauma that affect the wellness of individuals and their families. A longer-term goal of the practice is to facilitate generational healing through quality and effective care. THW addresses generational healing by providing psychotherapy as it relates to each client's mental, physical, and spiritual health. In addition to the holistic nature of Ms. Sadora's practice, THW is rooted in nature-based experiences that are inspired by both her professional experiences in outdoor behavioral healthcare and her personal experiences in nature.

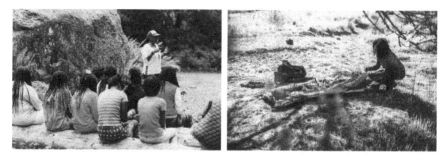

A CAMP TALK   LAYING OUT THE TENT

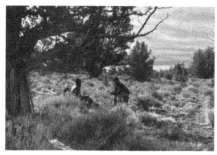 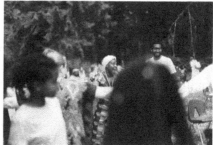

OUTDOOR TALK THERAPY SESSION   SMILES ABOUND IN THE GROUP SESSION
Photo credits: Judith Sadora

Beginning 2017 as an ecotherapist working in the outdoors, Ms. Sadora was impressed by the research illustrating that being outside in nature has positive outcomes related to the mental health of youths and young adults. Then, in 2019, working with wilderness therapy programs, she witnessed beautiful transformations in clients' lives and was amazed. Ms. Sadora appreciated the positive impact that nature-based practices had but identified a lack of inclusion. She noticed that the wilderness therapy programs were predominately run by White, cisgender, heterosexual males, with methods and ways of practice that did not consider other cultures.

Upon deeper reflection, Ms. Sadora recognized that her introduction to nature-based practices was founded in the worldviews, structures, and narratives of Western Euro-American culture. Thinking critically, she found that the existing practices excluded many people who lacked physical or economic access to nature-based practices. She noted that the narratives for "how one is supposed to be in nature and look while being in nature" excluded large swaths of the people in her community. She also observed that the existing narratives ignored the history of colonialism and lacked acknowledgment of its impacts on generational trauma. Furthermore, they failed to recognize the loss of human connection to nature caused by colonialism and the consequential deterioration of wellness. Something needed to change.

Ms. Sadora shared how she has personally grown from these reflections:

My relationship with the outdoors and how it informs the work I do has evolved in many ways and is deeply connected to culture, spirituality, and my ancestral identity. This evolution has been with the help of resources and leaders who shaped my decolonizing lens towards nature (see Murray-Browne [2022] for further information on resources). I am very mindful of my own worldview around my relationship with nature, unlearning the individualistic and conquering narratives that are easily found in Western Euro-American culture. Those narratives, as well as many systemic barriers, have been used to gatekeep who has access to lands and nature. And those narratives have both overshadowed and attempted to erase the narratives of Indigenous cultures, which have been in relationship with nature for centuries. These same Western Euro-American narratives and worldviews have shaped not only how many of us think one should connect with nature, but also the language we use to describe nature, the dress/gear we expect to see or wear in nature, how we communicate with others while we are in nature, and how we perform in nature.

My way of being in my personal life as well as my practice is to be in community. Being out in nature does not have to only be an isolated and individual experience that promotes solitude. I am able to tap into my own ancestral lineage as a Nigerian woman and connect with others on land. I am able to find movement and dance in African traditional practices that my ancestors used in community for a spiritual connection with nature and others. I am able to experience the wonder of music and rhythmic instrumental beats out in nature that allows me to connect with my divine power. I get to reconnect and center a relationship with nature that has been recorded for centuries among Indigenous peoples throughout the African Diaspora and among the global majority across the world.

With appreciation for the power of nature-based therapies and a recognition of its exclusions, she set forth on a new mission: to create change. Ms. Sadora's practice at THW centers on four pillars: culture, nature, community, and spirituality. Research shows that adventure programming with Western Euro-American perspectives struggles to meet the needs of other cultures (Chang *et al.* 2016). Ms. Sadora's mission as a systemic therapist is to slowly create change that supports other cultures and identities in nature-based therapy. She is dedicated to raising her critical consciousness through improved historical knowledge, connections with nature not centered on the Euro-American experience, engagements with local and national communities of people to create a sense of belonging, and deeper understanding of what spirituality means to her and its connection to self, others, and nature.

The core of Ms. Sadora's current practice with clients, whether out in nature or through telehealth, merges elements and concepts of reconnecting to nature and reconnecting with identity as the foundation. In addition to addressing mental health, THW provides care for spiritual health, identity reclamation, and community integration. She primarily works with adolescent youth (predominantly youth of color), adult Black women, and organizations in the community that support Black and/or African communities. Her practice aims to support clients of color, especially those who identify as Black or African, to reconnect with their culture and identity. Often the therapeutic work is toward identity reclamation and community building. The work with community organizations is often with nature-based programs centered around Black and African culture to help youth engage with nature from a wellness, identity, relational, and spiritual perspective. Ms. Sadora finds that building a relationship with nature is often a new experience for the youth with whom she works. She sees that this experience has sadly been erased in Western American society through systemic barriers and the process of objectifying people and land. As a consultant, Ms. Sadora works with existing nature-based programs and teaches the facilitators how to be more effective when working with families in nature, especially families of color.

Ms. Sadora shared a story from a recent collaboration with a local organization: an Ethiopian camp led by mostly Ethiopian adult counselors. She designed and ran an interaction workshop for the camp in the summer of 2022 in Mt. Hood, Oregon. The four-day workshop was organized for a group of 56 transracial adopted teens between 13 and 18 years old. One of the activities Ms. Sadora created involved the teens moving around in the outdoor space while engaging in deep and intentional conversations about class, race, ethnicity, spirituality, religion, sexuality, gender, and education. The teens felt so safe within the outdoor space that they shared stories they had never shared before. The teens talked about the qualities, characteristics, and attributes that make up who they are and how those things relate to a connection within nature and their identities. In another outdoor activity, the teens participated in a coffee ceremony, wore Ethiopian garments, and danced to Ethiopian music.

Ms. Sadora works with one of the teens, who is adopted and Ethiopian, outside of the camp in her practice at THW by providing individual counseling. After the camp experience, Ms. Sadora found that the processing they did together was powerful. The teen shared that they felt a deep connection spiritually that made them feel that they belonged and had an identity that was not connected to being Black as their race. Instead, they acknowledged that race is a social construct and felt more connected to their Ethiopian culture and identity as a whole. It is wonderful that these kinds of nature-based experiences have facilitated an improved sense of belonging, spirituality, and mental health.

When discussing benefits and challenges of outdoor practice, Ms. Sadora shared:

> Benefits look different for different people and cultures. It's really about what being outside means for people. As an Afro-Haitian woman, being outside means connection to God, ancestors, and community. Those connections increase my sense of belonging and rootedness in identity. Research shows interconnectedness to nature involves the experience of belongingness and that nature reflects the inner aspects of self and provides unconditional acceptance of self-discovery (Noar and Mayseless 2020). How I experience belonging is greatly connected to how I engage with the outdoors. When I was first assimilating to the way Euro-American society told me I should connect to nature, I felt disconnected to my identity and didn't feel like I belonged. This is why I deliberately engage Black and African kids in nature that centers their culture.

Ms. Sadora has found that the challenges of going outside are related to access, safety, and a lack of resources. But she also shared that these challenges are overcome by adjusting programming and keeping things simple. "Taking it outside" can be achieved in the simplest ways that do not require many resources—by simply going outdoors.

Ms. Sadora's advice is to educate ourselves on our perceptions and our community's histories. She shared a few questions to think about related to

our biases and knowledge gaps. "Who has access physically and economically to nature? How is someone supposed to *be* in nature? How is someone
supposed to look while being in nature? What communities of color used
to commune with the land and outdoor spaces where we live and work?"
She also offered a few specific examples of how we can reflect before taking
it outside:

> When working with clients and taking them outside, deconstruct what we
> think this is supposed to look like and invite our clients to share any connec-
> tions between culture and nature that they may have. Be open to what our
> clients may share too! Maybe their way of connecting to nature is tending
> an ancestral garden, playing basketball at the park with their friends, taking
> a cleansing bath in the river, doing ceremonies and rituals with community,
> connecting with herbs and medicinal plants, or playing music and dancing
> around a campfire. Our clients may not connect to nature by submitting
> or "conquering" a mountain, going on a long backpacking trek, roughing
> it in primitive ways, or wearing expensive name brand gears to look "out-
> doorsy." There are so many biases and narratives we hold about what we think
> something is supposed to look like, not considering where those narratives
> originated from, so my advice is for each practitioner to do their own work in
> deconstructing their relationship with nature and how they commune with
> it, before taking clients outside.

References

Chang, T.H., Tucker, A., Norton, C., Gass, M., and Javorski, S. (2016) 'Cultural issues in
    adventure programming: Applying Hofstede's five dimensions to assessment and
    practice.' *Journal of Adventure Education and Outdoor Learning 17*, 4, 307–320.
Murray-Browne, S. (2022) 'Courses.' Kindred Wellness. Accessed on 2/12/22 at www.
    shawnamurraybrowne.com/courses
Noar, L. and Mayseless, O. (2020) 'The therapeutic value of experiencing spirituality in
    nature.' *Spirituality in Clinical Practice 7*, 2, 114–133.

The Whole Person: Mind and Body Effects of Nature
Social-emotional: *Feeling*

Much of the research on the positive health outcomes from nature-based interactions focuses on the *social-emotional benefits*. Some of these general findings
include that participating in nature-based experiences increased a person's
socialization and reduced their sense of loneliness and isolation (Anderson 2019;
Brown *et al.* 2004; Irvine *et al.* 2021). Engaging in social nature-based activities

such as community gardening and walking groups enhanced participants' sense of belonging (Hawkins *et al.* 2013; Ireland *et al.* 2019). A provider serving individuals experiencing any type of marginalization or exclusion may find these results particularly important, noting that nature can serve as a moderating factor for the detrimental effects of loneliness and isolation.

NUGGET OF NATURE: THE EFFECTS OF LONELINESS

As articulated by U.S. Surgeon General Vivek Murthy, the effects of loneliness on a person's mortality are equal to that of smoking 15 cigarettes a day and are more detrimental than being obese or living a sedentary lifestyle (Scheimer and Chakrabarti 2020). Specific to adults and older adults, loneliness and social isolation are associated with depression, anxiety, cognitive decline, cardiovascular disease, respiratory conditions, lower immunity, and premature mortality (Courtin and Knapp 2017; Holt-Lunstad 2017; Landeiro *et al.* 2017; Malcolm, Frost, and Cowie 2019; Singer 2018; Smith 2012). In addition to the personal costs, the consequences of loneliness and social isolation cost the U.S. government $6.7 billion a year in medical expenses (Flowers *et al.* 2017).

Loneliness and social isolation may also lead to poor sleep quality and decreased occupational performance in social participation, health management, functional mobility, activities of daily living, and instrumental activities of daily living (AOTA 2017; Shankar *et al.* 2017). Social isolation—as understood as a lack of social participation—could also be considered a form of occupational deprivation (Whiteford 2000).

Many studies have identified a relationship between increased time involved with nature and stress reduction (Corazon *et al.* 2019; Coventry *et al.* 2021; Lottrup *et al.* 2013; Marselle *et al.* 2019; Shuda *et al.* 2020). Strong evidence finds that active and passive experiences with nature, such as walking in or viewing it, decreases depression, rumination, and anxiety, and improves health-related quality of life, sense of self-esteem, and resilience (Adams and Morgan 2018; Birch, Rishbeth, and Payne 2020; Bratman *et al.* 2019; Coventry *et al.* 2021; Pouso *et al.* 2021; Rogerson *et al.* 2020; Tillmann *et al.* 2018). While the prescriptive "dose" of daily or weekly nature exposure varies throughout the body of research, from 20 minutes a day to two hours per week, what is undisputed is that we feel calmer and restored during and after nature experiences (Barton and Pretty 2010; Klotz, McClean, and Yim 2020; Rogerson *et al.* 2020; Shanahan, Bush *et al.* 2016; White *et al.* 2019).

THIS MUCH I KNOW—GABACCIA

Growing up as a brown girl in México, I was constantly discriminated against because of colorism in my community. I remember locking myself in my grandmother's bathroom to cry about not having porcelain skin, wondering why God, who everyone kept saying was good, had then punished me with melanated skin. The bleaching lotions never worked, and by my teens, I had learned to live with self-hatred and self-consciousness about the color of my skin. Cut to a hunting trip with my dad when I was 14. We arrived at the hunting ranch on a chilly and starry night. I remember looking up to see the Milky Way for the first time. I felt so small. But I also felt very special witnessing and realizing the universe's immensity. We spent five days in the Mayan jungle tracking jaguars for fun and tracking deer to hunt. I felt happy and peaceful being out there amidst the smell of humid greenery and sheep and wild hogs. When I came home to my diary retelling my grand adventure, I realized that for the first time in my life, I hadn't had to compensate for being brown. I could be myself without worrying about having perfect hair, grades, or anything to "make up" for having dark skin. For five whole days, I had just been me. Nature did not care that I had dark skin; she had made me this way, and she had reminded me that I have a safe place to just be.

Cognitive: *Thinking and knowing*

Starting in our early childhood and throughout life, interaction and connections with nature support cognition. Learning, memory, attention, and focus are some aspects of cognition that nature and health researchers explore. Beginning with preschool, primary, and secondary school education, bringing learning outside, or ensuring that throughout the school day children and adolescents can go outside for recess and physical education, is important. Getting outside is positively related to improved cognitive function as is clearly shown by improved test scores, attention, focus, and memory (Mygind *et al.* 2018; Norwood *et al.* 2019; Thorburn and Marshall 2014; Wade *et al.* 2020).

In adulthood and older adulthood, the moderating influences of nature experiences, particularly those that involve physical activity, continue to support cognition. For example, test scores on a cognitive performance test improved after walking in nature, as compared to walking in an urban setting (Bailey *et al.* 2018). Similar improvements in cognition have been noted with comparing social visits outdoors versus staying indoors (Saadi *et al.* 2020). For older adults, particularly those with limited physical mobility, going outside less than once a week is associated with decreased cognition (Harada *et al.* 2016). What is evident from these studies is that being outdoors and engaging in physical activity supports and enhances cognition. The implications for studies such as these are important on a population-health level because if we can get children and adults outside and moving, not only will they experience improved social-emotional health, but also they may be "smarter."

THIS MUCH I KNOW—BEN AND NICK

Two young nature enthusiasts shared their thoughts about being outside.

- Being outside is the best. When spring comes, we can go into the pool. It is very cold, but we go in anyway. I like to warm up in the sunshine and eat snacks outside. Sometimes we have a picnic. Mommy does not like to be outside. Daddy, Jax, me, and my brother like to spend lots of time outside.
- Being outside makes me feel a little bit nervous, but I like it. It makes me nervous of birds trying to catch me and bees trying to sting me. I like the fresh air and going on a hike. One day I helped Daddy build a swing set. Now my brother and me can play on it and do parkour.

Physical: *Moving and physiology*

Participating in physical activity in nature is well documented to improve physical health, including mobility, strength, and physiological markers such as blood pressure, heart rate, and cortisol levels (Coventry *et al.* 2021). At a level of population health, where the location one lives does matter, access to nearby public green spaces increases the rate of physical activity, along with improving social-emotional health and wellbeing (Sugiyama *et al.* 2018). Again, we return to the finding that living near nature is a determinant of health.

CASE NARRATIVE: Kathryn Palano

Thank you to Kathryn Palano, PT, DPT, MPH, NCS, for her help in preparing this narrative.

In her seven years of physical therapy practice, Dr. Palano has treated people whose function and mobility have been significantly impaired by complex medical conditions—many due to largely preventable chronic diseases. The toll these chronic diseases have had on their physical and mental health drove her to feel as though what she was doing was too little too late. Dr. Palano wanted to have a wider-reaching impact on the quality of their lives, and potentially work to prevent the medical decline prevalent in so many of her clients. This led her to enroll in a master's in public health program with a focus on parks and recreation.

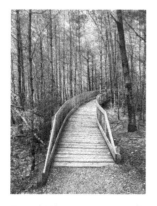

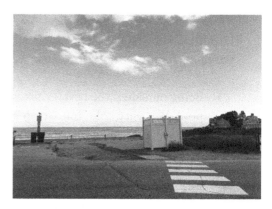

A GENTLE SLOPING BOARDWALK WITH HANDRAILS

MOBI-MAT TO THE SEA

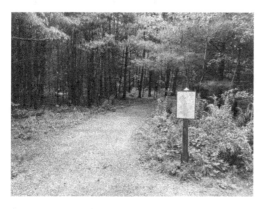

A LEVEL PATH WITH WAYFINDING SIGNAGE
Photo credits: Kathryn Palano

While Dr. Palano already knew being in nature relaxed her, the significant physical, cognitive, and emotional health benefits of nature exposure surprised her. While learning about these concepts and the limited application of nature's health benefits in our medical settings, she wondered why clinicians aren't leveraging these benefits to promote health and wellbeing. Therefore, she started intentionally incorporating nature into her clinical practice. Because Dr. Palano treats in both an outpatient clinic and an intensive home and community rehab program in Maine, nature-focused concepts are applied differently.

With her clients from the outpatient clinic, Dr. Palano educates them on nature's health benefits and strategies to increase daily nature exposure. If someone is unable to leave their home, she discusses with them strategies to bring nature to them—getting an indoor plant, sitting by a window with a view of nature or just making sure the window shades are open, sitting out on their porch, and listening to water or bird sounds. If they can safely leave their home, she recommends they walk outside on trails, sidewalks, parks, beaches, and other natural spaces with benches to soak in nature for their walking program. Not only do they receive nature's health benefits; they also practice walking in novel, complex, or challenging environments in their communities.

Dr. Palano shared that she can more easily incorporate nature into clinical care in her work with Rehab Without Walls (www.rehabwithoutwalls.com) due to the format and flexibility of this intensive home/community neuro-rehabilitation program. Being more intentional about integrating nature into practice has significantly elevated Dr. Palano's clinical care through the introduction of novel environments to facilitate therapy, changing the walking surface and incline to grade the activity, promoting relaxation during rest breaks, and, as the best outcome, making the sessions more enjoyable for her clients as well as herself. Two examples highlight these benefits.

The first example of how Dr. Palano sees the benefit of providing therapy outside is of a woman in her mid-40s two months post a right middle cerebral artery stroke (MCA cerebrovascular accident (CVA)) who presented with left hemiplegia limiting her functional mobility. As high-intensity gait training was indicated to promote neuro-recovery and functional mobility, and she expressed a love of being outdoors, the gait training was combined with being outside on her paved driveway as weather permitted. The client gradually progressed to walking short distances on the grass in her yard. As her stability, endurance, and confidence improved, collaboratively they decided she was ready for an outing to practice her mobility. They browsed a list of local accessible trails to choose the next therapy session location (https://mainebyfoot.com/wheelchair-friendly-trails). The client chose a local monastery with paved trails that she remembered excitedly from her past. Prior to the outing, they discussed what to expect from the environment and what equipment to bring, and researched the closest accessible restrooms. Luckily, the day of the outing was beautiful. Since the path was paved in some areas and had obstacles in other areas, the client had the opportunity to practice different aspects of walking. She practiced walking on uneven ground while maintaining stability and being accurate with left-foot placement. While walking on the more even, paved areas, a metronome provided her with auditory cuing to facilitate two-point gait pattern, increased walking speed, and improved symmetry of stance and swing phases. In addition, due to the novel environment, she had to practice maintaining attention on walking while also focusing on these other tasks. During rest breaks, she relaxed by focusing on her surroundings—the birdsong, birdwatching, the warmth of the sun, and the views of the river. Although the session challenged her, she was able to work at a higher intensity for longer because she was enjoying herself. This experience not only promoted neuro-recovery and improved her walking, but also increased her confidence to get out in her community.

The second client example is of a man in his early 60s with an incomplete cervical spinal cord injury due to a fall, with resulting tetraplegia and increased muscle tone. High-intensity gait training was indicated to promote neuro-recovery and functional mobility, and he was tired of being inside all day after spending a couple of months in a hospital. As a team, Dr. Palano and the client decided to take therapy outside. Gait training was initiated on his packed dirt driveway with a rollator. As his endurance, balance, and confidence grew, the next step was to have therapy sessions in the community. They met at a universally accessible trail (Hope Woods in Kennebunk, Maine), a beach with a ramp down to the sand, and a universally accessible trail at the top of Mt. Agamenticus. Each of these sessions focused on specific gait and community mobility goals—progressing from a rollator to a straight cane, walking greater distances before resting to improve endurance, walking on uneven ground, walking up inclines and down declines, negotiating ramps, and walking at quicker speeds with the use of a metronome. During rest breaks, they intentionally soaked in the natural surroundings to promote mental restoration and physiological relaxation. Not only did they (both) get many more steps in and practice walking on challenging terrain to facilitate a return to yard management tasks and other community mobility—they also had a lot of fun.

Dr. Palano shared that she has had the opportunity and privilege to bring many other clients outside in nature. By doing rehab out on trails, beaches, and other outdoor spaces, she feels that not only do her clients directly practice activities that will improve both their household and community mobility; they also become more aware of the accessible options in their communities and gain confidence to visit and recreate in these places outside of therapy in their daily lives.

On a larger, population level, the outdoors is not available to all people due to the lack of accessible outdoor natural spaces. The frustration that she hears time and time again from her clients was the driving force for Dr. Palano to focus on accessibility within the master's in public health program she had begun, focusing on parks and recreation. As she learned more about the major influence the environment and infrastructure have on health, physical activity, and wellbeing, she started thinking that we, allied and mental health professionals, must expand our reach into our communities to truly effect change in people's lives. If our clients are not able to participate in recreational activities or connect with natural spaces due to issues such as lack of access, are we living up to our obligations to them? Empowering them and focusing on behavior change strategies can only do so much. If the goals she and her clients set together are supposed to be attainable, but the environment makes them unattainable, she decided that she had to act and do something about it.

By focusing on the intersection of the natural environment and accessibility in her public health program and clinical experiences, Dr. Palano better understood the importance of equitable access to natural spaces for health and wellbeing, and strategies to become an accessibility advocate to have a wider reach in her coastal Maine town, where the beach is a large part of the fabric of the community. Unfortunately, many beaches are inaccessible, which is a social barrier in addition to a physical barrier for people with mobility-related impairments. Because of this, she reached out to her town to advocate for improved accessibility to the beaches. Dr. Palano started by speaking with people within her network to determine whom to contact. They recommended contacting the town's director of community development or town engineer. After speaking with the director, a group of people from the Departments of Community Development, Public Works, and Parks and Recreation met with Dr. Palano to decide on how to make the beaches more accessible and how to pay for the work. They chose to focus on the beach where it would be easiest to implement changes. After many emails, several meetings, and a site visit, there was change! A portable accessibility mat (www.mobi-mat-chair-beach-access-dms.com) was purchased and installed within six months of her initial email to the town. While not all her recommendations were implemented, the Mobi-mat enabled easier access from the parking lot onto the beach and from the beach to the water for all people.

As trusted healthcare providers in our communities, Dr. Palano shared that we all have the potential to be leaders in healthy, active communities. Ensuring our clients can achieve their goals and live healthy, active lives extends our work from the clinic and into our communities. By being advocates for accessibility, we promote both our clients' and our communities' health and wellbeing.

Some of the earliest research, beginning in the early 1990s, related to the impact of nature on physiological health focused on shinrin-yoku, which is a Japanese term that translates to forest bathing. In forest bathing, the participant "basks" in the experience of being in the forest, experiencing it with all the senses. It is intended to be deeply calming and meditative; to be a counter to the stresses and responsibilities that people face daily. The concept of shinrin-yoku was officially introduced in 1982 by the Japanese Ministry of Agriculture, Forestry, and Fisheries (Park *et al.* 2010), but its roots likely date back several centuries. One of the earliest published studies of shinrin-yoku compared an immersive forest-bathing experience with a walk in an urban environment. Results of the study showed that the forest-bathing experience led to decreased cortisol levels, decreased heart rate and blood pressure, and increased sympathetic nervous system activity. Since this study was published, there have been many more studies of shinrin-yoku completed with various populations, and the findings support Park and colleagues' study, that forest bathing is transformative for both the mind and body (Hansen, Jones, and Tocchini 2017; Wen *et al.* 2019). The concept of forest bathing has, with necessary adaptations to meet clients' needs, the capacity to be an important component of therapy.

Across the lifespan, nature is a stimulus for physical activity. For example, children and adolescents are more physically active when they are outside; they play more and are more engaged in group activities (Johnstone *et al.* 2022; Mygind *et al.* 2019). For adolescent and young adult males, there is a positive relationship between physical activity, family participation, and being in nature, because when families are outside doing things together, physical activity increases (Puhakka *et al.* 2018). For adults and older adults, spending 120 minutes a week engaged in nature is associated with self-reported good health and wellbeing (White *et al.* 2019). Further, with adults, there is a relationship between increased time outdoors and reduced risk of chronic illnesses (Beyer *et al.* 2018). For example, the installation of outdoor gyms in public green spaces and provision of outdoor exercise programs have been found to increase physical activity for adults and older adults (Levinger *et al.* 2018; Oliveros *et al.* 2021), provided the equipment is safe and well maintained. With older adults, engagement in physical activity outdoors is associated with increased capacity to participate in activities of daily living and instrumental activities of daily living, which collectively help to maintain independence and sense of autonomy (Shimada *et al.* 2010; Sjögren and Stjernberg 2010). Based on this powerful evidence that connects the entirety of the person with nature, health, and wellness benefits throughout all stages of life, and ways they can be experienced—in subsequent chapters of this book, we explore in greater depth social-emotional, cognitive, and physical outcomes that people experience when nature is part of their lives.

CASE NARRATIVE: Park Rx America

Thank you to Robert Zarr, MD and Founder of Park Rx America, for speaking with us about his non-profit organization.

Park Rx America (originally DC Park Rx) began in 2010 as part of a larger national Park Rx initiative. DC Park Rx was the upshot of pediatrician Dr. Robert Zarr's desire to improve the health-related quality of life for his patients and their families in Washington, DC. In his practice, Dr. Zarr noticed that many of his patients—young children and their family members—were experiencing chronic health conditions at an alarming rate; he suspected that many of these conditions could be ameliorated with more time spent active outdoors. He worked to create Park Rx America to connect his patients and their families with nature through prescribed activities in nearby parks. Today, the tagline for Park Rx America, *Nature Prescribed*, tells it all.

While the goal of Park Rx America is to improve human and planetary health through sustainable interaction with nature, Dr. Zarr's organization has shifted to an informational platform for those interested in a nature prescription program, including clinical practitioners (providers) and patients. There is also a third portal for everyone else that includes, but is not limited to, land management and park agencies, interested volunteers, philanthropists, and requests for further information.

The website www.natureprescribed.org contains a virtual plethora of information and knowledge sharing. All the materials are available at no cost, which increases the equity and inclusivity of the program exponentially. The website is easily navigated and understandable and provides helpful evidence-based guidance for interested parties to use. There is no right activity that is "prescribed" in a nature prescription. In fact, one of the beauties of the prescriptions, be they facilitated by a provider, self-generated, or requested by a patient from their provider, is that flexibility is inherent in the structure. This ensures that each prescription is tailored to meet the unique needs of the clients/participants where they are and for whom the program is intended.

- The provider option, which for many readers may be most applicable, is used when developing nature engagement goals for individual client-(patient)-centered health outcomes. Through the provider portal, therapists and clinicians have the option to set up a prescriber account that enables them to write nature prescriptions and send reminders. We highly recommend that you watch Dr. Zarr's helpful step-by-step nature prescription how-to video after setting up your prescriber account (www.parkrxamerica.org/patients/ask-your-healthcareprovider.php).

- Not surprisingly, clinicians have determined that the most popular and well-received nature prescriptions are those that are flexible and align with client interests. Taking this option a step further, in Dr. Zarr's opinion, Park Rx America prescriptions can be the catalyst to create behavior change both in physicians and other healthcare providers and in their patients. A new behavioral routine that includes using nature prescriptions as one of many interventions to help patients improve their health thus becomes as common as prescribing medication or a home therapy program. The provider option can be used to coordinate with other programs and increase collaboration to enhance client outcomes.

- The patient option empowers people to learn about the health benefits of nature and then to ask their healthcare provider to write them a nature prescription. It is a great strategy for patients to self-advocate for something they feel passionate about. Another option in this portal is for a patient to write their own nature prescription. A self-prescription template is provided in the patient portal.

- Pertaining to everyone, nature prescription programs are diverse and ever-evolving, often including collaboration between park and public land agencies, healthcare providers, and community partners.

Dr. Zarr eloquently shared why we must care for ourselves and for the planet. He said:

It is imperative to develop a relationship with the outside world and even bigger, with the planet. That's where it all starts, because if you don't have a relationship with it, why on earth (no pun intended) would you want to keep it right, to preserve it, love it, cherish it, and protect it? The same goes for caring for ourselves.

Please take some time to explore the incredible wealth of information on natureprescribed.org and consider signing up for the Park Rx America newsletter at www.parkrxamerica.org/learn/signup.html. No matter what type of outdoor program you may be considering, there is information on the website that will be invaluable to you.

Where and How Nature Can Be Included in Clinical Practice

How the benefits of nature accrue can be conceptualized in three categories or levels (Pretty 2004), which happen to seamlessly track with facilitating therapy outside or bringing therapeutic nature inside. The first level is viewing nature (Pretty 2004), as through a window, in a painting or sculpture, or simulated via virtual reality (Browning *et al.* 2020; Rose *et al.* 2021; Soga *et al.* 2020; Ulrich 1984). Recall that biophilia is a human predisposition to connect with nature (Wilson 1984). Nature is an important part of the human experience. Taking biophilia a step further, biophilic design is intended to "create spaces that are inspirational, restorative, and healthy, as well as integrative with the functionality of the place and the (urban) ecosystem to which it is applied. Above all, biophilic design must nurture a love of place" (Terrapin Bright Green 2014, Section 3.1). Applied to indoor therapeutic spaces, which are **the first category or level**, biophilic design includes clinics with windows that look onto nature. It involves arranging equipment so that clients can look out of the windows while receiving treatment. It also means having nature inside, as plants, live flowers, a water element, and/ or ambient nature sounds. Nature images and art are also ways to make a space more biophilic. Virtual reality, often facilitated inside, is an emerging area of interest for nature and health researchers as evidence indicates that virtual-reality nature experiences moderate levels of alertness and sense of belonging and connection with others (Anderson 2019; Calogiuri *et al.* 2018; Rose *et al.* 2021).

CASE NARRATIVE: P.R.O.D.U.C.E.

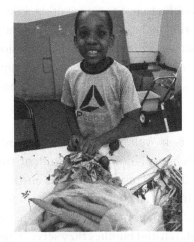

P.R.O.D.U.C.E
Providing Remarkable Opportunities Dedicated to Unearthing Children's Education

Student's Name:_____

Teacher: _____

FARM FRESH PRODUCE

"Fun Food Facts"
- Carrots are an excellent source of Vitamin A, providing more than 200% of your daily requirement in just one carrot.
- Carrots are not only orange! They can be white, yellow, red, and purple!
- Carrots were first grown in the area around Afghanistan in 900 AD.

PREPPING AND BAGGING PRODUCE FOR DISTRIBUTION TO CLASSMATES

THE OFFICIAL P.R.O.D.U.C.E. LABEL, COMPLETE WITH INTERESTING FOOD FACTS

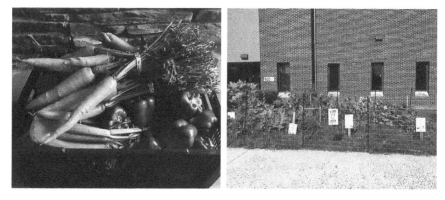

AN ARRAY OF FARM FRESH PRODUCE   THE P.R.O.D.U.C.E. GROWING GARDEN
Photo credits: Lauren Telesmanic and Antonio Fotino

Thank you to Lauren Telesmanic, OTD, OTR/L, Supervisor and Founder, and Antonio Fotino, OTD, OTR/L, Staff Occupational Therapist, from the P.R.O.D.U.C.E. program for helping to prepare this case narrative.

The P.R.O.D.U.C.E. (Providing Remarkable Opportunities Dedicated to Unearthing Children's Education) program is a new addition to The Arc Greater Hudson Valley, New York, Educational Learning Experience program, whose mission is to "support people with unique abilities to live as valued and contributing members of the community." The specific mission of the Educational Learning Experience is:

> to enable persons of all ages with disabilities to live as contributing, valued members of the community by promoting Inclusion, Independence, Individualization, Productivity, and Self-Determination. Among the education department we strive to establish a strong foundation that promotes learning through our effective teaching methods, while providing a positive support system for students, staff, and families.

Launched in July of 2019, P.R.O.D.U.C.E. is well aligned with the Arc's overall and Educational Learning Experience missions. It is a student-run program that provides fresh produce to the students and families enrolled in the education program. The overarching initial goal of the program was to create a partnership with a local farmer's market to support, advocate for, and enhance the quality of life for the children and families they serve in the education department at the Arc. By partnering with a local farmer's market, P.R.O.D.U.C.E. obtains fresh fruits and vegetables via donation for weekly distribution so that students and their families have easy access to healthy, nutritious food. School-age students participate in the program by sorting, cleaning, and labeling produce for distribution.

The inspiration for Dr. Telesmanic to create P.R.O.D.U.C.E. came to her, as good ideas often do, as an "Aha!" moment. She shared:

> While in a meeting discussing a student and his difficulties in the classroom including attention and behavior, it came to me that this student, along with most of our students, often comes to school with lunches that have low nutritional value. This is often a result of the availability of low-cost canned or packaged and highly processed foods. The children we serve are at risk for learning and social-emotional delays due to their home environment and socioeconomic status.

Thinking back upon her remarkable efforts, Dr. Telesmanic reflected that by "implementing this program, the children and families gained access to nutritious, fresh food options that may not have been previously afforded to them, therefore contributing to improving their health and wellbeing." Meeting the P.R.O.D.U.C.E. program's initial implementation outcomes included:

- establishing a lasting partnership with a local farmer's market to obtain free fresh produce
- establishing a free, healthy food program for the children and families in the education department of the Arc
- providing education to the children and families on the importance of good nutrition for brain development, and overall health and wellbeing
- promoting life skills for students who participated in the program
- promoting occupational justice for the children and families at the Arc.

P.R.O.D.U.C.E. is facilitated indoors and outdoors. Because the Arc is in upstate New York, where weather conditions can be rough and make for a shorter growing season, the program is offered year round, thanks to the addition of a greenhouse for when inclement weather prevents being outside. The students and staff take care of the garden and the kitchen area used to prep the produce for distribution. The accessible garden, which is 25 feet wide and 14 feet long, was collaboratively designed by Dr. Telesmanic, Dr. Fotino, and a teacher at the Arc. The site was selected based on being in a level area on the campus that is accessible for students and staff, sun conditions for optimal growing, and convenient access to a water source.

While adolescents are the primary participants in P.R.O.D.U.C.E., children, young adults, and all their families are also included as part of the program.

The diagnoses of students served at the Arc include developmental delays such as autism and Down syndrome, seizure disorders, learning disabilities, social-emotional delays, bipolar disorder, major depressive disorder, PTSD, anxiety disorder, attention deficit hyperactivity disorder (ADHD), disruptive mood dysregulation disorder, and reactive attachment disorder. Accordingly, the program goals are designed to address physical and mental health, education, and social justice.

Run by Dr. Telesmanic and Dr. Fotino with help from teachers and teacher's aides who assist with planting and supporting students in their responsibilities within the program, P.R.O.D.U.C.E. is facilitated in small groups of up to ten students or as a one-on-one intervention. It is open enrollment, so students can join any time. Typical sessions last between 15 minutes and an hour. There are no set numbers of sessions, as weather, classroom schedules, and student needs vary throughout the year. Interventions that are included in the gardening component of P.R.O.D.U.C.E. include watering, weeding, digging, raking, tilling with non-motorized tools, and soil removal. All interventions for gardening can be adapted to fit any child's ability level. Students use different types of garden tools depending on their ability and skill level. For the farmer's market's produce-donations portion of the program, interventions include cleaning, cutting, bagging, and delivering vegetables to classrooms. All interventions other than cutting are adaptable to align with each child's ability level. Students are matched with their "jobs" based on their abilities, individualized education program (IEP) goals, and, very importantly, their interests. Collaboration with classroom teachers, speech therapy, occupational therapy, and physical therapy are also an important part of the job assignment process so that it can best meet the students' needs and to be most appropriate.

Materials needed to run the garden portion of the program include fencing and fence posts, shovels, buckets, rakes, picks, hoses, watering cans, hand garden tools, plants and seeds, and gloves. The farmer's market program requires produce and materials to prepare them such as knives, gallon-sized zip-top bags, towels, gloves, paper to make labels and "fun food facts" for the produce bags, scissors to cut out the labels, writing tools, a kitchen sink, worktables, tablecloths, a wheeled cart, cleaning supplies, and aprons. For those wondering what "fun food facts" might be, it is an interesting tidbit of knowledge about a fruit or vegetable. Students whose IEP goals include handwriting and scissors skills are often given the job of filling out or cutting out the labels, examples of purposeful and meaningful therapy.

Families are made aware of P.R.O.D.U.C.E. through flyers and consent forms. Outreach to the local farmer's market is done via in-person meetings and phone calls. Obtaining the startup P.R.O.D.U.C.E. program materials transpired through a combination of donations, using existing items already available at the Arc, and via purchase. Due to the generosity of donations and using available materials, the remaining startup costs for zip-top storage bags for produce, fencing, and posts were less than $350. Presently, the annual cost is a mere $70 for zip-top storage bags. However, if materials break or need to be replaced, additional costs will incur. The P.R.O.D.U.C.E. program is now funded through grants and the occupational therapy department budget.

Stories tell much and we are happy to share a few about P.R.O.D.U.C.E. We learned that while watering and weeding the garden, one student was so happy to be participating that he said, "This was one of the best days! The entire classroom did such a great job with sharing gardening tools with each other and working hard to make their garden section look as good as they could." A teacher shared their joy of "seeing the smiles on the students' faces every day as they work in the garden and pick the fruits and vegetables as a direct result of their hard work." And finally, Dr. Telesmanic said that one day, after all the students went home and some staff members stayed to talk about their day and the vegetables growing in the garden, several of them discussed how much they enjoyed the garden as it provided a calm, peaceful place to be with the students. Learning, socializing, doing, and being outdoors—what more could we ask for?

Dr. Telesmanic and Dr. Fotino want us to know that one of the benefits of taking it outside is the increased sensory enrichment that students gain from being out of the classroom. Outdoor gardening experiences also give each student the opportunity to see the fruits of their labor pay off daily. The harder they work on maintaining the garden, the better the fruits and vegetables grow and taste! While benefits far outweigh challenges, the reality is that weather plays a significant role in the amount of time the students spend outside. Due to the high heat index during the summer, students have limited opportunity to do afternoon gardening activities. If it rains, they are unable to go outside at all. Mother Nature calls the shots.

When asked to offer advice about providing therapy outside, Dr. Fotino told us to take weather into account. Some students may have difficulty in the heat for extended periods of time, and some students may not be able to be in the sun due to certain medications. Photosensitivity is a real issue that must be considered in any outdoor therapy program. Dr. Telesmanic's advice is:

Absolutely consider it! Think outside the box! Changing the environment can make a tremendous difference in a student's level of participation, motivation, and happiness. Students are indoors for most of their school day, so a chance to be outside is a gift.

Indeed, being outside is a gift that everyone needs and deserves. Another thought offered by Dr. Telesmanic is that "This was one of the best programs I have ever created and implemented and that having the support of administration and key staff was key to starting and maintaining the program." We agree.

The second level is being outside in nature, but the reasons for being outside may not be to improve health and wellbeing (Pretty 2004). Nature is the background for engaging in activities such as walking or cycling to work, dog-walking, playing on a climbing structure, reading on a garden seat, or talking to friends in a park (Lee, Song, and Lee 2022; Rishbeth and Rogaly 2018; Souter-Brown, Hinckson, and Duncan 2021; Woodward and Wild, 2020). Applied to therapeutic outdoor program models, this includes deliberate selection of spaces that will enhance the therapeutic capacity of interventions. Nature is the important environment— rather than the "star" for facilitating therapy outside.

CASE NARRATIVE: Willow Family Wellness OT Services

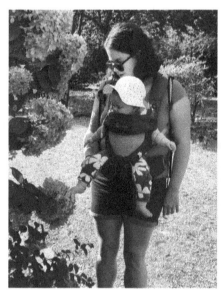

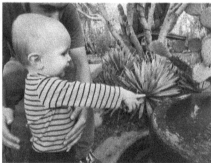

MOTHER AND BABY IN NATURE
Photo credit: Amy Wagenfeld

DO YOU SEE WHAT I SEE?
Photo credit: Shannon Marder

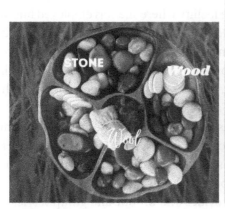

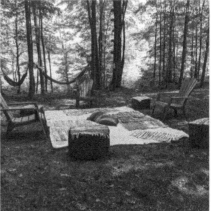

Nature fidgets
Photo credit: Amanda Hall

Forest therapy space: a gathering area
Photo credit: Amanda Hall

Thank you to Amanda Hall, MSc. OT, OT Reg. (Ont.), PMH-C (Perinatal Mental Health Certification), RYT (Registered Yoga Teacher), Owner of Willow Family Wellness Occupational Therapy Services (Willow Family OT), for contributing to this case narrative.

Being a mother is a complex and life-changing role. New mothers can sometimes feel intimidated by taking themselves and their baby outside, but Ms. Hall at Willow Family OT is challenging that hesitancy and taking mothers outside for therapy. The mission of Willow Family OT is "to provide quality and compassionate care to women and their families while maintaining their dignity, strengthening their hope, and discovering their resiliency to live the life they want." Willow Family OT gives mothers a space to "grow and survive in difficult conditions, thriving in and nourishing the surrounding environment despite hardships it may endure to survive"—much like a willow tree. By supporting new mothers and their growing families, Willow Family OT's nature-based interventions are unique in that they are bespoke to each client's needs and range from ergonomic education to social-emotional support.

Willow Family OT's story has a poetic beginning, as Ms. Hall was inspired to provide a nature-based therapy program while on maternity leave after the birth of her first baby. She was both dismayed by the lack of postpartum services available and invigorated by her time in nature. Ms. Hall became aware of gaps in maternal healthcare and access to wellness services, such as education on postpartum recovery, screening for postpartum mood disorders, knowing how to safely participate in physical activity postpartum, and maintaining pelvic floor health. At the same time, she felt motivated by her passion to be outdoors. Ms. Hall initially considered facilitating a nature-based program at the complex care facility where she was employed but was concerned about potential limitations that would be imposed by the facility regulations. Despite regulations and limitations, Ms. Hall knew that access to nature matters and that somehow she needed to be involved with helping others to reap its benefits. In her case, she found her purpose by leaving her previous job and starting Willow Family OT to work with mothers.

Launched in 2018, during her inspirational maternity leave, Willow Family OT is located on Ms. Hall's 147-acre family farm in Ontario, Canada. Her farm is situated on traditional Anishinaabe and Haudenosaunee lands, and she works to be respectful and openly acknowledge the land's heritage in her practice. Willow Family OT provides one-on-one and group services to women who are pregnant or postpartum. Services are individualized to meet each mother's goals, which frequently relate to physical health and recovery from birth, postpartum mental health, and adjusting to the demands of motherhood. To serve her clients, Ms. Hall has completed the OT Pioneers Course for pelvic health (run by Lindsey Vestal), level 1 cognitive behavioral therapy (CBT) training, CBT and Mindfulness training, CBT for perinatal mood disorders training, and CBT for physically distressing symptoms training. Ms. Hall shared that the most common physical health recovery needs are related to mothers learning to pace themselves when engaging in physical exercise, strengthening their pelvic floors, and ergonomic body positioning when caring for their babies. Typical postpartum mental health needs are addressed using strategies such as mindfulness practices, CBT work, adjusting expectations, building self-regulation and coping skills, and asser-tiveness training for self-advocacy. A common need related to supporting the role transition into motherhood is establishing routines in preparation for returning to paid employment.

One-on-one services are facilitated outside and/or indoors, depending on the mother's comfort level. If one-on-one services are provided indoors, Ms. Hall infuses as much nature as possible into sessions including providing smooth stones, pinecones, wood slices, and sheep fleece to "fidget" with, and facilitating sessions in a space with nature-based artwork and an abundance of natural light to evoke a sense of being outdoors. Typically, during the first one-on-one session, Ms. Hall works with a mother to develop intervention goals and a plan to work towards achieving them. These goals are tailored to each mother's unique motherhood story.

To illustrate Willow Family OT's one-on-one services, Ms. Hall shared Lisa's story. Lisa (a pseudonym), a 34-year-old mother, was three months postpartum with her first baby when she contacted Willow Family OT due to concerns that her baby was not enjoying tummy time and she was worried about her baby's development. During the initial discovery call, Ms. Hall determined that Lisa had high levels of anxiety and was experiencing low mood, more than usual. Lisa felt she had been failing her baby as she did not encourage tummy time as often as she thought she should, due to her baby's negative reaction. The result was both Lisa and her baby experiencing increased stress.

Lisa identified that she was comfortable with being outdoors, so the initial in-person session was planned to be in the farm's forest therapy space. When Lisa arrived for her initial session with her baby, she expressed some apprehension owing to the novelty of the space as she had never participated in any form of healthcare outside. Once settled into a space under the tree canopy, Lisa became more comfortable. Ms. Hall first completed the Edinburgh Postnatal Depression Screen, a standardized postpartum mood disorder screening tool. Lisa was then invited to lay her baby on a blanket covering the forest floor as the therapy session continued. Then, Ms. Hall led Lisa in a grounding and mindfulness exercise, which focused on breathing and the overall multisensory experience of being in the forest. She invited Lisa to relax her body, releasing the tension she was holding, allowing the forest floor to support her body. As she sensed how her body felt, she was invited to close her eyes or lower her gaze, and tune in to what she could hear (birds, leaves rustling), to feel the wind and sun on her skin, and to inhale deeply to smell (trees, forest, moisture). She was encouraged not to label these experiences and instead just recognize that they are there and allow herself to let go of control over the situation, allowing her mind to turn off, to hold no judgment if her mind wanders, and allow herself to simply exist with no demands. Following the mindfulness exercise, Ms. Hall and Lisa collaboratively developed Lisa's occupational profile, determining where barriers to occupational engagement were occurring, and determining her level of satisfaction with her current routine and time use.

Ms. Hall shared that what occurred in the first session with Lisa was a very typical conversation that generally happens indoors, but moving it to the forest seemed to elicit an increased sense of calm and focus when discussing emotionally provoking topics. During the session, attention was periodically brought back to her baby, who was showing interest in the wind blowing through the tree canopy. It was clear that Lisa's baby was tolerating being on the ground, possibly because they were distracted by the sensory experiences provided by nature. Lisa commented that this had been one of the longest periods her baby had been content out of her arms.

The session progressed into assessing how Lisa was working on tummy time with her baby. Education and strategies were shared and practiced within the forest therapy space. Hammock therapy was integrated into the tummy time education, and Lisa was invited to lie in one of the hammocks in the forest therapy space. Once comfortable, Lisa's baby was laid on top of her, chest to chest. This supportive tummy time position is typically done on a couch, bed, or floor at home, but in the forest it was done in a hammock. Sitting or lying in a hammock has been found to help regulate the parasympathetic nervous system and can be very effective in aiding self-regulation (Dodson 2004; Grabherr, Macauda, and Lenggenhager 2015; Miyazaki 2018). When used in this way, Lisa was able to practice self-regulation strategies, which resulted in a period of co-regulation with her baby. In addition, she was practicing a supportive tummy time position with minimal stress to her or her baby.

While Ms. Hall may facilitate one-on-one sessions inside, group sessions are always held outside or virtually (clients are encouraged to participate outside if participating virtually). In-person groups are distinct cohorts of six mothers who meet weekly for 7–8 weeks. In-person groups begin with a gentle and accessible hike into the farm's forest therapy space. The farm's forest therapy space was created in 2018 when Ms. Hall established a 100 feet × 250 feet clearing in a forested area of her farm. She also utilizes an additional 40 acres of forest with walking trails and a one-acre waterfront field on the property for her work. Ms. Hall furnished the forest therapy space with various seating options such as hammocks, tree-trunk stools, and Adirondack chairs that offer mothers choice and autonomy to select one that best fits their needs. Once the group is assembled, Ms. Hall typically facilitates grounding activities with babies in their mother's lap and then gentle yoga-based movement and stretches. During this movement time, mothers may choose to place babies on a soft canvas tarp covering the forest floor or in a wicker bassinet so that they are free to complete the movement exercises without a babe in arms. What follows is a storytelling-format check-in where mothers share a high and a low point from the previous week to build connection with one another. The unique stories that mothers share and hear help to build a supportive community. Ms. Hall then leads the group in a developmentally appropriate interactive song time with the babies before transitioning into the weekly discussion topic that pertains to the mothers' needs. These topics may include supporting pelvic floor health, managing expectations and big emotions, optimizing sleep, and ergonomic babywearing (slings and front carriers). The group concludes with more interactive play-songs and continued conversations among mothers.

Ms. Hall launched virtual groups in 2020 in response to the COVID-19 global pandemic to foster community. Virtual groups are open enrollment, and clients, including mothers and their partners or spouses, are welcome to join at any time. The virtual group is structured the same way as the outdoor group but meets for 30–45 minutes every other week for eight-week rotations. Discussions focus on topics such as wellness, coping strategies, loneliness, and other concerns mothers may identify. During each virtual group meeting, Ms. Hall encourages mothers to spend more time outdoors in a way that is accessible and manageable for themselves and their family. On days dominated by sleep deprivation, when getting outdoors is a daunting task, Ms. Hall recommends opening windows and curtains, and sitting in the sunlight, all of which can have a positive impact on mental health. As a registered Park Rx America provider, Ms. Hall can prescribe time outdoors, which can provide a way for clients to be accountable for changes in their daily routines and schedules when incorporating more time in nature. For more information about Park Rx America, please see the case narrative earlier in this chapter.

All group members have individualized goals based on their priorities. While sessions are scheduled for 60 minutes, they often extend to 90 minutes owing to the valuable conversations that ensue between mothers. In addition to Ms. Hall, occupational therapy students and volunteers support the groups' facilitation. Volunteers typically consist of university students who have an interest in occupational therapy. Ms. Hall provides students and volunteers with training so that they can assist her with checking in with the mothers about any concerns or successes they are experiencing. This training typically occurs over a couple of meetings (virtually or in person) to determine the volunteers' interests and abilities to support the groups. The volunteers and students sit in on a group session to observe before assisting.

Ms. Hall also facilitates an outdoor watercolor painting group for new clients. While the group is designed for new mothers, it is open to anyone, including non-mothers. This group runs periodically as a one-time event over the spring/summer months. The group is focused on understanding and dismantling perfectionist tendencies as a means to increase occupational satisfaction. Ms. Hall provides participants only three colors and two brushes. She encourages participants to use a small amount of paint and a lot of water so that the water takes control of the painting, symbolic of giving up control and perfectionism. After painting, participants discuss perfectionism and what they like and/or dislike about their art, and thoughts that might be driving their dislikes. The group's aim is to help mothers see that imperfections are natural, addressing a crucial mental health component of women's and maternal health. Participants are encouraged to share their paintings while building connections to their participation in daily activities, satisfaction with performance, and self-imposed expectations. A natural outcome of this process is finding common humanity among other women and mothers as a step toward increasing a sense of self-compassion.

While no funding was needed to rent or purchase a space for the outdoor program, initial costs included manual labor and a great deal of time to clear the forest therapy space, create furniture and seating from fallen trees, and build other structures such as chalkboards, which can be used to work through a thought record, practice journaling, or other behavioral therapy components. Ms. Hall created a website, set up an electronic patient record system, and purchased other furniture, such as multiple wicker bassinets, cushions, hammocks, hammock chairs, picnic tables, Muskoka chairs (https://muskokachair.com), and a canopy for cover when needed. Ongoing operating costs are related to property maintenance, art supplies, and any additional materials needed for therapy.

As the program was readying for launch, Ms. Hall marketed Willow Family OT by posting on social media; sharing via word of mouth; connecting with the Kingston and Area Pregnancy and Postpartum Professionals Network (KAPS); an interprofessional community organization for maternal health in the Kingston, Ontario area); and cold-calling television and news stations to ask them to bring awareness of her program to their listeners. Clients are referred to Willow Family OT by local perinatal professional community members, such as doulas, physiotherapists, social workers, and family health educators. Clients' needs often relate to physical, social, emotional, and cognitive dysfunction or barriers that affect their role as a mother. Services provided through Willow Family OT are funded by insurance if there are extended health benefits available through employers, or as a fee for service, as the Ontario Health Insurance Plan (OHIP) does not provide coverage for private organizations.

Ms. Hall is an adjunct professor within the occupational therapy program at Queen's University at Kingston. Advocating for occupational therapy's role in maternal health, she is working with students to assess the effectiveness of the interventions that are being done at Willow Family OT. She is also developing a maternal-health nature-based tool to measure the impact that time in nature can have on daily occupations and a card sort tool for mothers to identify meaningful outdoor occupations.

Ms. Hall explained that a key component of her work with mothers is curating a space where mothers feel safe and comfortable. She relies heavily on nature for this. She shared that a mother was able to view the forest and the mothers' group as a safe space to share her complex birth story and to become aware that she had missed something significant that felt like a loss.

Ms. Hall also identified that having babies present in the groups is helpful to increase bonding moments between the mothers and babies. In one case, a new mother was finding it challenging to relate and bond with her new baby, who was not yet developmentally able to reciprocate the love that she was giving or felt she was expected to give. This mother loved her baby but was also clouded by depression and learning how to bond with a colicky baby who was not yet smiling or cooing in response to their mother's love. As this mother sat in the forest, with her baby laid out in front of her on the forest floor, she noticed her baby seemed to be focused on the movement of the tree canopy on this windy day. For this mother, it was a moment of realization that her baby is more aware of their surroundings than she realized and is receptive to her love, attention, and efforts, thus allowing for a glimmer of hope that her connection with the baby will grow as they are able to share a reciprocity of awareness and love.

Experiencing nature provides a multitude of benefits for new mothers, but it also deals real challenges. For Ms. Hall, these are weather, public transportation access to the farm, and payment issues. Her farm is not located on a public transit route and services are not covered through OHIP; therefore, those mothers who may most need the services are most likely to not be able to receive them. To address the accessibility issues, she is looking to partner with community agencies with public transit access so that the nature-based occupational therapy services she provides can be offered to a wider range of mothers. Programs are in the development phase to run one of her group sessions in a public park within city limits, to increase accessibility for mothers who cannot easily get to the farm, as well as creating student-led opportunities to enhance maternal-health service delivery models through local community health centers.

Ms. Hall demonstrates that mothers can benefit from connecting with other mothers in a therapeutic outdoor environment through an innovative occupational therapy program such as Willow Family OT. For more information about Willow Family Wellness Occupational Therapy Services, please visit www.willowfamilyot.com.

References

Dodson, M.J. (2004) 'Vestibular stimulation in mania: A case report.' *Journal of Neurology, Neurosurgery & Psychiatry 75*, 168–169.

Grabherr, L., Macauda, G. and Lenggenhager, B. (2015) 'The moving history of vestibular stimulation as a therapeutic intervention.' *Multisensory Research 28*, 5–6, 653–687.

Miyazaki, Y. (2018) *Shinrin Yoku: The Japanese Art of Forest Bathing*. Portland (OR): Timber Press.

The third level is active participation and conscious involvement with nature (Pretty 2004), such as gardening or farming, hiking, camping, and outdoor adventure programs (Howarth *et al.* 2020; Littman *et al.* 2021; Tidball 2018). This category represents outdoor programs that directly engage clients with nature, such as digging and planting, beekeeping, and immersive exploration. Examples of all three of these categories or levels of therapeutic engagement with nature are shared as case narratives throughout the book.

CASE NARRATIVE: Outdoor Kids Occupational Therapy

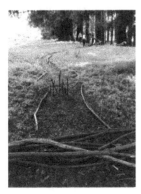

TRAIL BLAZING

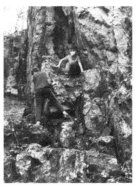

CLIMBING TO NEW HEIGHTS

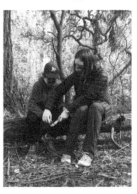

WHITTLING IS A TIME-HONORED ACTIVITY WITH THERAPEUTIC CAPACITIES

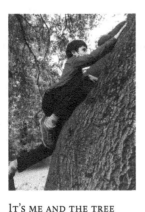

IT'S ME AND THE TREE OUTDOORS

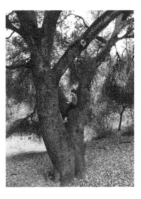

AND THE TREE LOVES ME

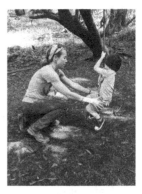

SENSORY-BASED THERAPY

Photo credits: Outdoor Kids Occupational Therapy

Thank you to Laura Park Figueroa, PhD, OTR/L, CEO of Outdoor Kids Occupational Therapy, for contributing to this case narrative.

Outdoor Kids Occupational Therapy (OKOT) is a nature-based occupational therapy practice started in 2015 in Oakland, California, by Laura Park Figueroa. OKOT offers occupational therapy groups in local parks or nature areas for children with challenges in the areas of motor skills, sensory integration, social skills, or mental health. Occupational therapy goals are established collaboratively by the OKOT therapist and parents to address areas that are most important to the family. Groups are run on a school-year schedule, with most children joining in September and attending the same group through May so group cohesion can contribute to the therapy process. Progress on goals is reported to families in December and June. In the summer, week-long camps are offered depending on staff and volunteer availability. OKOT is a fee-for-service program with scholarships available for low-income families that are provided through grant funding from a local philanthropic organization. The grant funding is also used to pay OKOT staff, purchase therapy materials, and cover the costs of park permits where the occupational therapy groups are facilitated.

Groups are run by an occupational therapist and supported by two volunteers, typically occupational therapy students. Groups can accommodate five to six children between the ages of four and ten years old and include children who are receiving occupational therapy services and those who are participating as peer playmates. Weekly group sessions last for 90 minutes to two hours. Peer playmates may be children who have received occupational therapy services in the past or are typically developing. Peer playmates do not have occupational therapy goals.

Each session begins with a review of the day's schedule in a Connection Circle led by an occupational therapist. During Connection Circle, children are encouraged to share with one another through emotional check-ins and mindfulness activities. The daily schedule is reviewed, and the group then transitions to a main therapy activity such as building with natural materials, snack and meal preparation, a craft, or a nature-focused scavenger hunt. Time is built into the schedule for ample opportunity for free play during which the therapists and volunteers seek additional opportunities to support children's individualized therapy goals through the context of play. For instance, a therapist may step in to provide verbal guidance or sensory supports when children experience conflict with one another during play.

OKOT uses the ConTiGO approach, which is an operationalized and evidence-based treatment approach developed by Dr. Figueroa. The intention of the ConTiGO approach is to empower pediatric therapists to take their work with children outdoors and into nature as a means to experience improved health and wellbeing for themselves and their families. ConTiGO is an acronym for Connection and Transformation in the Great Outdoors. *Connection* refers to the foundational belief that connection with other people and with nature is essential for children's long-term health and well-being. *Transformation* refers to the provision of outdoor therapeutic services that are evidence-based, informed by theory, and guided by the therapist's clinical reasoning. *Great Outdoors* refers to therapy sessions taking place in uncultivated nature spaces, and therapists partnering with nature in the therapeutic process. Formal research has not yet been conducted; however, an article on the ConTiGO approach was published in 2020 in the AOTA *Special Interest Section Quarterly Practice Connections* (Figueroa 2020). The complete reference for this article can be found at the conclusion of this case narrative.

The therapists at OKOT find many benefits to offering therapy outdoors. When in nature, children are freer to explore and play using all their senses. Nature invites children to spontaneously engage in play and exploration that leads to improved ability to adapt in daily life. In nature, children develop social connections with each other through shared experiences such as finding animals (both alive and dead). OKOT therapists are well versed in using as many found nature objects as possible during sessions. This approach enables children to build confidence and competence through novel experiences such as building forts from sticks in the woods or, as appropriate, using real tools such as hammers or knives. Therapists at OKOT have also observed that children with sensory differences quickly become more comfortable with messy play in nature. Some children with tactile sensitivities have also become more willing and motivated to wear a jacket and long pants as a precursor to going out to play and, as an outcome of therapy, became more independent in activities of daily living at home.

The staff at OKOT identify many benefits for facilitating therapy outdoors. As nature is anything but static and predictable, there are seemingly boundless opportunities to experience amazement and awe, and out of necessity, to be flexible and adapt to constant change when outside. This mindset parallels the contours of daily life. At OKOT, when children experience conflict with others, it is framed as an opportunity for growth. One parent expressed that their experience at OKOT was the first time any therapist had framed conflict *not* as a negative experience to be avoided in life, but as an opportunity to grow and learn from. This perspective is important to consider as it is a natural tendency to intervene and try to "fix" conflicts as quickly as possible.

In addition to the myriad benefits of outdoor therapy, Dr. Figueroa acknowledged that there are challenges that must be considered. Permits are required to use public parks, which may be restrictive, costly, and time-consuming to complete. For instance, public land may have strict regulations associated with it about where and how children can play in the nature setting. Some parks and recreation departments in large urban areas go to great lengths to protect the land by establishing regulations, and they may not permit children to touch water, climb trees, or pick up sticks or stones. Advocacy is an important consideration for setting up an outdoor therapy practice, and therapists may find they need to advocate for children's rights to play in these areas, while also taking care to protect the land, the park, and the environment. Alternatively, if a therapist is using private land, zoning variances may be required to legally use the land to provide services. Contracts should be established with the landowner to ensure understanding about how the land will be used for therapy services.

When asked to share some practical advice with practitioners, Dr. Figueroa encouraged "thinking like an entrepreneur" to grow programs to best serve a targeted client base. She encourages practitioners who want to take their work outdoors to define exactly who they want to serve with their nature-based program, and tailor their program to meet their participants' unique needs. Last, but certainly not least, Dr. Figueroa shared that practitioners need to be able to clearly communicate the value of their programs to potential participants, create systems to make the program run smoothly, manage finances to ensure the program is sustainable, and, if applicable, be prepared to lead a team that provides quality services.

Dr. Figueroa's innovative work in developing the ConTiGO approach demonstrates that, as healthcare professionals, our clinical work has the capacity to grow and flourish when therapy is facilitated outdoors. For more information about OKOT and the ConTiGO approach, please visit www.outdoorkidsot.com.

Reference
Figueroa, L.P. (2020) 'Nature-based occupational therapy for children with developmental disabilities.' *AOTA Special Interest Section Quarterly Practice Connections* 5, 3, 2–5.

Diversity, Equity, Inclusion, and Justice

As healthcare providers, it is incumbent upon us that we uphold the ethics set forth by the professional organizations we are associated with while providing care (see Chapter 2). As healthcare practitioners interested in taking therapy outside, it is also imperative to consider how diversity, equity, inclusion, and justice relate to health outcomes and access to nature. We recognize that there are shortcomings in the current healthcare and education systems in the U.S., but we also acknowledge that there are improvements we can facilitate as providers.

Because we serve unique and varied communities, it is important to consider all aspects of our client population, not just common symptoms or diagnoses. There are four major concepts to consider beyond symptoms or diagnoses— diversity, equity, inclusion, and justice—and in addition, ultimately, how they correspond to accessing and experiencing nature. Here, we describe the terms and how we broadly relate them to healthcare or other community and educational practices. *Diversity* refers to the different cultures, backgrounds, and demographics of a group. It encompasses the variety of experiences and thoughts within a population. *Equity*, in a generic sense, is fairness—here it refers to strategies, systems, and supports used to help people and communities achieve a goal or outcome. Importantly, equitable strategies are based on the population's needs, rather than predetermined supplies or generic allotments. *Inclusion* refers to ensuring that all people are included and feel seen or represented. Representation, thoughtful word choice, and reflective activity design are important to inclusion. *Justice* refers to how people are treated in the pursuit of providing fair access to care. Justice is achieved when all members of a population are included and considered, and receive appropriate and good care. These concepts work together to ensure that our clients and communities are receiving necessary, appropriate, and ethical care. The concepts of diversity, equity, inclusion, and justice are helpful and important in evaluating nature-based practices and ensuring that programs are appropriately tailored and individualized, as well as accessible.

NUGGET OF NATURE: THE OUTDOORIST OATH—PLANET, INCLUSION, ADVENTURE

The Outdoorist Oath (The Oath) is a non-profit community-focused organization that launched in January 2022. It was created with the belief that individual outdoorists (people) hold the power, privilege, and opportunity to collectively shape the future of the outdoors. It is directed by Gabaccia Moreno and was founded by Teresa Baker, José González, and Pattie Gonia. The Oath's purpose is to educate and unite all people with a shared commitment to act on and advocate for:

- planet
- inclusion
- adventure.

With a vision to "foster a whole-istic community of outdoorists collectively shaping the future of the outdoors," The Oath provides an educational foundation and framework for individuals to investigate questions such as: How can I be a better steward of the landscapes I use? How can I play a part in making the outdoors feel more inclusive to all individuals? In what ways does my everyday life support the protection of natural places for years to come? Visit www.outdooristoath.org to learn more about how you can be a part of this innovative organization and how it may align with your outdoor therapy practice.

We want as many people as possible to experience the health benefits of nature! We say this because while it has been said that "nature is the great equalizer" (Heyerdahl n.d.), this is not the case. Inequitable access to nature has intersectional associations with race, class/socioeconomic status (SES), gender, and ethnicity (Ibes, Rakow, and Kim 2021; Jennings *et al.* 2017; Larson *et al.* 2021). There are fewer outdoor recreational amenities and parks that are safe and accessible in lower-SES neighborhoods, which is both an occupational and environmental injustice (Rigolon and Flohr 2014). Askew and Walls (2019) identified that a lack of positive nature-based early childhood experiences, historical trauma, and personal safety concerns was also associated with inequitable access to nature. According to the Center for American Progress, people of color and low-income communities are more likely than White people or high-income communities to live in a nature-deprived area (Rowland-Shea *et al.* 2020). Despite current injustices and inequalities, we hope you become empowered and inspired to use nature as a tool to support your diverse community's needs, providing inclusive, equitable, and just care.

NUGGET OF NATURE: CONSIDERING UNIVERSAL DESIGN

Universal design, developed by architect Ron Mace and colleagues at North Carolina State University in 1997, is the "design of products and environments to be usable by all people, to the greatest extent possible, without the need for adaptation or specialized design" (NC State University 2019 [1997]). Above and beyond the standards required of the Americans with Disability Act, universal design contains seven principles: equitable use, flexibility in use, simple and intuitive use, perceptible information, tolerance for error, low physical effort, and size and space for approach and use. These seven principles are intended to coalesce into products, services, and environments that improve the quality of life for everyone.

There are ways to think about incorporating universal design into outdoor spaces. As a healthcare practitioner, it is an exciting role to work with design teams to advocate for inclusive design. Below are some definitions and examples of how universal design might be applied to creating new or renovating existing outdoor spaces.

1. Equitable Use: The design is useful and marketable to people with diverse abilities.
    Example: Accessible swings on a playground to meet the needs of a wide range of children.
2. Flexibility in Use: The design accommodates a wide range of individual preferences and abilities.
    Example: Provide left handed and right handed gardening tools or select tools that work equally well with either hand.
3. Simple and Intuitive Use: Use of the design is easy to understand, regardless of the user's experience, knowledge, language skills, or current concentration level.
    Example: The intention of a garden is easy to understand.
4. Perceptible Information: The design communicates necessary information effectively to the user, regardless of ambient conditions or the user's sensory abilities.
    Example: Provide multiple modes for locating trails in a park.
    Example: Provide information about grade (slope) and sensory information about the trails.
5. Tolerance for Error: The design minimizes hazards and the adverse consequences of accidental or unintended actions.
    Example: Paving is level and the joint spaces between pavers is less than 1/8" to avoid catching cane tips and heels.
6. Low Physical Effort: The design can be used efficiently and comfortably and with a minimum of fatigue.
    Example: Paving options such as concrete, asphalt, or rubberized surfaces require less physical effort to navigate over than wood chips.
7. Size and Space for Approach and Use: Appropriate size and space is provided for approach, reach, manipulation, and use regardless of user's body size, posture, or mobility.
    Example: Provide wide trails so that two wheelchair users or two baby strollers and their caregivers can travel in tandem.

North Carolina State University (2019 [1997])

Adapting to Different Environments: If You Cannot Take It Outside, Consider Bringing the Outside In

As previously discussed in this chapter, Ulrich and colleagues found that views of nature were restorative and led to improved healing (Ulrich 1984; Ulrich *et al.* 1991). Newer research conducted during the COVID-19 pandemic supports these findings (Corley *et al.* 2021; Soga *et al.* 2020). With that in mind, we provide you with several ideas for promoting nature-based interventions in alternative environments. Ideally, your program will be designed in collaboration with your clients, and the physical environment will match their needs while maximizing time outdoors. But that may not be feasible as various factors, including client status, staffing, and physical environments, may limit being outside. Further, program delivery must be flexible and responsive to any current situation, and the space may change week to week. Fortunately, successful nature-based programs can be delivered in a variety of environments: indoors, outdoors, a combination of indoors and outdoors, in an outdoor space that has built structures and walkways, in an outdoor space free of any built structures, and virtual environments. With proper planning, any environment can support your program's success. Table 3.1 contains ideas to consider when adapting a nature-based therapy program for a variety of environments.

Ideally, your program is a hybrid of all three environments (outdoor, indoor, and virtual as needed), but reality is what it is, and you as innovative practitioners will adapt to what is required. Applying the above considerations to a specific program could look like this.

If facilitating an indoor container-herb-gardening therapy group at a skilled nursing facility, grow lamps will likely be needed. Plants will need to be located within comfortable reach for sitting and standing. There will need to be an ample supply of gardening tools, many of which are commercially available and adapted or modified by you (refer to Chapter 7, Nugget of Nature: Caring for Mind and Body—A Simple Way to Adapt a Garden Hand Tool). A water supply will be helpful. The workspace will need to accommodate tables and seating and spaces for wheelchairs. Flooring will need to be kept as free from plant material debris as possible. If the program is outdoors, the same considerations for planting materials and garden tools are needed, and a major decision will be whether the plantings are in ergonomically sound raised beds that enable wheels and knees to be directly under the planter or a series of accessible planters. Planning where to work and how to do so most comfortably is key. If there is a virtual element to the therapy group, plants and maintenance items will need to be distributed to clients and placed where they will not only thrive but are easily accessible for clients to tend. Setting up and teaching clients to navigate the virtual meeting platform may be the biggest challenge for a virtual therapy group.

Table 3.1 Considerations for delivering a gardening program in alternative environments

Program delivery indoors		
Changes to consider	**Potential benefits**	**Potential challenges**
• Try to use the same nature-based materials you would use outdoors (e.g. leaves, sticks, flowers, rocks). • Equipment needs may be different. Consider using smaller containers/planters that would be more appropriate for indoor use. • Consider the level of mess you can accommodate indoors and find materials to contain it such as tarps and shower curtains. • Think about the stimuli clients would experience if outdoors (e.g., sounds, wind, smells, sun) and consider incorporating these stimuli indoors by opening windows or doors.	• Increased control of all aspects of the environment, such as: – access to water and toilets – flooring – lighting – temperature – ventilation – noise level. • Participants may attend more consistently, as they will not be subject to the weather conditions during programming. • If incorporating nature into the services you currently deliver, starting indoors could be a smoother transition for clients.	• Some programming, such as wilderness backpacking, may not be adaptable to indoors and cannot be marketed the same way as an outdoor program. • Reduced physical access to nature may minimize healing effects of nature, such as reduced stress and restored attention (Hawkins *et al.* 2013; Kaplan 1995; Ulrich *et al.* 1991).

Program delivery outdoors		
Changes to consider	**Potential benefits**	**Potential challenges**
• Consider where equipment will be stored, such as tables, chairs, and all the associated gardening equipment. • Provision of shade. • Different herbs may be considered if growing totally outdoors. • Consider terrain and accessibility, either looking for more accessible spots or making changes to the space provided.	• More access to nature may improve healing benefits of nature, such as reduced stress (Hawkins *et al.* 2013; Kaplan 1995; Ulrich *et al.* 1991). • Some clients may be more comfortable outdoors and more likely to attend the therapy sessions.	• It may be impractical or unsafe if there is no access to toilets and water or shade. • Working at tables may be challenging on uneven surfaces. • Closer supervision may be required for clients who may wander.

Virtual

Changes to consider	Potential benefits	Potential challenges
• Location of plants may need to be modified from the facility/clinic. Consider: – keeping some plants with the practitioner – delivering plants and materials to clients' homes, if possible. • If the virtual therapy session is intended as a group model, consider alternative ways to promote conversations, perhaps using breakout rooms, white boards, or through chat functions.	• Reduced considerations for transportation as clients will not have to travel to the garden site. • Clients will see plants growing in their homes.	• To be in compliance with HIPAA rules, the cost of a virtual meeting platform may be prohibitive. • Technology and connectivity requirements can be onerous and may discourage or inhibit participation. • Simulating working together in a virtual community setting may be challenging. • Each client's home environment is different for their respective plants, and individual plants may have different growth patterns, which may impact how the clients engage and participate. • In a virtual group model, sharing tools and materials is not possible.

Wrapping It Up

The bottom line is that being in, interacting with, and connecting with nature improves social-emotional health, makes us better thinkers, and makes our bodies and internal systems stronger and more robust. A growing body of evidence overwhelmingly tells us that we, as biophilic individuals, need nature to be part of our lives. As healthcare practitioners, applying the expansive evidence into development of an impactful, client-centered outdoor therapy practice can be revelatory. There is also every possibility that you, the practitioner, will also thrive when you take it outside.

CHAPTER 4

Children and Families

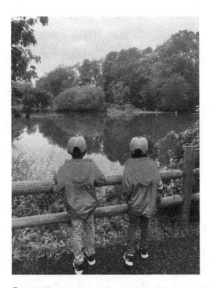

Soft fascination
Photo credit: Rose Adams

Introduction

Childhood begins at birth and ends with the onset of adolescence at about age 12–13 years. While childhood begins at birth, a developing fetus is vulnerable to outside influences such as maternal physical and mental health, maternal nutrition, and *teratogens*, which are environmental factors such as chemical exposure, smoking, and alcohol consumption that may impact the health of the fetus (Chaudhary and Sehgal 2019; Gaillard, Wright, and Jaddoe 2019; Leimert and Olson 2020). The stages associated with the time between birth to about age 13 are often referred to as newborn, infancy, toddler, preschool, and school age. During childhood, and throughout life, the major areas of development are categorized as social-emotional, language, cognitive, and physical/motor. There are many milestone charts and tables available online to track a child's development, including an updated version on the U.S. CDC website (2022b). Interested readers are encouraged to examine several and compare the ages at which developmental skills are typically understood to emerge. For the purposes of description, we separated the areas of development, but in reality, development of each area is connected with the others.

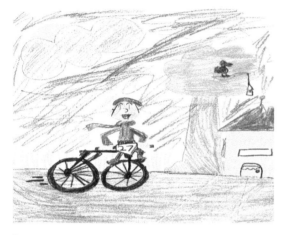

I LIKE BIKE RIDING IN THE COOL AIR!

Social-Emotional Development and Health in Childhood

Social-emotional development is a challenging term to define, so let's first look at its two component parts and then piece it together. Social development is about a child being able to understand the "values, knowledge, and skills" needed to participate in meaningful ways on microsocial (family), mesosocial (school), and macrosocial (community) levels (Kirk and Jay 2018, p.474). A child's social development relies upon their emotional development, which is the ability to recognize, understand, and regulate their emotions (Kirk and Jay 2018). There is strong synergy between the social skills required to build relationships and the emotional skills needed to sustain those relationships. The importance and implications of social-emotional development and health across the lifespan cannot be underestimated, according to Halle and Darling-Churchill (2016): "as children continue to develop social and emotional skills, they gain the confidence and competence needed to build relationships across settings, problem solve, and cope with challenges" (p.9). Social-emotional health is the bedrock of resilience.

Early in life, children begin to develop social-emotional competencies, most often through the interactions they have with their primary caregiver (Behrendt *et al.* 2019) such as singing, reading, and cuddling. Historically, the mother typically filled the role of primary caregiver (Ainsworth 1979; Lewis and Feiring

1989), but more contemporary research literature tends to avoid stereotyping with whom a child develops this pivotal first relationship and instead refers to this relationship partner as parent/caregiver (Hornor 2019). A first pivotal relationship could be with a father, mother, grandparent, aunt, uncle, nanny, or other significant person. A responsive caregiver who is available to consistently comfort the child, to help them regulate, to talk with them, and to be their secure and consistent "rock" of support—or, in attachment vernacular, "secure base"—lays the foundation for resilience, confidence, and healthy relationship building (Bowlby 2008 [1988]). Throughout childhood, children develop a set of social-emotional skills and strategies that enable them to understand and manage emotions, set and achieve goals, appreciate the perspectives of others, feel and show empathy for others, establish and maintain relationships, make responsible decisions, handle interpersonal situations constructively (Kirk and Jay 2018, p.474), and support relationship management (Scorza *et al.* 2015).

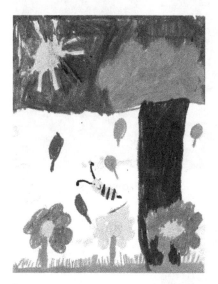

JUMPING INTO LEAVES

NUGGET OF NATURE: NATURE YOGA

Yoga is an evidence-based practice for people of all ages that is beneficial for the body and mind (Cartwright *et al.* 2020). It is becoming increasingly popular with children to help self-regulate, alleviate anxiety, and to move their bodies (Nanthakumar 2018). Yoga can be practiced anywhere—inside or outside—and can be an engaging activity for children or as a caregiver–child activity.

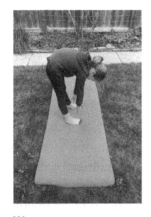

WATERFALL POSE

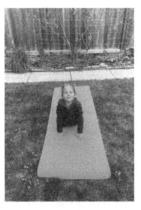

UPWARD-FACING DOG POSE

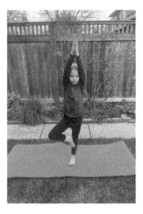

TREE POSE

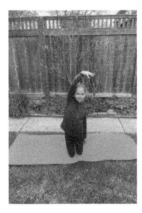

RAINBOW POSE

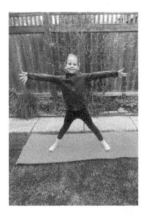

STAR POSE

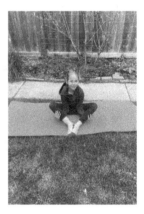

FLOWER POSE

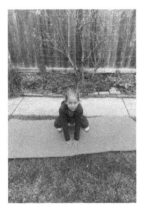

FROG POSE
Photo credits: Ryan Durkin

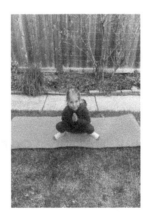

LITTLE SPROUT POSE

Materials you will need

- Yoga mats, small blankets, or bath towels

Steps to facilitate the activity

1. Use the photos provided with this Nugget of Nature or consult books and/or Internet sources as guides for children's nature-focused yoga poses.
2. Spread out enough mats/blankets/towels so each child has their own space with room around each mat for arms and legs to move without touching other children.
3. Share with children that yoga is a very ancient activity and when we do yoga, we may be very quiet when doing some poses such as "tree" or sometimes make noises like a soft "ribbit" when doing frog pose.
4. Explain to children that everyone has their own way of doing yoga and however they do it is just fine.
5. Tell children that you might help them with a pose if you think they might be hurting themselves.
6. Start the session by asking the children to lie on their backs with their arms and legs spread out like a starfish and ask them to slowly breathe in and out to the count of three for five repetitions.
7. Introduce one pose at a time, demonstrating and holding the pose for at least ten seconds so the children can take time to process what you are doing. Use words to describe your actions as needed.
8. Invite children to assume the pose as best they can, with your hands-on intervention as needed to correct any postures that could be physically harmful for them.
9. End the yoga session by having children (again) lie on their backs with their arms and legs spread out like a starfish and ask them to breathe in and out to the count of three for five repetitions.
10. Ask the children to roll onto their left side and then slowly sit up, stretch their arms up above their heads, and then lower them and clasp their hands together over their heart, and say aloud, "Namaste."

How to make the activity easier

- Modify the poses so that they can be done in a chair.
- Use only one or two poses per session.

How to make the activity more challenging

- Invite children to invent and share their own nature-inspired yoga poses.

Communication and Language Development in Childhood

We communicate through physical gestures and touch, spoken words/sounds, and/or written words, icons, and pictures. For children, communication begins early and happens often. A typically developing infant will cry when they are hungry or tired, need a diaper change, or want attention. An attuned caregiver responds promptly, and thus the earliest dyadic communication loop begins. When a caregiver talks and sings lullabies to their infant and repeats the sounds they make, these are lovely early conversations that set the stage for the explosion of language that typically occurs towards the end of the first year.

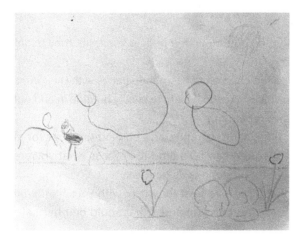

BEING OUTSIDE WITH MY FAMILY IS THE BEST

Language development represents a combination of the constructs of speech (the sounds), language (comprehension of words, sentences, and ideas), and communication (verbal and nonverbal use of language to interact with and convey ideas to others) (Visser-Bochane *et al.* 2020, p.421). Children understand (receptive language) words before they can say (expressive language) them (Kobaş *et al.* 2022; Stolt *et al.* 2016). This results in the earliest forms of communication typically manifesting as gestures, behaviors, and expressions of needs. As communication skills develop, children become more adept at expressing their needs, holding conversations, and learning to interpret nonverbal cues. Social-emotional development and language/communication development are entwined, as social relationships are sustained through communication.

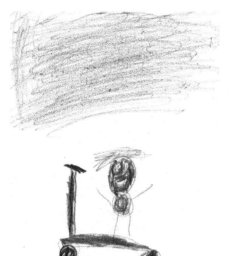

RIDING ON MY SCOOTER

Cognitive Development in Childhood

Cognitive development encompasses thinking and reasoning and entails acquiring, organizing, and using knowledge to solve problems (Gelman 1978). With age and experience, the quality of cognitive development advances. We often view play as a child's way to work through developing cognition (Ginsburg, Committee on Communications, and Committee on Psychosocial Aspects of Child and Family Health 2007; Robertson, Yim, and Paatsch 2020). Children increase their ability to understand more advanced concepts as they acquire command of simpler skills such as searching for an object hidden under a blanket as a precursor to solving puzzles, problem solving how to take off a sock before being able to button a jacket, and identifying letters in readiness for learning to read. Like all other areas of development, cognitive development relies on interplay between social-emotional, language and communication, and physical/motor development. For instance, we cannot assemble puzzles without motor skills or engage in hide-and-seek without the requisite social skills.

NUGGET OF NATURE: PRODUCE PEOPLE

Creating "people" out of pieces of produce is a fun way to learn about fruits and vegetables and may also be a useful activity for a feeding group. Best of all, children can eat their produce person when the activity is over.

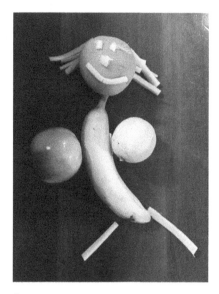

A DELICIOUS AND NUTRITIOUS PRODUCE PERSON
Photo credit: Nari Chung

Materials you will need

- Fresh fruits and vegetables
- Fresh herbs
- Raisins
- Knife
- Food processor or grater
- Cutting board
- Posterboard or other heavy-duty paper cut into 18" squares
- Toothpicks (optional)
- Bags
- Markers

Steps to making a produce person

1. Cut the heavy-duty paper into approximately 18" squares.
2. Thinly slice or shred some of the fruit or vegetables for use as hair or facial features. Jicama (Mexican potato/turnip), carrots, or peppers will work well.
3. Provide every child with the same selection of produce and herbs.
4. Invite children to arrange their produce and herbs on their work surface and make a produce person. Encourage them to rearrange and arrange as much as they need to make a person they are most satisfied with.

5. If using toothpicks, children can fasten the sliced or shredded vegetables onto their produce person's head.
6. Ask children to tell you or others in the group about their produce person— who it is and what is special about them.
7. Take photographs of each child's produce person and be sure that their caregiver receives a copy of it.
8. Carefully wash each child's produce and invite them to eat it and take home what they do not eat.
9. Talk about the fruits and vegetables, what colors they are, their shapes, what they taste like, whether they have seeds, etc.
10. Pack up the leftover produce in bags labeled with the child's name on so that they can take it home.

How to make the activity easier

- Provide hand-over-hand assistance to arrange the produce.
- Limit the number of pieces of produce to use.

How to make the activity more challenging

- Use tweezers or small tongs to pick up and place the thinly sliced or shredded vegetables on the produce person.
- Place produce in a paper bag and ask children to identify each piece of produce by touch before removing it from the bag. Also consider using the non-dominant hand to do this task.

Physical/Motor Development in Childhood

Physical and motor development is about how movement skills are acquired and progress in the body. Physical and motor development starts with reflex integration to allow for purposeful movement, developing postural control to support active movement, and gross and fine motor skill development to play and learn about the world. Like all other areas of development, physical and motor development is influenced by internal factors such as genetics and external factors and contexts such as prenatal care, socioeconomic status, and maternal physical and mental health.

Gross motor skills, such as crawling, standing, walking, and running, are initiated with and supported by the larger muscles and joints of the body. The larger muscle groups and joints, such as the shoulder and hip/thigh, are located proximally (closer) to the center of the body, and the smaller muscles and joints such as the fingers and toes are located distally (further) from the center of the body.

Gross motor development typically precedes fine motor development. For instance, before an infant can grasp a piece of cereal from a highchair tray, they need to be able to have the trunk control to sit upright and to have the shoulder stability needed to reach for the cereal. The interested reader can find the typical progression of gross motor skills in a developmental milestone listing (e.g., CDC 2022b).

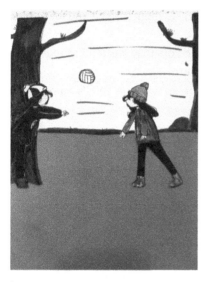

I LIKE TO PLAY VOLLEYBALL OUTSIDE WITH FRIENDS

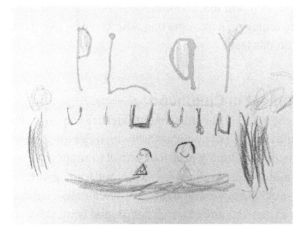

I LIKE TO PLAY OUTSIDE AND DO AN OBSTACLE COURSE—IT'S FUN

Fine motor skills are refined movements done with the fingers, such as grasping that piece of cereal from the highchair tray. Fine motor skills involve grasp, manipulation, and release (Strooband *et al.* 2022; Valevicius *et al.* 2018). Skilled use of the fingers starts with larger and less coordinated hand and wrist movements, like using the entire hand as a scoop to retrieve the piece of cereal from the highchair tray, and progresses to being able to use smaller and more precise movements, like using the tip of the thumb and index finger to grasp the piece of cereal (Brook, Wagenfeld, and Thompson 2016). Skilled hand use enables humans to use and manipulate tools such as pencils to write with and forks to eat with. An integral part of the entwined relationship between social-emotional, language and communication, cognitive, and physical/motor development is that we use our hands to touch, feel, understand, and communicate with the world around us.

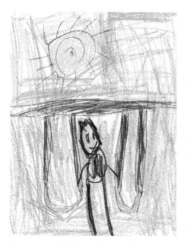

PLAYING ON THE SWINGS

NUGGET OF NATURE: SCAVENGER HUNT

A scavenger hunt is like going on a spy expedition to look for things in plain sight and other things that might not be so easy to find. Its benefits are broad and include physical activity, sensation, learning, communicating, and cooperation. And most of all it is fun! A table that includes a sample list of items to find and their holistic qualities follows at the end of this Nugget of Nature. Expand on this list and explore on.

Materials you will need

- Heavy paper, small chalk boards, or white boards
- Pencils, chalk, or erase markers
- Stickers (optional)
- Camera or smartphone
- Collection bag (optional)

Steps to facilitating a scavenger hunt

1. Decide where the scavenger hunt will commence. It could be anywhere that is safe and has nature. Note: If your scavenger hunt is to be facilitated by looking out of a window rather than being outside, prepare a list of things that your client will be able to see from the window, such as birds, trees, grass, flowers, clouds, etc.
2. Create a list of items to be found. The list can be written words, photos, icons, drawings, and/or an audio list.
3. Copy the list into whatever format that works best for your client to participate in their scavenger hunt.
4. Decide how found items will be checked off. It could be dictating to you, a tick mark with a pen, piece of chalk, dry erase pen, sticker, photograph, etc.
5. Prepare to go on a scavenger hunt!
6. Provide copies of the scavenger hunt list.
7. Once at the site, explain that there are items to be found and that when they are found, you would like them to be ticked off the list or stickered, or you will help take photos of each item (if help is required).
8. Set and discuss a time limit, if appropriate.
9. Encourage gentle touching and exploration of the scavenger hunt items.
10. It is the least optimal option to collect the items in bags, but if that is necessary, please compost the nature materials after the activity is over.

How to make the activity easier

- Include only two or three items to be found.
- Be consistent as to the location of items, such as only on the ground, waist level, etc.
- Assist clients with identifying items and ticking them off the list.

How to make the activity more challenging

- Include a list of ten or more items to be found.
- Vary the location of items, such as on the ground, above shoulder height, waist level, etc.
- When the scavenger hunt ends, encourage your clients to create stories about their experience. It could be a written story, a narrated story, drawings or paintings, a video, or a clay sculpture.

Table 4.1 Scavenger hunt items and benefits

Scavenger hunt item: simple	Scavenger hunt item: complex	Move	Think and communicate	Sense
Tree	• Tree with many branches • Pine tree	Hug the tree trunk Reach up and "touch" the highest branch	What color is the bark? The leaves? Does it have flowers?	How does the bark feel? How tightly can you hug the tree? What does the tree smell like?
Rock	• Smooth rock • Shiny rock • Round or square rock	Squat down and pick up the rock and/or turn the rock over in your hands and move it between your right and left hand	What shape is the rock? What color(s) is the rock?	Is it smooth or rough? Dark or light? Does it have a smell?
Pinecone	• Small pinecone • Medium pinecone • Large pinecone	Reach up to the pine tree with both hands to touch a pinecone If there are pinecones on the ground, scoop them up and make a pinecone tower on the ground, a tabletop, bench, chair, or wheelchair tray	What shape is the pinecone? How many pinecones do you see? Where are the pinecones?	Is the pinecone rough? How does it smell? Can you hold it in your hand without squishing it?
Leaf	• Leaf with pointed edges • Heart-shaped leaf • Round leaf	Dance like a leaf waving in the wind	What color is the leaf? How many leaves can you find? Are there big and little leaves?	How does a leaf feel when you stroke it with your fingers? Does a leaf have a smell? Can you hear the leaves rustling in the breeze?
Cloud	• Lacy cloud • Puffy cloud	Use your finger to trace the clouds in the sky	What color are rain clouds? What do you think clouds feel like?	What shapes can you see? Can you see clouds shaped like animals?
Flower	• Pink flower • Flower with yellow petals • Lots of flowers on a single stem	Gently pinch the flower petals without pulling any off the stem Bloom like a flower (keep your arms close to your body and then raise them out to the sides and up towards the sky)	Count the petals on a flower What color flowers did you find? What shape are the flower petals?	What does the flower smell like? Are the petals smooth and silky or are they sticky?
Puddle	• Shallow puddle • Puddle on a sidewalk	Splash in the puddle, right foot first and then the left Toss small pebbles into a puddle	How big is the puddle? What color is the water in the puddle? Why are there puddles?	What sounds do you hear when splashing in the puddle or tossing pebbles into them?

Therapeutic Benefits of Nature: Children and Families

Nature-based experiences can, even in utero, positively impact how children develop social-emotionally, communicate, learn, move, and become lifelong lovers and stewards of nature (Dzhambov, Dimitrova, and Dimitrakova 2014; Mulholland and Williams 1998; Runkle *et al.* 2022). In this section, we explore the literature that links nature with childhood development and family enrichment. Many of the findings add an extra layer of authenticity and evidence that you might want or need for setting up your pediatric outdoor therapy program. We also share some incredible examples of child- and family-focused outdoor therapy programs and how they have changed the lives of those they serve. We can only assume that not only are children and families the beneficiaries of this therapy outside, but so too are the practitioners who are also reaping the benefits of being outdoors.

But first, take a moment to reflect on your childhood and your outside play. Perhaps a tree was transformed into a castle, or flowers and grass became ingredients for a delectable soup, and the empty lot in your neighborhood was a magical island where a ship had been marooned and children made all the rules. These fun and creative play schemes are examples of how nature-based play positively impacted our childhoods. Outdoor play contributes to children's overall development and health and wellbeing, but today's children are not spending enough time outside, and this is negatively impacting their development and overall health, including increased rates of obesity, attentional issues, and depression (Beery and Jørgensen 2018; Kuo and Faber-Taylor 2004; Wyver *et al.* 2010). Refer to Table 4.2 (see p.122) as well as the American Academy of Pediatrics' (2007) position statement, which recommends children spend a minimum of 30–60 minutes a day engaged in free play, much of which can and should happen outside. When considering why children spend insufficient time outside, the reasons may include barriers to physical access to outdoor nature and play spaces for children and their families with disabilities, perceived lack of time, caregiver perception that play is not valuable, and safety concerns. We can be part of the movement to change this paradigm and assist clients to access nature and the opportunities for connections—connections of the imagination, profoundly meaningful connections to places, and connections between people.

CASE NARRATIVE: TimberNook

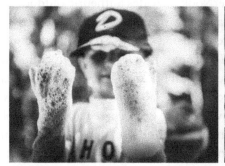

SUPER-SUDSY SENSORY PLAY

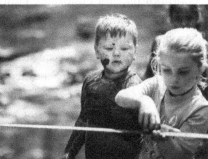

SENSORY-RICH EXPLORATION

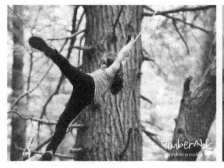

DEFYING GRAVITY

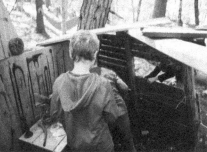

COOPERATIVE SOCIAL CONSTRUCTION

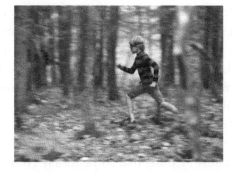

NATURE BRINGS OUT THE BEST IN CHILDREN
Photo credits: TimberNook

Thank you to Angela Hanscom, MOTR/L, Founder of TimberNook, for helping to prepare this case narrative.

Imagine a therapy world where children are outside, playing together, getting dirty, and having fun. TimberNook, a leading therapy organization, makes this happen through its mission "to restore and enrich the occupation of outdoor play for children." TimberNook provides authentic outdoor play experiences for children and teenagers. At the heart of every TimberNook program is the "experience." An example of a TimberNook play experience is after listening to classic story *The Three Little Pigs*, children build their own life-sized "little pig" homes out of real bricks or bales of hay. They can find sticks out in the woods and create an elaborate obstacle course over giant mud puddles for the big bad wolf to traverse. These nature-based play adventures engage the muscles and senses, and use higher-level thinking skills as children experience the story through authentic play. It also offers a child-directed opportunity, where children can participate at their own level, often eliminating the need to upgrade or downgrade by an adult.

Loose parts are fundamental to running a TimberNook program. The play environment is staged using loose parts such as tires, milk crates, planks, bricks, pallets, sticks, ramps, and other unique materials like feathered masks, transparent curtains, Mardi Gras beads, paint, giant canvases, fake jewels, pulleys, tools, and kitchenware to inspire hours of creative play in the woods with other children of mixed ages. Providers and teachers often seek out donations from their community for many of these items. They may also find a lot of these materials at thrift stores or garage sales. Each play experience is unique and provides new opportunities to learn, adapt, transform, and connect with others.

For any practitioner looking for the inspiration to start small and local and dream big, Ms. Hanscom started running nature-based programming in 2010 in her backyard in Barrington, New Hampshire. Out of this initial effort, TimberNook was created in 2013 to share the concept and program with children in other parts of the world. Since then, home base has become one of their training facilities. There are now TimberNook sites located throughout the United States, Canada, Australia, and the United Kingdom.

Knowing the back story is often compelling, and TimberNook is no exception. A series of events happened in Ms. Hanscom's life that set her on this path. It was never "her idea," but something that authentically evolved due to an incredible need—not just in her community but all over the world! The first thing that set her on this journey was observations in an outpatient pediatric therapy clinic setting. She was noticing a rise in interesting sensory issues such as an intolerance to wind in the face, displeasure with getting hands messy, and decreased strength. Most interestingly, children were apparently becoming clumsier. At the same time, her daughter was entering kindergarten. The expectations in her school were far from developmentally appropriate, and she started coming home saying, "I hate school." They had taken play out of kindergarten and replaced it with academics and testing. Ms. Hanscom knew she was not alone in her concern as a parent about the unrealistic academic demands on young children.

Inspired to help her own daughter and the growing need in her community, Ms. Hanscom created and implemented a small therapeutic nature-camp program in her backyard. The "roots" of TimberNook are revealed! Ms. Hanscom shared that she was only going to do it for a summer. Little did she know that this was the beginning of something far greater than she ever could have imagined.

Every year, she would agree to run summer camps for "one more year." Fast-forward a couple of years, and Ms. Hanscom found she could not meet the growing demand on her own. For example, an occupational and physical therapist reached out to ask if they could replicate the program, noting it to be "unique for our profession." Realizing this was a "gift" that needed to be shared, she decided to license the program and share with others. In 2014, she wrote an article called "Why Kids Fidget and What We Can Do About It" on her blog. It went viral and got picked up by the *Washington Post* (www.washingtonpost.com/news/answer-sheet/wp/2014/07/08/why-so-many-kids-cant-sit-still-in-school-today). Then the *Washington Post* article too went viral. Ms. Hanscom started writing for the *Washington Post* and many of her pieces continued to have a great reach. That is how TimberNook quickly became an internationally recognized program. Her widely acclaimed book, *Balanced and Barefoot: How Unrestricted Play Makes for Strong, Confident, and Capable Children*, was published in 2016 by New Harbinger Publications. It is a must-read.

In addition to being in nature, and based on a mainstreaming model, children of different abilities, interests, ages, and backgrounds come to TimberNook and play together in a natural social environment. This scaffolding helps to create an authentic, real, "natural" environment, where more advanced children often model more advanced language, social-emotional, and problem-solving skills to their peers. In effect, this peer modeling helps to influence the group dynamics and promote healthy change in children whose developmental skills are still emerging.

TimberNook is facilitated outside in a large group format that typically includes 20–25 children, with each group functioning as its own cohort. The ideal TimberNook teacher-to-child ratio is about 1:6. Deeply immersive, TimberNook sessions in the woods typically last for three to six hours. In the school setting, they run for about two hours. This length allows for group cohesion, problem solving, and great opportunities to play in the best place of all, outside. Children and providers are out in the snow, rain, and warmer weather as TimberNook programs are run year-round. To enable year-round participation, TimberNook training includes providing education to the school and parent communities on the importance of proper gear for children to wear, no matter the season.

Most TimberNook sites are on privately owned land, but a few are on public land. The programs typically take place in woodlands located away from buildings. There are a few structural additions to the otherwise untouched woodland such as a rope swing, fire pit/circle, and other such elements. The rest of the materials are loose parts that can be moved in and out of the woods such as wooden planks and tires. Program maintenance varies.

Ms. Hanscom's location is on her property, so it is self-managed. Typically, the host site manages the property, but the TimberNook providers take care of the outdoor classroom maintenance. Some TimberNook providers do not own the property where they facilitate the program but work with a "host site" such as a farm, orchard, or wooded schoolground. As part of TimberNook training, providers learn how to create and prepare an inspiring outdoor environment where it is safe for children to have hours of outdoor play opportunities. The outdoor therapeutic classroom is usually a few acres or more and ideally is immersed in the woods. Wooded sites provide shade and a sense of being immersed in woodland play. Many TimberNook sites also have access to natural sources of water such as giant puddles, vernal (seasonal) ponds, streams, and/or a river, which provide wonderful opportunities for rich water and mud play.

The main goal of TimberNook is to inspire children and teens to play independently and creatively. The therapeutic and educational benefits of the program are vast and limitless. The program challenges everything from executive functions such as being able to initiate a play idea and then execute that play scheme, to dealing with social-emotional skills like frustration tolerance and being mentally flexible with other children's ideas, to sensory integration and physical activity. The program also offers hands-on learning experiences. For instance, giving children the opportunity to work and play together to create a giant ball run in the woods by using gutters, tubing, and duct tape encourages them to use advanced problem-solving skills, practice physics concepts, and test out their leadership skills.

Both providers and schools receive ongoing professional development, curriculum support, branded marketing materials, website access, and connection to other providers/schools and the TimberNook conference. TimberNook is a credentialed AOTA (American Occupational Therapy Association) provider; therefore, occupational therapy practitioners can use training hours, both initial and ongoing, towards their licensure hours.

In 2017, a TimberNook initiative was established so that schools were offered the opportunity to become a TimberNook Certified School and to provide the program as part of their curriculum. The hope was to use this approach to make TimberNook more accessible to all children. The TimberNook play experiences are also linked to national standards for children aged 4–14 years. The teachers train in the TimberNook approach and offer two-hour blocks of "TimberNook time" during the week. Teachers receive ongoing curriculum and professional development to increase carryover and richness of the program. A list of schools (both public and private) that have become certified can be found at www.timbernook.com/timbernook-certified-schools-and-curriculum/teacher-training.

TimberNook providers pay roughly $8500 for the licensed program and the eight-day training. This also covers a protected exclusive territory for implementing the program. Certified schools pay $10,000 for the license and onsite training to offer the TimberNook program for their school community. This covers training of four teachers. Some of the certified schools and providers receive grant funding to pay for their training. Public schools have used Title 1 grant funding from the U.S. government, and parent teacher organization (PTO) money to obtain training.

Typically, there is at least one provider who runs the program for liability reasons and to maintain the richness of the program along with trained support staff and counselors. TimberNook providers are professionals and/or organizations that are licensed to use the TimberNook program as a small business opportunity. They have access to everything from TimberNook summer camps to forest programming, and even TimberNook birthday parties. Many providers are occupational therapists; however, there are educators, passionate parents, therapy clinics, and non-profit organizations that also hold a license to provide TimberNook programming to their community. TimberNook takes private pay for their programming. The cost is kept reasonable and within the market of high-quality forest and camp programming. An example cost for a week of camp for one child is $325 for a 9.00 a.m. to 3.00 p.m. program, Monday to Friday. Some providers will take sponsorships and provide scholarships for a few children to attend their program.

When facilitated at schools, there needs to be at least one trained teacher or therapist helping to run the program. Support staff are frequently trained by the trained teacher. Additional support staff are often college students—most commonly occupational therapy students. Some of the locations take fieldwork students as part of their learning experience. While the actual program is not facilitated virtually, some training can happen via video conferencing; ideally, though, it is all about being outside and in nature as a key part of training.

TimberNook has been involved with several research projects, and the result of a recent one was development of an observational tool to assess social-emotional, executive functioning, and overall richness and benefits of the play experiences at TimberNook. For additional information about research that has been conducted about TimberNook, please see www.timbernook.com/our-approach-outdoor-experiential-learning-play/our-timbernook-emotional-social-physical-growth.

In terms of marketing, most TimberNook providers use Facebook as their primary method of sharing current research and the neurological benefits of outdoor play. Many also use Twitter and Instagram. Additionally the website (see below) helps parents to learn about what and why they offer this type of programming. However, the programs have always sold themselves mostly via word of mouth from excited children and families.

Words from the source are often the most meaningful, and the two stories below, which are from parents of TimberNook campers, are no exception. The first story was shared during the COVID-19 pandemic.

Hi Angie, Thank you for yet another wonderful day at TimberNook! I wanted to share how impactful your program is for our son, Philip. I know we discussed how he had multiple tics that developed during remote learning last spring. They were with him all day and night and impacted his day "big time." They went away after three hours of TimberNook this past July. And they didn't come back. We now homeschool Philip for this very reason but try to stay connected to his teachers/classmates. Last Thursday, the children at his school were first invited back to the outside grounds, where they did social connection types of things while masked and all of the rules that are necessary for the public-school setting. He was there for one-and-a-half hours. He was with familiar children and familiar teachers, outside of his familiar school.

I picked him up, and he was absolutely exhausted and drained, and needed me to read to him for like three hours afterwards to unwind, and then take a long bath. It was so upsetting to observe his body moving so out of control again. It seems that he enjoyed being there, but he said it was way too long and he can't put into words what they did. He was paying attention to all the details and trying to understand the environment/new rules/etc. Long story short, after one-and-a-half hours, he climbed into my car and the tics were back for the first time since TimberNook camp in July. We focused on a lot of deep play and no-pressure activities, and they were slowing down. I noticed when I picked him up from TimberNook this past week they were gone again! After TimberNook, Philip is tired, but energized, and so happy/content. Like his body can settle in. He bubbles into the car and describes so many exciting things about his day. He goes on and on about it. Today he said, "It was just so fun. It was the best!" For our family, TimberNook is what is grounding Philip and helping him function as the child he truly is, during a time when so much has changed in his world. See you next week! Cindy

Another parent shared:

My daughter just finished a week of camp at TimberNook. After completing her first year of pre-kindergarten, I was left feeling that the system we placed her into, albeit well-meaning, stifled her gifts and often failed to recognize her uniqueness and penchant for all things nature. One week of Timber-Nook brought my daughter back to life in so many ways. Her eyes opened wide again, and she couldn't wait to arrive at camp each and every day. What y'all are doing is a true gift.

The providers at TimberNook also have been greatly impacted and inspired by the work they do. Occupational therapist Kate Davis shared:

I think that TimberNook values experiences over activities, because they tap into a child's highest potential, and this is where you really captivate and "transform" a child. The ability to generate new ideas is a difficult skill to teach children, and the only way to really tap into that is to give them an open-ended opportunity, a set of materials that sparks interest and the freedom to experiment.

TimberNook provider Christa Thomas said:

Rarely are children ever given the opportunity to just be themselves and do what they want to do—explore their own interests. At TimberNook, children get a different experience. They get one that will make lasting impressions on who they are and what they are capable of. We provide an escape for children... I'm so proud to be part of something so magical. My heart just about explodes every time I see a child smile with pride as they accomplish something new.

As with any program, there are benefits and challenges. Ms. Hanscom said that the hardest part is often finding a location to run high-quality programming. Another barrier is a provider/practitioner with limited business knowledge and/or experience. For this reason, she often recommends that anyone who trains with TimberNook have a business mentor in place before starting.

You can get a free business mentor from the Small Business Association here in the United States. The advice they provide is invaluable. The benefits far outweigh the challenges as children thrive in TimberNook, and so do the providers.

When asked to provide some advice, Ms. Hanscom told us:

> Nature offers the ultimate sensory experience for children. The more immersed in nature you are, the greater the therapeutic potential. My recommendation is to find a space, preferably in the woods, for programming and/or therapy. It is ideal if you can leave things out there such as a fire pit, swing hook ups, and loose parts to make life easier for the practitioner. I also highly recommend having a storage unit somewhere on property to increase ease of accessing materials.

Sage advice indeed for any outside therapy program. For further information about TimberNook, please visit the website at www.timbernook.com.

Reference

Hanscom, A.J. (2016) *Balanced and Barefoot: How Unrestricted Play Makes for Strong, Confident, and Capable Children.* Oakland, CA: New Harbinger Publications.

Feeling in Nature: Social-Emotional Development

Natural environments and shared time in nature provide opportunities for social interaction and connection within families (Rantala and Puhakka 2020). A parent/caregiver-and-child interaction is more "responsive and connected" when it happens in an outdoor environment compared to inside (Cameron-Faulkner, Melville, and Gattis 2018, p.10). For instance, neighborhood parks can offer children and their families opportunities to be in nature, to nurture their connections with each other, to engage in fantasy play, and to celebrate the awe of nature (Harris 2016). For outdoor therapy practices that are intended to be family focused, take heed of its social connectivity potential!

Playing outside should not be a luxury or privilege, but a necessity and key ingredient for healthy development. Outdoor nature play is important for children's social-emotional development as it provides opportunity for restoration and relaxation and escape from stressors of daily life (Chiumento *et al.* 2018). The attention restoration theory (Kaplan and Kaplan 1989), discussed in Chapter 3, is applicable to children's social-emotional development. Nature exposure, such as walking in a park or gazing out of a window at a tree canopy, is a positive counter to engagement in prolonged and highly focused tasks such as seated classroom learning. For children, an important way to experience attentional restoration is through recess. According to a 2013 American Academy of Pediatrics policy statement, "Recess promotes social and emotional learning and development for children by offering them a time to engage in peer interactions in which they practice, and role play essential social skills...including negotiation, cooperation, sharing, and problem solving"—all invaluable lifelong tools (Council on School Health *et al.* 2013, p.184). The term "recess" may conjure up different images, such as playing games like jacks, four-square, or hopscotch on an asphalt surface, navigating a sensory path, playing on a playground with swings, slides, and climbing apparatus, or a natural play space with unstructured elements such as logs, rocks, and trees. This imagery is important and here is why.

There are demonstrated links between the physical qualities of an outdoor space and children's emotional self-regulation (Moore, Morrissey, and Robertson 2021). Outdoor spaces that children perceive to be crowded, dirty, and loud can be distracting and lead to untoward behaviors (Ismail *et al.* 2017). On the other hand, outdoor spaces that are open and less crowded provide opportunities for children to experience agency, to place attachment, and to hide (prospect and refuge) (Moore *et al.* 2021, p.949). These same spaces that support play also enhance a child's sense of wellbeing, relaxation, and happiness. Other elements such as trees, plants, and objects to climb on and explore are not only rich in sensory opportunities but also provide children with a sense of peace and calm, and an early appreciation of nature (Nedovic and Morrissey 2013). Providing children with early and frequent nature exposure is a matter of occupational and environmental justice leading to improved health and wellbeing, and learning to love and sustain our planet.

The Nature Communication Connection

Research finds that exposure to nature can positively impact a child's language development. Being outside provides children with unique experiences, play situations, and novel objects that promote language development (Flannigan and Dietze 2017). According to a study by Norling, Sandberg, and Almqvist (2015), the outdoor environment acts as a stimulating language-learning environment by providing additional freedom and activity choices, increased interaction between children, increased discussion with peers and caregivers about how the outside world works, and increased play opportunities.

Learning color names when flowers are in bloom, words that express size and shape, and animal sounds can happen spontaneously when children and the adults in their lives are outside (Honig 2019). Working together to construct a fort or cubby house from loose parts, such as branches and twigs, stones, vines, and whatever else can be found, involves the give and take akin to the most complex of negotiations to create an optimal space to occupy. Planning the recipe and gathering the ingredients to make "mud stew" and sharing it with peers involves communication and social interaction. While pretend cooking and block building can happen indoors, the sheer spontaneity and opportunity to expand the creative process increase exponentially when children cook, build, and play outdoors.

CASE NARRATIVE: Christopher Griffith Monroe, Metro Music Therapy

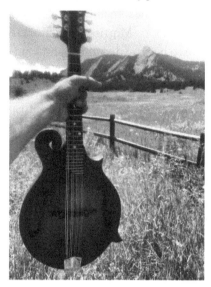

NATURE IS THE ULTIMATE MUSE
Photo credit: Chris Monroe

Thank you to Chris Monroe, MM, MT-BC, NMT, Staff Therapist at Metro Music Therapy for helping to prepare this case narrative.

Music therapist and nature enthusiast Mr. Chris Monroe is on staff at Metro Music Therapy, Inc., (MMT) and recently completed his master's degree in music therapy at Western Michigan University in Kalamazoo, Michigan. Mr. Monroe has provided music therapy sessions outdoors in clients' backyards, at day programs, and residential facilities. Practicing in Denver, there is often a majestic mountain view in the background when facilitating therapy sessions outdoors, thus increasing the nature factor. Being a very sunny city despite any chill in the air, sunshine makes being outside desirable.

Metro Music Therapy (www.metromusictherapy.com) was founded in 1997 by Lori Sanders, MM, MT-BC, NMT Fellow, who now serves as its President. Metro Music Therapy is a private practice located in Denver, Colorado, that provides evidence-based in-home and facility-based music therapy services for clients aged 2–100+. Music therapists at MMT work with individuals experiencing a wide range of conditions and disabilities including, but not limited to, autism spectrum disorder, cerebral palsy, Down syndrome, developmental delay, mental illness, traumatic brain injury, multiple sclerosis, and stroke, and those in hospice care. Goals and outcomes typically focus on physical, communication, cognitive, and psychosocial/affective skills to improve and increase functional abilities and activities of daily living that are important to clients and their families. Music therapy sessions are facilitated in small and large groups and one-on-one. Up to 20 people can participate in a group, with sessions lasting 45 minutes. Individual sessions are typically an hour long.

Mr. Monroe uses items such as a guitar, guitar pick and strap, keyboard, paddle drums and mallets, tambourines, shakers, bells, cabasa, disco taps, scarves to wave with the sound of music, and other small classroom instruments in his practice. For those unfamiliar with some of these instruments, a cabasa is a percussion instrument made with loops of steel ball chain wrapped around a wide cylinder, which is attached to a long handle. Latin in origin, it was originally made from a hollow gourd covered with a beaded net or strung with small shells. The cabasa is intended to be rolled or shaken. Disco taps are metal discs that wrap around a foot/shoe to depict tap dancing sounds. As is the case with many therapy organizations, the practitioner or the company itself is responsible for obtaining and maintaining these materials.

Sessions offered through MMT are only administered outdoors if a client is interested and the outdoor space is accessible and safe. For example, when working with clients at their home, the yard needs to be fenced to avoid elopement or running away risk, and the weather should be conducive to being outside. Sometimes parents participate in sessions with their children. We learned that a family's backyard trampoline can be the perfect place for a music therapy session as Mr. Monroe uses music to provide a sensory-based session that includes bouncing, dancing, music improvisation, songwriting, and active instrument play. For instance, while one client, a young boy, was bouncing on the trampoline, Mr. Monroe played 'Rocky Mountain High' by John Denver on his guitar, and the little boy suddenly entrained his bouncing to the beat of the song, started dancing, and displayed highly positive facial affect—smiling, laughing, and random, loud vocalizations. It is also worth mentioning that the spectacular view from this little boy's backyard was of the Rocky Mountains. Therapy outside with a view—what could be better?

Other outdoor music therapy interventions Mr. Monroe shared that he has done include musical improvisation through West African drumming (using djembes) with clients. This intervention encompasses a musical conversation in a call-and-response format by using musical elements such as rhythm, tempo, melody, harmony, dynamics, form, phrasing, and timbre to interact with each other. Mr. Monroe suggested that there seems to be an overall heightened sense of freedom while playing the drums outside. You can hear the instrument carry far past the distance of the four walls indoors. It also can be captivating to observe how the sound might reflect off different surfaces or travel through the surrounding outdoor environment. There are many other music interventions that address outdoor themes and/or knowledge while using music as the primary tool.

Mr. Monroe told us that he can always make an intervention more challenging by increasing the complexity of the music by manipulating specific musical elements such as rhythm, form, dynamics, tempo, harmony, phrasing, and melody, adding more verbal or gestural prompts/cues, and providing the client with more leadership opportunities within sessions. To make activities less challenging, Mr. Monroe says that he gives the interventions more structure and organization by using fewer prompts and simplifying the tasks. For instance, rather than responding to one specific lyric or word within a song that may occur many times, Mr. Monroe might have the client respond to the chorus section of a song that occurs just two or three times.

He has found that music, in general, makes his clients feel better and provides a unique way to work towards non-musical goals and objectives. Mr. Monroe has used music, specifically songwriting and singing, with a client with two traumatic brain injuries to express himself about snowboarding. This client was only able to speak three to five words at a time but could sing familiar songs in entirety. By the end of his music therapy sessions (three months), he was able to write lyrics, create a background accompaniment on GarageBand, sing the entire song, and record this entire product to have a physical hard copy CD of his song.

As to sharing advice, Mr. Monroe suggests the following. Always be aware and knowledgeable of your outdoor surroundings before you head outside with a client. Know prior to going outdoors if your client tends to wander and if they are capable of finding their way home or to safety if they get lost. Understand how you might use your environment to your benefit, such as a fenced backyard if your client does tend to wander. Think about correct gear for outdoor terrain and weather. Allow time for free exploration within limits to provide clients with the opportunity to experience the environment on their own terms. Have a safety contact just in case, and always tell a colleague where you are planning to "take it outside" with a client, particularly if it is remote. Aside from therapeutic skills, Mr. Monroe feels that an appreciation of nature and taking it outside is also needed.

Mr. Monroe believes that there are many potential benefits to providing therapy services outdoors as it provides a higher sense of spatial freedom and increased imagination overall. There is also the potential to experience a heightened feeling of relaxation with nature sounds in the nearby environment. Being outdoors may also reduce boredom for clients as it is never static; there is always something different or out of the ordinary happening—passing clouds, temperature shifts, the smell of rain in the air, and the sounds of birds. These same benefits may also become challenges as some clients can become distracted by external stimuli outdoors as it deviates from their regular routine or schedule. They may also wander or lose focus. Another challenge may be that there is less structure than an indoor setting, so sitting on the ground, tree stump, or rock might need to be acceptable.

Past and present outdoor experiences matter to Mr. Monroe and are likely the catalyst for him taking it outside with his music therapy clients. Growing up, he attended fine arts camps in the northern woods of Michigan, and outside of camp he performed with bands and orchestras in outdoor settings. He loved playing music outdoors. His experiences at the camps and performing outdoors also involved recreation, as he always camped and found ways to participate in outdoor leisure activities. Presently, he is an avid hiker and outdoor person living to travel and see new ways of life. He has traveled and hiked extensively around the American West, Midwest, Hawaii, New Zealand, Australia, Scandinavia, Germany, France, Belgium, the Caribbean, Iceland, Canada, and parts of Mexico. Most recently, he hiked the Tahoe Rim Trail (TRT), a 171-mile trek around Lake Tahoe located on the California/ Nevada, and completed the 93-mile Wonderland trail around Mt. Rainier in Washington. Mr. Monroe enjoys landscape photography as it keeps him traveling to new places, staying physically active, and going outdoors. Several of his images are included throughout the book.

There has been a small body of research conducted on the impact of music therapy outdoors, which are fascinating reads and a source of evidence that validates taking therapy outdoors. The articles that Mr. Monroe recommends are:

- Adams, D. and Beauchamp, G. (2018) 'Portals between worlds: A study of the experiences of children aged 7–11 years from primary schools in Wales making music outdoors.' *Research Studies in Music Education* *40*, 1, 50–66.

- Pfeifer, E., Fiedler, H., and Wittmann, M. (2019) 'Increased relaxation and present orientation after a period of silence in a natural surrounding.' *Nordic Journal of Music Therapy 29*, 1, 75–92.
- Yamasaki, T., Yamada, K., and Laukka, P. (2013) 'Viewing the world through the prism of music: Effects of music on perceptions of the environment.' *Psychology of Music 43*, 1, 61–74.

Nature as Teacher: Supporting Cognitive Development

Nature-based learning can be motivating, interesting, and enjoyable (Kuo, Browning, and Penner 2018). Learning in nature settings also tends to mediate discord between social, cultural, and interpersonal differences that can interfere with classroom or group cohesion (White 2012). The outdoor learning model is gaining popularity, perhaps in part because of parental and educator awareness of the seriousness and chronic impact of what Richard Louv (2010) identified as childhood nature-deficit disorder in his highly acclaimed book *Last Child in the Woods* (Bates 2020).

There has been a surge of interest in green schoolyards, forest school models, and outdoor classrooms. Support for increased interest in outdoor learning has brought exciting research findings. Aligned with attention restoration theory, outdoor learning spaces tend to be quieter than indoor classrooms and infuse a sense of calm for learners (Kuo, Barnes, and Jordan 2019). In nature environments, preschoolers can learn about size (different sizes of leaves), shapes (a circular, triangular, and square stone), "same and different" (a plant in bloom and the same just about to), beauty (a rainbow after a storm and a brilliant sunset), and patience (a tadpole slowly developing into a frog). These concepts may be abstract, yet, in nature, learning takes on a flow of its own (Honig 2019).

Learning in or nearby nature can be intrinsically motivating for children as it enables them to be more available to take in and retain information and enhance their engagement with the materials (Hobbs 2015). Nature and nature-based interventions have other benefits related to school-aged children's cognitive development, including better academic performance, enhanced attention, increased engagement and enthusiasm in school-related tasks, and improved behavior and focus (Bates 2020). A study comparing the effect of identical lessons facilitated in the classroom and outside (same teacher for each group, same lesson, same approach) found that students who learned outside were statistically more engaged than the children who received their lesson inside (Kuo *et al.* 2018).

CASE NARRATIVE: The Therapeutic Forest

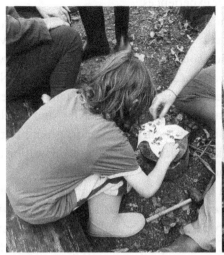

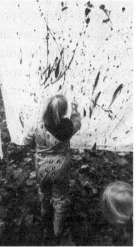

METICULOUS ATTENTION TO THE TASK   ARTISTRY AT ITS BEST

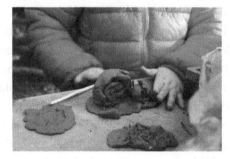

CREATING WITH CLAY
Photo credits: The Therapeutic Forest

Thank you to Hannah Broughton, Co-founder and Managing Director, and Caspian Jamie, Co-founder, Speech and Language and Land Lead Therapist, at The Therapeutic Forest for helping to prepare this case narrative.

Where do you feel the most like yourself? For many people, it is outside. Ms. Broughton saw it in her work as a child development specialist at a school for autistic children. Ms. Broughton and Mr. Jamie believe that the outdoors have enormous therapeutic potential, particularly for children and young people who have additional needs and challenges. They started The Therapeutic Forest in December 2017 and envisioned it to be a space where children could feel authentically like themselves and engage with therapists in a very relaxed way. Services are provided using a play-based and child-led approach. This service model also allows for families to build relationships with the therapy team and chat honestly about their experiences.

The Therapeutic Forest is primarily held in Rawtenstall, Lancashire, in the United Kingdom. It is a social enterprise that is funded by grants as well as profits from continuing education courses. The Therapeutic Forest serves both children and adults. The special education needs and disabilities (SEND) program serves children and focuses on using outdoor play to build children's speech, language, and communication skills, and social skills, and develop coping tools. The Therapeutic Forest partners with support groups in the community and advertises on social media. Currently, there is a waiting list that families can register for on their website.

Therapeutic strategies created by the clinical psychology team are provided weekly to clients and caregivers. The program lasts for 6–8 weeks with a group of 12 children with a variety of diagnoses including learning difficulties, autism, developmental delay, cerebral palsy, Down syndrome, ADHD, and genetic disorders. Parents/caregivers also participate in the program. Sessions last 1½–2 hours and are facilitated by an interdisciplinary group of 15 staff members including three Therapeutic Forest School Leaders who have gone through the Certificate in Therapeutic Skills for Outdoor Leaders qualification. The qualification is delivered by an interdisciplinary team made up of two speech and language therapists, five clinical psychologists, one speech and language therapy assistant, one occupational therapist, one play therapist, and one yoga teacher (www.thetherapeuticforest.org/courses).

Sessions are held outdoors at existing venues with accessibility and risks assessments completed in advance of the sessions. Interventions are child-led and play-based. For example, a child may choose to splash in the stream instead of sitting in the circle. The speech and language therapist may join in and pour water near the child to work on joint attention and other skills while also incorporating the parents and caregivers in the session by inviting them to model strategies such as intensive interaction. The therapist reinforces a child's positive attempts at communication and often gets parents involved, modeling strategies that promote communication so they can use the same approach at home. The speech therapist may then try to scaffold social interactions with other children to support social skill development. The play therapist may work with children with clay or introduce a game, gently encouraging children to express their feelings and share them with those around them. The occupational therapist may set up an activity with slacklines (similar to the concept of a tightrope) designed to support gross motor skills, or join children for a craft activity that supports fine motor skills.

Like other interventions, parents/caregivers are also included in the mental health component of the program. The psychologists introduce weekly strategies to parents to help them to support their child and take care of themselves. The psychologist facilitating the session talks about this strategy around the firepit and makes themself available to parents to converse throughout the session. Strategies are evidence-based and designed to help parents/caregivers build new coping tools. Parents/caregivers are given space to talk to each other, creating a sense of community. Siblings are also invited as a way to help them better understand each other. Parents/caregivers often comment that this is the only activity that siblings can attend and access together.

Materials and equipment are provided by therapists and coordinated among the team. Dr. Alexia Barrable and her team at the University of Dundee have developed a range of tools to help measure participant progress. From intake, children and their parents/caregivers are seen as individuals. Parents complete an "About Me" profile prior to sessions and have phone calls with families to put in place a plan of support for each child. Staff at The Therapeutic Forest see the success of this approach as children and their parents/caregivers have reported that their children are recognized and accepted for who they are and understood at The Therapeutic Forest. One parent reported:

> My son enjoyed so many of the different activities which had been adapted so that he could access them, even with his difficulties. The staff were so enthusiastic and really brought warmth and excitement to the sessions for all the children. The specific training and professionalism of each staff member shone through and added a learning element for the parents and carers too.

Another parent shared:

> [My daughter] can't wait to get to these sessions and asks about coming...she loves telling me about what she has done at The Therapeutic Forest, something she doesn't do readily often. We also notice she is a little calmer. She has learned some (calming) techniques at The Therapeutic Forest which we have been able to use at home, and will be passing this on to her schoolteacher to use. Thank you so much for providing this service; we were dreading the summer holidays and not knowing how to keep her entertained... The Therapeutic Forest has been amazing.

Through these stories, we can see that children are truly able to be themselves outdoors with the support of The Therapeutic Forest and their dedicated staff.

The Therapeutic Forest provided multiple virtual programs to continue to support clients and provide them with activities outdoors during the COVID-19 pandemic. For instance, Woodcraft for Wellbeing is a virtual program that began in the spring of 2020, which combines mindful nature activities with therapeutic strategies to support adults with mild to moderate mental health difficulties, and support the mental health and wellbeing of frontline workers during the COVID-19 pandemic. Within the first six months of the pandemic, Woodcraft for Wellbeing served 1050 adults. Examples of the weekly mindful nature-based activities provided include mindful walking, therapeutic nature photography, and mindful bushcraft.

Additionally, the clinical psychologist introduced participants to a weekly virtual evidence-based tip to support mental health and wellbeing. One participant said:

> My whole wellbeing has changed over the past six weeks, and this is directly down to doing these sessions with The Therapeutic Forest. I am happier, more focused, and have become more able to achieve the things that are ahead of us, moving forward in this environment.

Another reported that:

> [The program has] given me structure and a focus during lockdown. A positive outlook and a feeling of being in control at a time when it would have been easy to get lost in pandemic panic and negativity. I now have strategies to use to keep me feeling more mentally healthy.

One participant shared that their personal struggles during the COVID-19 pandemic included their husband receiving a cancer diagnosis, having surgery canceled, and being unable to work due to his immune system. They said:

> The program was on a weekly basis, which gave me something to look forward to each week for six weeks. I would enjoy the activity and take part in doing it in my garden. The photography course was something I never would have looked at—but it would seem taking pictures of flowers in my garden and the birds in the trees was so calming! The wellbeing information from Dr. Aadahl was absolutely brilliant...mindful walk, muscle relaxation, mindfulness on an object, and so on...these are massively helping me.

Access to the program is freely available at www.thetherapeuticforest.org/woodcraft-for-wellbeing.

For children, a variety of virtual programs were provided during the COVID-19 pandemic, including virtual foraging sessions and virtual forest school sessions. Some equipment was sent out to children to continue participating in nature-based activities with the speech and language therapist online. A series of adapted yoga videos accompanied by visuals and signing were created for children with communication difficulties. The Certificate in Beginners Nature Photography, led by the speech and language therapist, was designed to be suitable for children with a range of additional needs. The certificate program can be accessed at www.thetherapeuticforest.org/certificate-in-beginners-nature-photography-for-teenagers-with-send.

In addition to benefits expressed by participants, Mr. Jamie has also found that "taking it outside" frees children to talk more openly about their feelings and experiences. He told us that initially he noted that autistic children seemed to find it easier to engage when talking side by side, but since then he has learned this is true for many children and adults. Sitting side by side, particularly when engaging in a shared task, can remove pressure and allow people to talk more openly about their feelings and experiences.

He recalled in his own work that playing in a sand table with a very shy child allowed him to share information about what her family had done over the weekend without him even asking. Mr. Jamie has also discovered that the outdoor environment allows individuals to engage as equals as there is less of an expectation to sit still and be quiet outdoors. He shared that "behavior that might be seen as destructive indoors might be an invitation to play outdoors." The outdoors also allow for child-led and play-based approaches, naturally engaging and rich with sensory experiences. Although there are multiple benefits, Ms. Broughton also recognizes the challenges. It requires more organization and planning such as making sure everyone is dressed appropriately, travel time to the venues is considered, equipment is available, and shelter and risk assessments are considered. Ms. Broughton's advice to practitioners is to work in a multi-disciplinary way when considering taking it outside. The Therapeutic Forest provides us with a rich look into how outdoor therapy services can be provided in person and virtually, as well as encouraging other practitioners to do the same through their courses. Courses can be found at www.thetherapeuticforest.org/courses.

Regarding academic performance, a randomized controlled trial study of outdoor learning involving more than 3000 students demonstrated that students who learned outdoors increased their knowledge acquisition, compared to students who learned in traditional indoor classrooms. Perhaps even more exciting, the greater the amount of time spent learning outside, the bigger the academic gains

(Wells *et al.* 2015). Might this also translate to clients meeting therapy goals when intervention happens outside?

Taking it a step further, schools with a high rate of outdoor vegetation perform better on academic achievement tests as compared to schools with lower rates of vegetation, even when factoring in socioeconomic status (Kuo *et al.* 2019). Research also shows that having the opportunity to learn in nature reduces rates of absenteeism. Being outside may make coming to school seem more worthwhile (MacNaughton *et al.* 2017). This is exciting!

As Alice Honig (2019) so beautifully shared, "The fresh air of outdoors is like a 'mental floss' that can help clear out children's cobwebs of grumpiness and feelings of confinement" (p.668) and ready them to be optimal learners. Learning outdoors means learning differently. The sensory experience of being outside is amplified, seating is different, and the walk from the indoor classroom to an outdoor classroom provides a brief attention restoration and physical activity break. And as Steven Moss (2012) eloquently wrote, "children who learn outdoors know more, understand more, feel better, behave better, work more cooperatively and are physically healthier. Not a bad result from simply changing the location where they are being taught" (p.9). It is not a far reach to change the last phrase to "changing the location where they are *receiving therapy*" with similar expectations.

Let's Move: Physical Development

When children explore nature, it is often a highly sensorimotor experience (Beery and Jørgensen 2018). Being in outdoor environments is a natural place for children to develop and practice motor skills. Being outside provides the extra space to move about freely and enrich motor skills such as balance, coordination, and body awareness (Harris 2016). Many children find it irresistible to roll down a hill, hide behind trees, jump from rock to rock, or balance along a fallen log. Hills, trees, and rocks are not only fun, but also great learning tools. Interestingly, a year-long study comparing the motor skills of preschool-aged children found that children whose childcare facilities' outside spaces were flat playgrounds had poorer balance, agility, and motor control as compared to children whose childcare facilities' outdoor spaces were contoured and had rocks and trees (Fjortoft 2001). A more recent study confirming the 2001 Fjortoft study, by Sääkslahti and Niemistö (2021) found that children who engaged in more outdoor play had greater motor competence. What comes "naturally" to children is, in fact, beneficial to their physical and motor development.

CASE NARRATIVE: Bearfoot OT

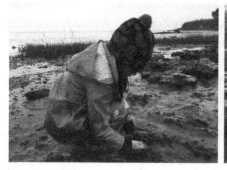

MUD RULES

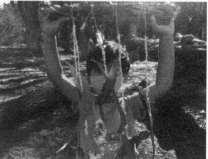

FOUND OBJECTS FROM NATURE
MAKE THE BEST MOBILES

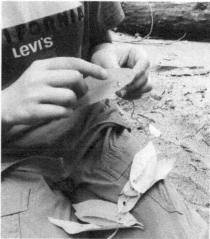

JOY, JOY, JOY
Photo credits: Bearfoot OT

THREADING LEAVES

Thank you to Marika Austin, MS, OTR/L, Founder and Lead Clinician of Bearfoot Occupational Therapy for helping to prepare this case narrative.

With its mission "to provide child-centered outdoor pediatric therapy services in order to help children be successful and thrive across contexts," Bearfoot Occupational Therapy (OT) represents a unique alternative to traditional indoor clinic-based services. Bearfoot OT offers individual occupational therapy services, social groups, and therapeutic summer camps to children aged 1–13 in the San Francisco Bay Area of California. All services are provided completely outdoors at specified public sites, acting as Bearfoot's different "offices" around San Francisco and Marin. In addition to providing services outside the four walls of a clinic, Bearfoot OT also packages their services in a way that challenges the traditional model of once-weekly therapy. Individual occupational therapy sessions are only offered as bundled fee-for-service quarterly packages. This bundle includes built-in caregiver communication to ensure families receive the essential elements of therapy to address all areas of concern a family may have. By bundling the services, Bearfoot OT moves away from the model of therapy that relies on one therapy session a week to help support a child and their family, and instead creates a model that prioritizes support in between sessions as well. Through this quarterly therapy package model, Bearfoot OT also receives compensation for these additional pieces including in-person sessions, phone consultations, and an online platform to increase communication with families and caregivers. The model addresses the problem often encountered in pediatric therapy in two ways. First, it builds in essential support beyond the therapy session. Second, it compensates the business and the therapist for the work done outside of the therapy session, which is usually uncompensated. Collaboration with other providers is also improved owing to all the services included in the bundle, as families often use the consultation service to bridge communications between Bearfoot OT and school or other providers.

Before founding Bearfoot OT, Ms. Austin spent many years working in clinics and schools, all the while acknowledging an ever-growing intuition that the children she worked with could be better served if they were working on their skills outdoors. This intuition was inspired by her childhood days growing up on a sheep farm in Maryland, where she spent hours and hours outside exploring, climbing, getting dirty, and playing in the stream. As she was providing occupational therapy services inside, the nagging thought that "this would be better outside" continued to grow, and after a couple of years it was impossible for her to ignore the thought. So, she left her indoor jobs and started Bearfoot OT.

Bearfoot OT works with children, aged 1–13 years old, and their families. Their services are provided for children with and without formal diagnosis. The typical formal diagnoses include—but are not limited to—ADD/ADHD, autism, dyspraxia, dyslexia, fragile X syndrome, anxiety, and depression. While the individualized children's goals are wide-ranging, all relate to increasing skills to help them be successful and thrive across contexts. Individual therapy sessions are 50 minutes long and delivered once a week, and caregivers are welcomed into the sessions. Social group services and therapeutic camps are offered in a group setting with distinct cohorts of six children (maximum). Group sessions are 90 minutes long and meet weekly, while summer camp meets for four hours a day, Monday through Friday.

In addition to the in-person services, the bundled packages include three consultations per quarter.

At the start of 2022, Bearfoot OT had three occupational therapists on staff. Therapy groups are also staffed by thoroughly vetted volunteers and occupational therapy graduate students (both Level 2 and Level 1). Bearfoot OT therapists work with clients toward improved physical health, motor skills, mental health, sensory integration, and social skills. The cornerstone of their services is facilitating "the just right challenge"—therapists work to make activities easy enough to engage in but challenging enough to be fun and promote growth. Clients and therapists engage in activities that address motor skill development and sensory processing such as climbing trees, swinging, building forts, playing in the ocean, completing obstacle courses, and doing nature crafts.

All Bearfoot OT services are provided outdoors and on public property. Ms. Austin uses various criteria to select sites: available parking, adequate cell phone service quality, and access to running water, trees to climb, natural bodies of water, natural shelters and accessible bathrooms. In addition to the above criteria, Ms. Austin shared that the process to obtain permits to operate in public spaces is also considered. When seeking permits, consideration is given to how the land can be used, such as permission to climb trees and play in water, the level of administrative complexity required to gain the permit, and cost.

In addition to public land, staff members, and volunteers, it takes equipment and money to make Bearfoot OT operate. The supplies and equipment used for sessions varies depending on the group, but all materials are brought in and taken out of the site by the therapist daily. Materials needed for all services include a swing and the hardware and ropes to hang it, first aid kit, craft supplies, cones, rings, and walkie talkies—tools for safety and materials that can be used in multiple ways and may inspire collaboration and social interaction between the children. The initial funding needed to start Bearfoot OT was around $5000, which went towards creating a legal entity, purchasing a business license, liability insurance, and permits, and acquiring startup materials. Bearfoot OT is funded through fee for service. Ms. Austin was generous with her business acumen and shared a list of costs needed to maintain Bearfoot OT: bookkeeping, a virtual assistant to help with scheduling, monthly subscriptions for communication platforms, electronic medical record program, insurance, payroll, workers' compensation, materials, testing materials, permits, and taxes.

Bearfoot OT's holistic and nature-based services are making big and positive impacts on the families they care for, and Ms. Austin shared some feedback from a couple of them. One caregiver shared:

Our family is so grateful for Bearfoot OT services. Our six-year-old has an expressive/receptive language and motor coordination disorder. Over time we've watched him grow and become more comfortable in his communication and social skills. We love Marika and Bearfoot OT because she meets the child where they are at developmentally and formulates creative strategies to help support them in their social journey. Marika and her staff provide a warm and welcoming environment outdoors. She has done a great job with integrating occupational therapy into nature. Being outdoors with other children (especially during the COVID-19 pandemic) has been so therapeutic for our child. She trains her staff in strategies to help bridge or connect children in their relationships. The groups have a low adult-to-child ratio which reassures me that my child is safe and provides ample opportunity for adults to provide a good level of attention to each child. We appreciate her timely feedback through video recordings and her progress notes. Because of my child's speech/language delay, he does not often describe the activities of his day or time during group. Marika's feedback allows us to get a peek into fun activities during group and provides practical suggestions of how we can help our child at home. She is dedicated to educating future occupational therapists and introducing them to the possibility of OT outdoors. Our son truly enjoys meeting and engaging with the staff throughout the sessions: it has helped him become more flexible with his social interactions. They are always motivated, positive, and happy to be with the kids.

Another parent shared:

My six-year-old daughter didn't even notice all the growth and development that occurred because she was having so much fun. Marika and her team provide the safest and most supportive environment for the kids to learn, grow, and PLAY! My child couldn't wait to walk out the house every morning for camp and she was super-bummed when it came to an end.

One last story to share sums it up well:

The ability for my kiddo to be outside in a play-based therapy group is absolutely amazing! It's so rewarding to see how much he loves it and is learning so many skills at the same time. He's so happy and confident. Having our son learn to regulate and embrace his power and energy through this playful guidance has been so beautiful to witness. And we especially appreciate all the extra info on how to support this work further at home.

This overwhelming validation for therapy outside is inspiration for all who are contemplating the shift from inside to outdoors in nature.

Many of the challenges Ms. Austin faces with taking it outside have been referenced above—such as the litany of tasks required to run a business, finding adequate public spaces that will accommodate the program's needs, and navigating the bureaucratic paths to get permits. However, the challenges pale in comparison to the list of benefits to taking it outside. Ms. Austin shared a portion of the benefits she sees each day in her work with children.

- Motor skill development accelerates outside since there are so many naturally occurring opportunities for practice. The seemingly simple activity of hiking to the beach for a therapy session has many gross motor aspects: balance, motor planning, strength, and endurance, to name just a few.
- Opportunities for risky play are wherever children find them, and research tells us that it is highly beneficial to engage in.
- Sensory opportunities are everywhere.
- Outside, you are not competing for space as you are in a clinic.
- When therapy is outside, families are better able to generalize the activities to their everyday lives because they are not dependent on specialized equipment.

In hopes to inspire more therapists to take it outside, Ms. Austin shared: "Take the leap and do it. You can start small and grow—people need the outdoors and creating a therapeutic space outside the clinic is so powerful." We couldn't agree more, and we hope that after reading this you consider taking the leap toward taking it outside. For even more inspiration, please visit Bearfoot OT's website at www.bearfootoccupationaltherapy.com.

Nature is also an ever-changing sensory tapestry. In nature, there are opportunities to touch tree bark, look at insects up close or see big trees hundreds of yards away, smell the sweet essence of cut grass or the stench of a skunk's "perfume," listen to the wind blowing through the leaves, taste (maybe!) plants, and to move, roll, climb, jump, bend, stretch, and learn about their body's capabilities and boundaries.

Being outside for an hour a day, on average, adds seven minutes of moderate to vigorous physical activity time, but also reduces sedentary time by 13 minutes, (reported) interpersonal issues by 31%, and social-emotional angst by 22%—findings that Larouche, Garriguet, and Tremblay (2016) reported in their nationally representative study of over a thousand 7–14-year-old Canadian children. Why are we not making daily time spent outside a global priority for children and youth? The WHO (2020) has made recommendations for children's physical activity. While these recommendations for physical activity are not specific to being outside, we share some simple ideas as to how it may be accomplished. Please see Table 4.2.

Table 4.2 Getting outdoors

Age range	Recommendations	Take it outside
Less than 1 year	"Be physically active several times a day in a variety of ways" and "not be restrained for more than 1 hour at a time"	Stroller walk to a nearby park or nature space. Lay a blanket or tarp on the ground and place the infant on the covering. This is free time—let the infant lead the play! If possible, find a shady or semi-shaded spot for this infant-directed play time.
1–2 years	"Spend at least 180 minutes in a variety of types of physical activities at any intensity, including moderate- to vigorous-intensity physical activity, spread throughout the day"	Set out a variety of push toys like carts and child-sized wheelbarrows. Short mounds or tiny slides to climb and roll down can be irresistible. Consider watering or caring for plants, as toddlers love pouring water and opportunities to be helpful.
3–4 years	"Spend at least 180 minutes in a variety of types of physical activities at any intensity, of which at least 60 minutes is moderate- to vigorous-intensity physical activity, spread throughout the day"	At this age, children may be interested in formal playgrounds (designed for the under-five cohort). Most important is to find outdoor areas that allow children to run, jump, climb, roll, push, and pull.
5–17 years	"Engage in at least an average of 60 minutes per day of moderate-to-vigorous intensity, mostly aerobic, physical activity, across the week... incorporate vigorous-intensity aerobic activities, as well as those that strengthen muscle and bone, at least 3 days a week...[and] should limit the amount of time spent being sedentary, particularly the amount of recreational screen time"	At this stage, children may have their first experiences with team sports. Bike riding, swimming, and free play outdoors are a few ways to increase physical activity.

Adapted from World Health Organization (2020)

Beyond physical and motor development, nature positively contributes to global health benefits. Parents of preschool-age children reported that their children slept better and experienced better overall health after attending preschools with outdoor environments with trees, hills, plants, open space, and play structures, as compared to children whose preschool had limited outdoor play experiences (Söderström *et al.* 2013). With decreasing rates of physical activity among children, greener schoolyards are a potential counter to this trend. A study of grade-school-aged children found that, for girls, schoolyards with a woodland theme, and, for boys, access to playing fields were positively correlated with staying physically active as they got older (Pagels *et al.* 2014). In support of these findings, when considering outdoor spaces for therapy programs, strive to find places that are nature-rich.

CASE NARRATIVE: OT OuTside and Messy Tot Group

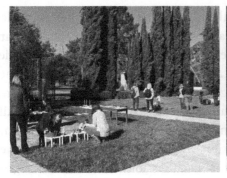
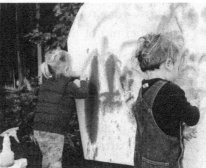

ANOTHER FABULOUS DAY AT MESSY TOTS   EXPERIMENTING WITH DIFFERENT PAINTING STRATEGIES

Thank you to Courtney Boitano OTD, OTR/L, BCBA-D, Founder of OT OuTside, for helping to prepare this case narrative.

When considering the value of taking therapy outside, we typically focus on how it benefits our clients. Dr. Courtney Boitano helps us remember that taking it outside is equally as beneficial for caregivers as it is for children.

Messy Tot Group is run by Dr. Boitano as one of the programs in her occupational therapy practice, OT OuTside. Located in San Jose, California, OT OuTside is a unique pediatric occupational therapy clinic that "inspires OTs and caregivers with easy, fun, and intentional ways to connect with children and share knowledge about the benefits of play, sensory experiences, and process art." The inspiration for OT OuTside was Dr. Boitano's time spent outside with her children. Messy Tot Group evolved from OT OuTside "to hold a space for caregivers to engage with their children through observation and learn about their child's sensory processing in a play-based, natural setting."

Messy Tot Group meets for an hour in 6–8 weekly sessions. They gather rain or shine, and regardless of the weather, the children and their caregivers love it. The group consists of 8–14 caregivers and their children who are between the ages of 18 months and four years old. The group meets in an outdoor space on private property that Dr. Boitano leases. She chose the location based on it being central for participants, its physical accessibility qualities (e.g., flat paths and curb cuts), its ease to set up activity stations, and access to running water. The materials needed to facilitate Messy Tots include tables, water tables, plastic storage bins, tarps, art supplies, pipettes, scooping and pouring toys, a parachute, easels, and a variety of sensory items and sensory bin fillers including shaving cream, playdough, beans, rice, corks, flour, and corn.

Messy Tot Group is open to all children and their families, regardless of whether or not they have a diagnosis. During the group, children and caregivers explore a variety of messy stations and engage in art activities. Messy Tot Group provides the structure to help each caregiver and their child find the "just right challenge" for engaging in activities together. It also allows caregivers an opportunity to practice the strategies and skills they learn in group as they become more confident with their parenting. They also participate in a circle time where they are invited to try a new food during the group's snack time. Each session concludes with a gross motor activity.

One parent expressed that the Messy Tot Group helped them "get comfortable with mess and see the value in exploring with all the senses. It radically changed the way I parent." Another reported:

> The highlight of our week is now Messy Tot Group, meeting with an OT committed to equipping us as parents to get down on the same level, to slow down, enjoy, play, and explore, all while [helping to nurture our children's] fine motor skills and coordination.

Messy Tot Group helped one parent "open her eyes to so many creative projects and unique uses of everyday items." Messy Tot Group provides a unique opportunity for parents to carry over what they learned in therapy.

When there is a will, there is a way. To those who are thinking about taking their practice outside, Dr. Boitano says, "Do it!" There are challenges, but these challenges can be overcome with planning and thought, says Dr. Boitano. Dr. Boitano reminds us that "outside" does not always need to happen in the most picturesque backdrop. Taking it outside can look different for everyone because we all experience it differently. What's important is to be outside as much as we can as part of our daily routine. For further information about OT OuTside, please visit their website at www.otoutside.com.

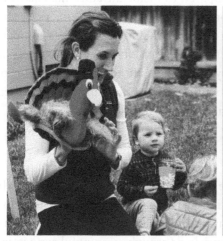
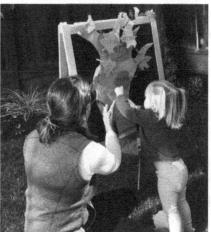

TURKEY TALK IS CAPTIVATING   LEARNING OUTSIDE COMES "NATURALLY"

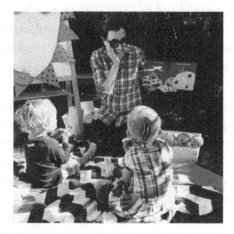

SHARING STORIES, SNACKS, AND SUNSHINE IN NATURE
Photo credits: OT OuTside

Home and neighborhood contexts also contribute to health, as certain attributes of a child's neighborhood are associated with increased time spent outside playing. These factors include access to yards, limited volume of traffic, moderate overall levels of greenness, lower levels of neighborhood disorder, and lower residential density (Lambert *et al.* 2019). These findings are crucial because families who live in residential areas may be able to both increase the green factor in their yards and become advocates for increasing the natural qualities of their neighborhoods. On a clinical level, selecting an outdoor space that is as quiet and green as possible can be a catalyst for increased engagement in therapy.

Lower rates of cortisol (the stress hormone) were noted when students learned in a forest school setting compared to inside a traditional classroom (Dettweiler *et al.* 2017). This is an important finding for therapy services, because if cortisol levels can be lowered when receiving therapy outdoors as compared to indoors, one hurdle to effective therapy intervention could be accomplished simply by the context in which therapy is provided. For those interested in conducting research, consider biomarker studies such as measuring cortisol, heart rate variability, and blood pressure when facilitating therapy outdoors.

Wrapping It Up

More research on the benefits of nature has been conducted with adults, but what has been published related to children is hopeful and positive. Research supports that children's social-emotional, language and communication, cognitive, and physical and motor development are enriched through meaningful connections with nature. This is important because development does not happen in a vacuum. All areas of development are intertwined and rely on each other to "build" a resilient child, adolescent, and, ultimately, adult. When we stop and reflect, the developmental tasks associated with childhood are impressive and breath-taking. More research is needed, including such topics as how nature enhances family connections and how our physiology changes when we are outside.

Louise Chawla, Professor Emerita in the Environmental Design Program at the University of Colorado Boulder, suggested two lines of research necessary to understand how nature buffers and mediates family relationships. Her questions include "How are children's experiences of nature influenced by their caretakers? Can children's playfulness and curiosity influence what their caretakers notice and feel?" (Chawla 2015, p.446). There are many areas of children- and nature-focused research that are worthy of exploration, and perhaps as part of a therapy outside program that will be something you pursue. But first things first. Understanding the evidence-based benefits of nature, healthcare professionals have been and continue to be inspired and empowered to provide services for children outside or to bring nature inside. Think of taking it outside as a viable therapeutic partner. The potential is endless.

NUGGET OF NATURE: FROM TRASH TO TREASURE— SEED-STARTING MINI GREENHOUSE

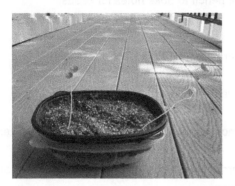

UPCYCLED GREENHOUSE IS A FIRST HOME FOR HEARTY NASTURTIUM SEEDLINGS
Photo credit: Shannon Marder

This is a simple way to make a seed starter mini greenhouse that makes good use of plastic rotisserie chicken containers.

Materials you will need

- Plastic rotisserie chicken container
- Drainage tray for the greenhouse
- Scissors or an awl
- Seeds
- Potting soil
- Bottle with spray-mister top
- Chopstick or pencil
- Bowl for seeds
- Tweezers
- Spoon
- Pots for transplanting
- Trowel
- If making multiple greenhouses, some type of labeling system to keep track of what seeds are in each greenhouse

Steps to making a mini greenhouse

1. Thoroughly clean the tray and clear plastic dome that the chicken comes in.
2. Carefully poke a few holes in the bottom of the tray for drainage (adult only).
3. Place the base of the greenhouse on the drainage tray.

4. Use a trowel to fill the tray with potting soil to its rim. Do not use topsoil as it is too dense, will not drain well, and will choke the seedlings.
5. Use the end of a chopstick or a pencil to poke holes for seeds.
6. Place seeds into a bowl.
7. Place a seed in each hole and cover with soil.
8. Gently mist the soil until it is very damp.
9. Place the cover over the tray.
10. Remove cover, mist, and replace the cover every few days.
11. Watch for germination.
12. When the seedlings are a few inches tall, gently remove them with tweezers or a spoon, being careful not to damage the roots.
13. Transplant the seedlings into larger pots filled with potting soil until they are ready for their final planting place.

How to make the activity easier

- Pre-poke holes for seeds.
- Plant larger seeds such as beans or peas.

How to make the activity more challenging

- Poke holes for the seeds with the non-dominant hand.
- Use tweezers to pick up and place one seed at a time in its hole.
- Place two kinds of visually different seeds in the bowl and have children sort or plant the same seeds in their own row.
- Calculate the number of seeds that can be planted based on spacing requirements on the seed packages.

CHAPTER 5

Adolescents

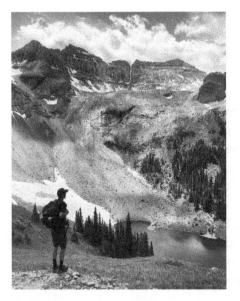

Finding solidarity with nature
Photo credit: Chris Monroe

Introduction

Adolescence is a period of tremendous development and change in preparation for adulthood and future health and wellbeing; it begins with the end of childhood, around age 13, and ends when a person enters young adulthood, around age 18 (Sawyer *et al.* 2012). It is divided into three stages: early adolescence 10–13 years old; middle adolescence 14–16 years old; and later adolescence, 17 and 18 years (Barrett 1996).

Shifting Social Situations

Complex interpersonal and environmental characteristics shape adolescent social-emotional development (Fletcher and Kim 2019). It is a social time when peer relationships and the acceptance, influence, and pressure that comes along with them become increasingly important as adolescents take on the important task of identity formation (Orben, Tomova, and Blakemore 2020; U.S. Department of Health and Human Services 2018). As adolescents place increasing importance on peer relationships over caregiver relationships, increased conflict may ensue (Allen and Waterman 2019). Despite the shift to increased valuing of peer relationships, from an ecological perspective an adolescent's development does not occur in a vacuum, and (like other stages of development), is influenced by their family, community, societal norms, and the qualities within the adolescent themself (Seaman *et al.* 2019).

THIS MUCH I KNOW—L. (AGE 14)

God created nature for a reason. He creates everything for a reason. I believe that He created nature as a healing tool. If you just look outside for a moment, you mostly see trees, maybe a few birds, and some flowers. But if you just looked a moment longer, you would see the beauty in it. The wind dancing along the trees, carrying leaves through ocean blue sky. Sometimes I like to imagine that I'm dancing along with them. Sometimes it does rain, fog, and storm; but that is just the wonder of it. It all depends on you, to make the most of it. Kids nowadays wouldn't make the most of it; I know that, because I didn't. It's just the way the bees pollinate the glowing flowers, or even the way the drop of tears from the clouds hit the window. I didn't get any of that, but now I do. This is what nature means to me; it means everything to me. Nature saved me from what I was in, and it can save you too.

Despite the tug towards peer influence, caregiver influence remains important in adolescence. A caregiver's provision of effective discipline while maintaining a high level of warmth, support, and closeness can positively impact social-emotional development and self-esteem, all of which influence wellbeing (Hunter, Barber and Stolz 2015; Murry and Lippold 2018). A high level of family-based nature activity (FBNA) during adolescence is one way to support social-emotional development (Izenstark and Middaugh 2022). Engaging in FBNA can relieve discord and increase communication between adolescents and their caregivers, as being in nature provides a positive distraction from responsibilities and "realities" (Izenstark and Ebata 2019). We will come back to FBNA later in this chapter.

THIS MUCH I KNOW—D. (AGE 14)

Being outside makes me feel peaceful. When I have a lot of homework and I need a break, I often take jogs to help center and calm myself. As I run through my local park, I see plants that don't have to be constantly moving and making decisions. And walking through a forest and looking up at the trees and their leaves strikes me as awesome—I imagine that the trees are wooden giants, slow but powerful.

The adolescent brain is different from either a child's or an adult's brain, so it experiences and interprets daily-life situations, particularly stressful situations, differently than a child or adult (Eiland and Romeo 2013). In fact, stress may be intensified during adolescence because of neurobiological, social, and environmental factors (Eiland and Romeo 2013; Jackson *et al.* 2021a, 2021b; Li and Sullivan 2016). Fortunately, nature-based experiences are increasingly being found to be an effective stress reduction intervention for adolescents.

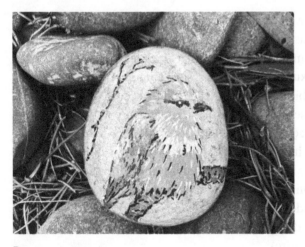

ROCK PAINTING
Photo credit: Amy Wagenfeld

Executive Functioning Development

Adolescent brains go through an intense period of growing new neural connections, pruning old connections, and strengthening other connections (U.S. Department of Health and Human Services 2018). What we see because of these neural changes includes the ability to understand concepts and skills such as abstract and logical thinking, advanced reasoning, meta-cognition, and enhanced learning (Anil and Bhat 2020; Larsen and Luna 2018). During adolescence, there is also marked growth and development within the frontal lobe of the brain, which enables increased decision-making capacity (Eiland and Romeo 2013). Note that frontal lobe development is not complete until young adulthood. Adolescents are additionally developing and understanding their own definitions of right and wrong and their unique sense of morality (Crocetti *et al.* 2019). It is, indeed, a very busy time in development.

THIS MUCH I KNOW—R. (AGE 17)
My favorite moments spent with nature often occur at night. Walking on the soft grass and passing towering trees, I feel strangely at ease knowing that I'm by myself. Gentle breezes carry the earthy scent of my surroundings across the path. If I'm lucky, the stars reveal themselves as a vibrant celestial glow. These moments of peaceful solitude bring me great joy.

Literally Growing Up

Puberty typically starts at the conclusion of childhood or during adolescence, and impacts physical changes inside and outside the body. One of the hallmarks of puberty is the release of hormones in the body that affect fertility and initiate the emergence of secondary sexual characteristics, such as larger breasts in females, facial hair for males, and pubic hair for both (Best and Ban 2021). Adolescent bodies also grow taller and heavier, and changes in facial structure occur (Blakemore, Burnett, and Dahl 2010, p.929). During the entirety of adolescence, girls typically grow about 9 inches and gain about 35 pounds, and boys gain about 42 pounds and grow about 11 inches taller (Özdemir, Utkualp, and Palloş 2016). Muscles and bones are ready to accommodate these changes to endure more weight and physical activity. During middle adolescence, males' voices typically deepen and girls have typically completed their physical growth, including starting menstruation (Allen and Waterman 2019).

Preparing to emerge into the world of adulthood, adolescence is a time to learn and grow social-emotionally, intellectually, and physically. Combined with brain development and hormonal shifts, adolescence is a highly sensitive period of life (Eiland and Romeo 2013). As providers of care, we have many opportunities to help adolescents learn the skills needed to begin to function independently from their caregivers and start making choices that may affect them for the rest of their lives.

Therapeutic Benefits of Nature: Adolescents

Most studies investigating the impacts of nature-based interventions are focused on social-emotional health, education, and physical health outcomes. Fortunately, the research overwhelmingly supports the use of nature and the outdoors to facilitate improved adolescent experiences and outcomes. For example, results of a survey of nearly 1000 adolescents, conducted during the first years of the COVID-19 pandemic, found that they reported experiencing increased physical and mental health by just being outdoors (Zamora *et al.* 2021). The researchers also learned that nearly 90% of these adolescents reported wanting to spend more time outdoors but were not able to do so because of various barriers such as busy schedules, barriers in the built environment, and COVID-19 restrictions (Zamora *et al.* 2021). Experiences matter: as we explore, nature can be a positive mediator in adolescent development. In fact, Wales *et al.* (2022) argue that outdoor environments need to be designed with both adolescents and younger children in mind, as wellbeing in adolescence matters because it is the bridge between childhood and adulthood.

Typical nature-based therapeutic interventions for adolescents are wilderness/outdoor adventure, recreation programs, park-based programs, and outdoor learning and school garden programs (Chawla *et al.* 2014; D'Agostino *et al.* 2019; Van Hecke *et al.* 2018; Vella-Brodrick and Gilowska 2022; Williams *et al.* 2018), all of which offer varying degrees of moderate to vigorous physical activity (MVPA). The most physically rigorous nature-based interventions are outdoor adventure programs. Successful outdoor adventure programs are facilitated in unfamiliar (to participants) outdoor environments, composed of activities that are physically and emotionally challenging, and have consequences that require collaboration with others; they are run as small groups and are facilitated by experienced and skilled instructors to ensure physical safety and provide emotional support (Mutz and Müller 2016). We would add that a successful outdoor program of any type must also strive to meet the highest standards of inclusion for all participants regardless of abilities, identities, or preferences.

As we explore some of the research, it will become evident that nature matters a great deal to adolescents, yet there is cause for concern. Adolescence is a life period often characterized by declines in physical activity and time spent outdoors (Lingham *et al.* 2021; Nigg *et al.* 2021; Piccininni *et al.* 2018). Not only are adolescents spending less time outdoors: less time outside is spent in nature than in previous generations (Kellert *et al.* 2017). While it is an easy oversimplification to blame contemporary lack of time in nature on adolescent addiction to screen time, there are other factors in this increasing nature disconnection including an over-abundance of scheduled afterschool time, overprotective caregivers, and concerns about safety (Larson *et al.* 2018).

CASE NARRATIVE: Monarch School of New England

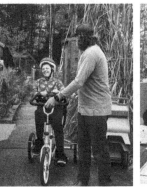
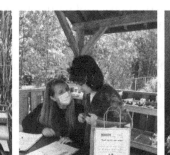
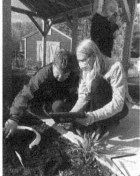

HAVING FUN BIKE RIDING   WORKING ON
                          COMMUNICATION
                          ACTIVITIES OUTSIDE

INTEGRATING TECHNOLOGY
INTO A NATURE-BASED
THERAPEUTIC ACTIVITY

Photo credits: Monarch School of New England

Thank you to Kathryn Perry, MA, OTR/L, HTR, for being the lead contact and for the following staff who actively worked with Ms. Perry to prepare the Monarch School of New England's case narrative. What an interdisciplinary team effort this case narrative represents!

- **Executive Director:** Diane Bessey, M.Ed., PT
- **Director of Community Engagement:** Amanda Gebo Martineau, MS, CCC-SLP
- **Occupational Therapists:** Kathryn Perry, MA, OTR/L, HTR; Britany LeBoeuf, MS, OTR/L; Lacey Fowler, MOT, OTR/L
- **Physical Therapists:** Erica Mann, PT, MPT, DPT; Jessica Roy, PT, DPT; Corry Pelsnor, PT, DPT; Jason Smith, PTA; Kelsey Motto, SPT
- **School Psychologist:** Jonathan Stearns, PhD(c), M.Ed.
- **Speech Language Pathologists:** Morgan Dorr, MS, CCC-SLP; Gina Henshaw, MS, CCC-SLP; Crystal Deguzis, MS, CCC-SLP
- **Teacher, Visually Impaired:** Desiree Casian, M.Ed., Ed.D.

Located in Rochester, New Hampshire, and incorporated as a non-profit in 1976, for over 40 years the Monarch School of New England (MSNE; www.monarchschoolne.org) has provided unlimited possibilities for students with special needs—supporting them to reach their greatest potential. It is a member of the New Hampshire Private Special Education Association, and its programs are accredited by the New Hampshire Department of Education.

The school currently provides services for children, adolescents, and young adults. Originally called the Child Development Center of Strafford County, the organization began as a volunteer-run playgroup in the late 1960s to meet a growing need to provide opportunities and support for children with disabilities. During that time, there were limited resources available for children with disabilities and their families in the community. As the organization evolved into a school in the mid-1970s, the school's founder, Carrie Foss, continued to demonstrate her leadership as a pioneer in this field, to provide opportunities for children with special needs, where there previously had been none. This is the foundation on which the school is built: people who see potential and are willing to step outside of the mainstream to make a difference in the lives of children, adolescents, and young adults with disabilities. Today, MSNE continues to embody this legacy as a renowned, non-profit, specialized day school for students with significant developmental, physical, medical, behavioral, and emotional disabilities between the ages of 5 and 21. Since its founding, over 300 students have graduated from the school.

The MSNE is now recognized across New England for excellence in academic, therapeutic, functional life skills, and vocational programming for students with complex disabilities. Rooted in the belief that every student deserves an environment in which they can thrive, students at MSNE have access to the same educational content as their peers in public school but are given modifications and adaptations to make learning meaningful, motivating, and functional. Therapy services, such as speech, occupational, physical, and behavioral therapies, are delivered using an integrated and collaborative approach to support access to the curriculum and increase independence in functional life skills. Students can develop healthy habits and lifelong leisure skills through inclusion in MSNE's innovative therapeutic and adaptive recreation programs in the community. The MSNE also offers an array of pre-vocational/vocational training programs in different career sectors. Students graduate from MSNE with a resumé of skills to prepare them for productive, meaningful employment to the greatest degree possible.

Students at MSNE are valued for their abilities. They are seen for what they can do, not what they cannot. The overarching philosophy at MSNE is the starting premise that every student has potential, every student can learn, and every student can grow and thrive, given a supportive environment and carefully designed supports to capitalize on their abilities and support areas for growth. As a program, MSNE strives to help students grow to reach their greatest potential, and to develop independence to the greatest degree possible. The MSNE provides unlimited possibilities for students with special needs, and the staff recognizes and embodies that it takes the support of a community to create such opportunities. Accordingly, the mission of the MSNE is:

> to support individuals with special needs so they can realize their greatest potential. In this nurturing environment, a comprehensively trained staff works one-on-one with each student, uniquely integrating both education and therapy, to ensure successful transitions to school and to the community.

Students attend the MSNE as an out-of-district placement from over 30 partner school districts across New Hampshire and southern Maine. Students at MSNE have a wide range of diagnoses. Examples include autism, traumatic brain injury, Down syndrome, cortical visual impairment, sensory processing disorder, neurological differences, rare genetic syndromes, cerebral palsy, and other physical impairments. Students are placed at MSNE when their needs cannot be safely or appropriately met in a public-school setting, or when there is a disconnect between their needs and the learning environment available within their home school setting. As an out-of-district placement, all students are referred to MSNE through the special education process beginning with their home school district. Placement is a team decision, made through the individualized education program (IEP) process. Once the determination is made that MSNE is an appropriate placement for that student, the sending school team and MSNE's staff work closely together for a smooth transition.

Programs and therapy sessions designed to address students' physical and mental health, sensory integration, and educational challenges are provided both indoors and outdoors. All 62 students participate in a variety of outdoor activities during the week, weather permitting. Program activities are provided both individually and in small groups, depending on the activity and the students' IEPs. Group size varies, according to the type of group. Each classroom has six-to-eight students, and each student has a one-to-one paraeducator. At times, an entire classroom may participate, but often the classroom is divided into smaller subgroups for group activities. The sessions are 30 minutes long and the number of sessions per week are provided according to each student's IEP. The programming and therapy take place on two sites: the MSNE Foss Elementary School, which is located on four acres, and the MSNE Regional High School and Vocational Center's eight-acre campus. Both sites are easily accessible for all. The elementary school has wetlands, a seasonal brook, woods, and open space. The elementary school nature trail was built by volunteers from the local United Way volunteer organization about 30 years ago. The playground was designed by playground specialists and built by staff and United Way volunteers in 2013. The original elementary school garden/greenhouse was designed and installed by an occupational therapist and a master-gardener volunteer 25 years ago. They were updated in 2016 with the addition of raised beds, sidewalks, and a gazebo.

The high school was originally a farm field and is open and sunny with woods in the distance. The new high school therapeutic garden was designed by a landscape architect who specializes in therapeutic gardens with input from MSNE staff, administration, and facilities personnel. The garden was installed in 2019–2020 by staff and various contractors from the community with the maintenance director having built many of the structures. The director of human resources oversees the facilities, including the outdoor spaces. The facilities maintenance director takes care of the overall grounds, with the help of an assistant. The therapeutic gardens are maintained by Ms. Perry, with the help of an assistant.

MSNE has 120 staff, including administrators, special education teachers, paraeducators, nurses, related service providers, and facilities maintenance staff, all of whom have a role in the year-round program. Therapy is delivered by all disciplines in various indoor and outdoor locations on school property (playground, nature trail, school gardens, parking lot, sidewalks, and an above-ground swimming pool in the summer) as well as offsite in the community (adapted skiing, hippotherapy, kayaking, field trips, work-based learning at outdoor job sites). Co-treatment is typical in both individual and group therapy sessions. During the COVID-19 lockdown, school was provided virtually, using the Google Classroom platform. Therapists uploaded activities on Google Classroom, provided therapy sessions via Zoom, and mailed pertinent materials to the students' homes. Prior to the COVID-19 pandemic, volunteers from a variety of programs periodically assisted with program delivery, under the direction of MSNE professional staff. Examples include peers from the local high school, mentors from the University of New Hampshire, international students from Friends Forever, specially trained adaptive ski volunteers, and specially trained hippotherapy side-walkers.

The materials needed for all programming are specific to each discipline, and each discipline orders what they need according to their budget. Each discipline submits an annual budget proposal in early spring for anticipated items needed the following school year. The MSNE board of directors approves or modifies the budget requests according to the financial status of the school. The Director of Community Engagement seeks funds to supplement programs through grants and fundraisers.

Regarding student funding, the United States Special Education Law mandates that all students must be provided a free, appropriate public education (IDEA Section 504). While applicable to all students, if that cannot be met within the home public school setting, when a student is placed at MSNE, the sending school district must pay tuition to cover the costs of educating that student out of district. There is no cost to students or families to attend MSNE. The sending school district also pays MSNE for any services outlined in the student's IEP that they require to access their education, such as speech, occupational, or physical therapy. The sending school district additionally assumes the cost of providing transportation to and from MSNE each day. As an out-of-district placement, MSNE does not directly receive town taxpayer money as a public school would for the school budget.

While the majority of MSNE's funding comes from a fee-for-service model with sending school districts paying for tuition and therapy service, due to the number of innovative programs and therapies that MSNE offers as part of its collaborative, holistic approach to education, costs for these opportunities are supported through fundraising. As a 501(c)(3) non-profit, MSNE engages in traditional development activities such as grant writing, working with individual and corporate donors, and hosting community events to help support the programs and therapies its students require. The MSNE also raises funds through individual and corporate donations and special events.

The MSNE staff are deeply committed to their work and attuned to the needs of their students. The stories below illustrate that taking it outside can take many forms and be truly impactful for the students; sometimes simply being outside makes a world of difference for a student and can be the sole difference between no participation at all and an engaging and meaningful session (all names are pseudonyms):

> The kids are happier outside, and when they're happier, they're more willing to participate in things that are difficult for them. For example, Blaine does not nod his head "yes" for me inside the school. The other day, we were outside, and we went around the corner and Lucas rode up in his mom's car. Blaine was nodding his head so much his walker popped up—his favorite things are vehicles, such as cars and lawn mowers.
>
> *—MSNE teacher*

> Being outside eliminates extra auditory stimulation such as sound bouncing off the walls in a small space. Sometimes when I take students outside, they can see things I didn't realize they could see because auditory distractions are reduced. I knew by his reaction that Billy could see that the doors to the shed were open, meaning that the lawnmower might be in use.
>
> *—MSNE teacher*

Job opportunities are key for students with visual impairment. The more things you can expose our students to the better, and if they love to be outside and that love can be shaped into a job opportunity, you will have success, and the sooner you find that out, the better you will be.

—MSNE teacher

One of our students, Taylor, could be sleeping for hours but as soon as I say it is time for gardening, his eyes open wide and he gets a huge smile on his face. I don't see him as engaged in any other activity as I do during gardening. One of his goals is use of a button-type switch to initiate an activity. When it comes to using the switch in gardening, I only need to cue him once, and he starts using it to activate a pouring cup attached to his tray on a flex mount to mix soil and add water and such. He is truly in his happy zone when it comes to gardening!

—MSNE school nurse

As part of my "check-in" with older students, I can connect and process with them while walking on Monarch's nature trail. This outlet provides us with opportunities to regulate our bodies. As the therapist, I can increase or decrease the walking pace or stop entirely to model for and benefit a student's regulation. A simple breeze, sun on the skin, bright and engaging colors, and endless nature-made fidgets are in abundance. It's a fun challenge and personal exploration to help students identify strategies in nature that can help them to independently regulate.

—MSNE school psychologist

There are many great ideas for therapeutic outdoor activities and how to make them easier and harder, which are shared by the MSNE team for you to consider as you create your therapy outside program. Most important to note is that all the therapeutic and educational activities are graded and adapted according to the student's physical, cognitive, sensory, and social-emotional abilities and IEP goals. For example, gradations for following directions may include following a picture or object cue schedule, following written directions, or watching a step-by-step "how to" video on a tablet. Physical and environmental adaptations may include special seating, using tools with built-up handles, use of solid visual backgrounds to reduce visual load, and working with plants that have specific sensory qualities such as smells or textures. When using adaptive trikes in the parking lot to follow motor directives such as "stop/slow/go" or "red light/green light," the challenge can be increased when students are taken onto the nature trail where there are slight turns, and they can go uphill and downhill. Other gradable outdoor activities (all facilitated outdoors at MSNE) including setting up an obstacle course using natural elements and equipment, exploration using the nature trail, structured and unstructured sensory exploration, interoceptive sensory observations such as "the cold rain makes my body feel cold," work-based learning opportunities such as gardening tasks and building, hippotherapy, and working on safety awareness in real (rather than contrived) settings such as the parking lot.

Following directions, vocabulary building, and social skills can also be enhanced when therapy happens outside. For articulation goals, auditory bombardment (saying words that have the target sound in them) is used by modeling vocabulary that is in the student's immediate environment. For example, if a student works on the /b/ sound while riding a bike (to target a physical therapy goal), the speech and language pathologist and physical therapist when co-treating may model multiple /b/ words, such as bike, bark, boy, bounce, bound, brake, bird, bee, brown, behind, before, and bump. This activity can be simplified by repeating the same words or modeling a lesser variety of words, by pairing the words with two-dimensional visuals, or by having the student stop the bike to practice the sound before riding again. This activity can become more advanced by having the student receptively identify the items that begin with /b/ and practice saying the words. To work on those sounds phonologically, the therapists can try to "trick" the student by saying words that sound like the targets and asking the student to tell them if they said the /b/ sound or not, which is a fun way for students to correct the therapists.

For social pragmatics, the playground is the perfect place to work on social skills. The playground provides an opportunity to practice the skills in a natural environment, rather than in a contrived scenario in the treatment room. If there are other students around—even better! Therapists can scaffold support and help provide structure or prompting to start the social interaction, then fade supports as needed to help the student navigate all the various social situations that arise on a playground, including wanting to ask a peer to play, needing to take turns on a swing, and determining how to help if a friend falls and gets hurt.

Therapy can be particularly effective for acting out memories or experiences, as well as role-playing individuals that are important to the student. The outdoor playground provides students with a physical, contextual structure to play and act, use their imagination, and process grief and trauma. The playground is also used for numerous motor activities such as practicing getting on/off swings, ascending and descending ramps and stairs, and climbing.

Sunlight and being outside offer many opportunities to practice using vision. On the nature trail, asking things such as "Do you see the light reflected through the trees? Do you see the stick on the ground? Reach down and feel it. How high do you need to lift your foot to step over the stick?" Outside, students practice wearing sunglasses and are taught to use auditory cues to know where they are on the property through the change in sound such as pavement versus leaves underfoot, and to listen for unexpected obstacles like people and cars. It is also helpful for students with visual challenges to practice navigating around unexpected things outside such as changes in terrain. Students can additionally practice accessing furniture/equipment such as benches and outdoor swings.

Activities are often selected to correspond with monthly school-wide academic themes, as well as the natural cycle of the seasons. For example, if an academic theme is Habitats/Biomes, students might harvest milkweed seeds from the garden and create Monarch butterfly "seed bombs" to sell in the school store. If the academic theme is the Revolutionary War, students might grow/harvest herbs used by the colonists to make "Liberty Herbal Tea" teabags to replace black tea.

Advice and thoughts are always welcome when considering a shift from indoor to outdoor practice, and the staff at MSNE were eager to share theirs. The physical therapy team suggested:

> Have fun and enjoy nature! Most students love to be outside, and you can tailor the environment to work on the goals you are trying to accomplish. There are many ways to incorporate opportunities outside into treatment sessions. Students often are happy to be outside and see this time as "play."

From speech and language pathologists we heard:

> Have fun and don't be afraid to think outside of the box. You can work on all the same goals that you have already written if you think creatively. You may find that a student presents very differently inside than outside, sometimes in a very positive way. You are going to be pleasantly surprised at how motivating going outside can be for some students.

The school psychologist said:

> Working outside helps me to regulate and center, so that I may provide attuned and active/engaging therapy. The fresh air, walking, and relaxing environment all work to benefit my health, as well as my students.

The teacher for the visually impaired indicated:

> If you're itinerant, it's helpful to have a designated space outside with a place to sit, potentially grassy. Children who have both visual impairment and gravitational insecurity want to sit for many reasons: they're close to the ground; there's nothing unexpected that will happen; sitting helps them know where they are in space. If the space is familiar and it becomes uncomfortable—for example, loud sounds can be interpreted as being close by, even if they're not outside—the child can direct the adult to move away. It's also helpful to have a trail for walking.

This teacher recommended having transportable ways to control light, such as hats and sunglasses at the ready. The teacher also discussed the benefits of having access to an awning for shade and allowing time for eyes to adjust to light changes. The horticultural therapist suggested:

> Have a designated area. Use a familiar sequence/structure for sessions with a clear beginning, middle, and end and to allow a few minutes for free choice/exploration outdoor activity at the end of a session.

And finally, occupational therapy staff shared:

> Do it! Find a way to get outside as much as possible for sessions! Set expectations prior to going outside, set aside a "toolbox" of equipment to take outside, but don't limit yourself and by all means use imaginative play to explore and create therapeutic experiences.

The MSNE staff came up with a collective list of what they find to be benefits and challenges associated with "taking it outside" with the students to learn and for therapy. Here is what they compiled, beginning with myriad benefits, summarized by one therapist: "There are endless benefits to therapeutically engage with a student outside." Well said!

Benefits:

- Students are often happier when they are outside.

- Using the natural environment for learning and therapy is helpful as it has better carryover to daily living.
- Natural environment teaching is motivating and fun for students (and staff).
- For all therapy targets, taking treatment outside of the therapy room is a great way to effectively generalize skills. For a student who can use a target sound during structured practice, sitting at a table in a quiet room with no distractions, the next step is to work on generalizing their skill to a different environment. Taking it outside provides the perfect opportunity to bridge the gap between the ideal treatment space for initially learning a skill and more real-life scenarios in which the student will be using what they have learned.
- As it promotes a more natural sensory environment with lighting and sounds, therapy outside naturally lends itself to natural, truly occupation-based experiences and allows for age-appropriate exploration and play.
- Soil contains a microorganism (*Mycobacterium vaccae*) that may reduce anxiety, which is a very good reason to garden. See reference below.
- Following on from this, when students are more relaxed, they are better able to work on their goals, sometimes without realizing that they are working. This often happens when they are outside.
- Movement of objects in the outdoor environment such as leaves fluttering and swings swaying stimulates vision, as does movement through the environment such as walking, riding a bike, and riding a horse.

Challenges:

- Unpredictable New England weather! It can be too hot, cold, windy, or wet.
- Due to our students who have trouble with thermoregulation and sensitive skin, temperature changes and the presence of stinging insects can be challenging when outside. For instance, for our students with seizure disorders, when it gets too hot, it is hard on them because they cannot safely be outside.
- Controlling the light is a challenge. One student hates the glare of the sun and refuses sunglasses. He says, "Turn it off!" An overcast day with a good temperature is ideal.
- Although rare, a student may dysregulate or continue to escalate once outside, resulting in a fight, flight, or freeze scenario. Recognizing

opportune times and locations to process certain emotional content is critical to student success and regulation, as well as individual safety. Processing our emotions can be difficult work!

- Some students and staff have "biophobia" to insects, snakes, and other natural phenomena.
- The greenhouse water lines are drained in the cold months, requiring water to be carried into the greenhouse.
- Uneven surfaces can be daunting for untrained staff to navigate when working with students who have mobility challenges.

What better way to wrap up this inspiring case narrative than with the words of MSNE's Executive Director, Diane Bessey, M.Ed., PT, who shared:

> We are so fortunate to live in a beautiful state with so many outdoor opportunities. Parents often have no idea how successful their kids can be outside, given a little adaptation, and it gives the families hope that they can do outdoor activities together. When our students participate in outdoor activities, it builds leisure skills that they can enjoy for a lifetime.

Reference

Matthews, D.M. and Jenks, S.M. (2013) 'Ingestion of *Mycobacterium vaccae* decreases anxiety-related behavior and improves learning in mice.' *Behavioural Processes 96*, 27–35. https://doi.org/10.1016/j.beproc.2013.02.007

Social-Emotional Connections with Nature and Improved Mental Health

Positive youth development and contact with nature is a relatively unstudied but fascinating area of research. Owens and McKinnon (2009) suggest that easy access to outdoor spaces that offer solitude and reflection, such as a backyard garden, religious center garden, or even a cemetery, helps adolescents with "positive identify formation, self-efficacy, and value formation" (pp.51–57), all of which contribute to positive youth development. Bowers, Larson, and Parry (2021) identified five "C" factors—"competence, connection, confidence, character, and caring"—(as well as a "sixth C" of "contribution") that shape positive youth development (p.2). In their self-report study of 587 diverse, low-income, middle-school children, aged 11–4, it was found that time spent in nature was positively correlated with increases in the six "C" factors. Like most nature and health researchers, their recommendation is that caregivers, practitioners, and teachers make every effort possible to encourage adolescents to spend time in nature to nurture positive youth development (Bowers *et al.* 2021). Mental health indicators such as resilience, health-related quality of life, stress reduction, and improved self-esteem are also positively associated with outdoor nature-based experiences (Tillmann *et al.* 2018) such as adventure camps and educational programs, as well as just getting outside to play.

Here is what some of the research tells us about the social-emotional benefits of outdoor adventure programs. Outdoor programs with a final expedition component have been associated with nurturing autonomy, particularly for female participants (Chang 2021). Tillmann *et al.* (2018) found evidence of increased resilience for adolescents who participated in outdoor adventure programs, resulting in increased sense of mastery and decreased emotional reactivity. Results of "The Journey," a 23-day outdoor adventure program for 76 adolescent boys found that emotional intelligence, specifically intrapersonal skills, and adaptability were both enhanced and sustained for three months post-program participation. Emotionally intelligent people manage daily life, health, and wellbeing by being realistic and flexible problem solvers with a high degree of self-motivation and optimism (Opper *et al.* 2014). In further support of the social-emotional value of outdoor adventure programs for adolescents and young adults, Mutz and Müller's (2016) study of the "Crossing the Alps"—a nine-day trek for 14-year-old adolescents across the Swiss, Austrian, and Italian Alps—reported that the experiences associated with the rigorous programming enhanced resilience, life satisfaction, physical health, overall wellbeing, and stress reduction. Outdoor summer camps that do not have a specific therapeutic intention have also been found to be effective in supporting adolescent social-emotional development. In an exploratory study conducted by Garst and Whittington (2020), adolescents attending a summer camp expressed "novelty, challenge, friend-making, tradition, achievement, positivity, and emotional safety" (p.306). These are exciting findings suggesting that nature supports social-emotional development and improved mental health in myriad ways.

For those working on a community level, mental health and youth development programming in parks may also help prevent violence among at-risk youth (D'Agostino *et al.* 2019). An afterschool park-based mental health program called Fit2Lead was designed to foster improved mental health among at-risk 12–17-year-olds. More than 500 adolescents participated in the program, and outcomes were measured over a two-year period. Results showed a reduction in arrest rates for areas adjacent to Fit2Lead programs, as compared to programs that did not offer a park-focused program. The results of the study indicated that "park-based programs may have the potential to promote mental health and build resilience, and also to prevent violence among at-risk youths" (D'Agostino *et al.* 2019, p.S215). There is no magic formula to definitively indicate how much time needs to be spent outside daily to maximize mental health, but what the research finds is that there is a positive relationship between adolescent engagement in MVPA and improved mental health. For example, in a year-long self-report study of 242 adolescents aged 14–16 years, it was determined that the amount of time and the higher levels of physical activity positively mediated their mental health status (Bélanger *et al.* 2019). Getting outside, being outside, and moving outside matter for good mental health.

NUGGET OF NATURE: EMOTION LOTION

This is a simple aromatherapy activity that blends nature with mental health. Making the lotion is a nice way to discuss emotions and problem-solve ways to control and express them through the herbal properties of the oils. This activity lends itself nicely to clients to reflect on how they can make behavioral changes.

Materials you will need

- Unscented body lotion
- Essential oils—see list below for specific properties associated with the oils
- 4-oz. plastic jars with screw top-lids
- Craft sticks or chopsticks
- Permanent marker

Steps to facilitate making emotion lotion

1. Have the client squeeze or pump lotion into the 4-oz. jar.
2. Encourage the client to smell the various essential oils and choose one, two, or three that they like.
3. Have the client add about 15 drops of essential oils to the lotion. If using two different oils, add about seven drops of each, or five drops of each if using three oils.
4. Have the client stir the lotion with a craft stick or chopstick.
5. Once the lotion and oil are well combined, screw the lid onto the jar.
6. Encourage the client to think of a name for the lotion blend and write it on the jar lid. One example might be "Peace and Quiet," a blend that includes lavender and ylang-ylang oils.

A safety note: Unless otherwise indicated, never apply essential oils directly to skin as they are very concentrated and cause skin irritation.

Below is a list of common essential oils and their properties, all of which have a unique scent and potential healing properties.

- Basil: Enhance mood, increase alertness, and soothe muscle aches.
- Bergamot: Relieve anxiety and soothe tired feet.
- Cedarwood: Ease stress and improve sleep.
- Cinnamon: Relieve stress and ease pain.
- Citronella: Relieve stress and fatigue.
- Clove: Pain relief.
- Grapefruit: Reduce stress, increase energy, and enhance mood.
- Helichrysum: Soothe body and mind.
- Jasmine: Relieve stress.
- Lavender: Relaxation and relieve insomnia.
- Lemon: Boost mood and energy, and relieve anxiety.
- Lemongrass: Relieve stress and ease anxiety.
- Neroli: Relieve anxiety.
- Orange: Boost energy, improve mood, and ease anxiety.
- Patchouli: Improve sleep.
- Peppermint: Boost mood and relieve pain.
- Rose: Ease stress.
- Rosemary: Enhance mental focus.
- Sandalwood: Relieve anxiety and improve sleep.
- Ylang-ylang: Relieve pain, reduce inflammation, and improve mood.

Information from: www.verywellhealth.com

How to make the activity easier

- Add oils to the lotion for the client or provide hand-over-hand assistance.
- Pre-label jars with names of lotions.

How to make the activity harder

- Discuss the herbal properties and invite clients to develop their recipe based on how they are feeling in the moment.

Improving the Provision of Education: Nature Makes Us Better Thinkers

Not only is nature itself an outdoor classroom, but also taking a formal class outside can have profound and positive impacts on students' learning capacity.

A meta-analysis by Fang *et al.* (2021) found that outdoor educational programs for adolescents resulted in improved self-efficacy, even when mental health status and length of intervention were accounted for as moderating factors. Another study reported that outdoor learning programs increased self-efficacy and decreased fear, as well as increasing reported connectedness with school and among peers (Williams *et al.* 2018). Any therapy provider is an educator—we are teaching our clients and their families and caregivers new skills, or practicing newly learned skills each time we meet—and nature has the power to help us enhance that learning experience!

If we can't take it outside, let's work to bring a bit of nature inside. Harkening back to Roger Ulrich's seminal 1980s study showing that views of nature improved inpatient outcomes, a mixed-methods experimental study involving high school students found that even a mere window view of vegetation from a classroom decreased both student heart rate and self-reported stress, whereas a classroom without windows did not (Li and Sullivan 2016). Location does make a difference, and if therapy cannot be provided outside, try to ensure that clients have a window view of green outside and/or plants inside.

Let's build on the value of nature views. A study by Determan *et al.* (2019) found that a physical learning space designed with biophilic principles led to reduced stress and improvement in standardized test scores. Students and teachers expressed positive perceptions of the biophilically designed classroom and felt "calm" in this nature-rich environment. Recall from Chapter 3 that biophilia is the innate predisposition we have that connects us with nature (Wilson 1984). Biophilic design is intended to "create spaces that are inspirational, restorative, and healthy, as well as integrative with the functionality of the place and the (urban) ecosystem to which it is applied. Above all, biophilic design must nurture a love of place" (Terrapin Bright Green 2014, Section 3.1). The intention of biophilic design is to enhance learning, creativity, and health, and to reduce stress (Terrapin Bright Green 2014). We need biophilic design to prevail wherever we work, learn, worship, play, and live.

Being in a biophilic-rich learning environment is vital, but so is going outside. The importance of taking breaks from cognitive tasks cannot be understated. A cross-over study of 16–18-year-olds looked at the impact of cognitive performance and wellbeing following three nature conditions: a one-hour lunch break in a small park, a larger park, and a forest. After each condition, wellbeing improved, but was sustained longest following time in a forest. While concentration improved after all conditions, the most significant gains in cognitive performance were achieved after time in a larger park (Wallner *et al.* 2018). For therapists and practitioners, seeking larger and more nature dense areas may be the most impactful environments in which to facilitate therapy.

CASE NARRATIVE: Leg Up Farm

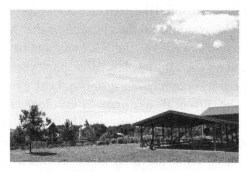

ACTIVE AND QUIET SHELTER SPACES EXPAND
THE POSSIBILITIES FOR OUTDOOR THERAPY

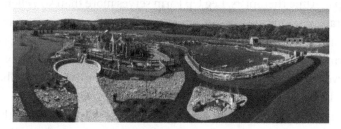

AN AERIAL VIEW OF LEG UP FARM
Photo credits: Leg Up Farm

Thank you to Maura Musselman, Director of Community Engagement, for contributing to this case narrative.

Located in Mount Wolf, Pennsylvania, Leg Up Farm is a unique interdisciplinary therapy clinic with a mission to "enrich the lives of individuals and families with special needs and unique challenges, through support and customized programs." It achieves its vision by providing traditional therapy services indoors as well as outdoor options galore. What makes Leg Up Farm unique is that it is the only pediatric therapy facility to offer physical, occupational, aquatic and speech therapy, behavioral health, therapeutic horseback riding and equine-assisted therapies, nutrition counseling, and a variety of educational and recreational programming all under one roof. Since opening, Leg Up Farm has provided therapy services to more than 3000 children and adolescents.

Poised with a vision and passion to do for others, Louie and Laurie Castriota set out to create a therapeutic riding center, merging their love of horses with their desire to give back to their community. Six months into planning, their daughter Brooke was diagnosed with mitochondrial disease, causing cognitive and motor function delays. Through their experience of trying to find the best treatment for Brooke, the Castriotas recognized the need for a comprehensive therapy center, which would provide coordinated therapy services that were both affordable and accessible for children with disabilities. Louie and Laurie seized the opportunity to expand on their initial plan. After many years of hard work, and thanks to the generosity of community members, Leg Up Farm opened its doors in April 2010. The current 18-acre property was donated to Leg Up Farm, and today the facility and property is maintained by the staff. Leg Up Farm's pediatric therapy program serves clients with disabilities and unique challenges from birth through age 21. While providing care to clients with a wide variety of diagnoses, Leg Up Farm's therapy services are directed towards meeting each individual's unique mental and physical health challenges. Staffed by 13 full- and part-time therapists, Leg Up Farm serves more than 500 clients each year. Therapy sessions are one-on-one, typically last for 45 minutes, and are provided year-round. During the early part of the COVID-19 pandemic, all the Leg Up Farm therapy programs were offered virtually, demonstrating yet another high level of flexibility and commitment to providing the best possible services for its clients and their families.

Leg Up Farm provides therapy in a unique way, catering sessions to the interests of the child and wrapping their actual therapy around them. They can accomplish this because of the huge variety of therapy spaces that they have onsite. In addition to unique and engaging child- and adolescent-centric indoor therapy spaces, Leg Up Farm has the benefit of also having wonderful outdoor spaces to use for therapy sessions. These outdoor spaces include a large barrier-free playground that enables access for all to climb, play at heights, wheel, run, walk, swing, touch, look, be curious, and explore, no matter their abilities or challenges. There is also a music garden with accessible outdoor musical instruments and a large therapeutic koi fish pond, which clients can enter to feed the fish by hand. There is a wide, flat, paved walking path that meanders around the outdoor areas that clients can use to learn to ride bikes, scooters, and practice ambulation. During warmer months, most clients want to "play" on the playground, which looks different for each child or adolescent, depending on their needs and goals. Play could be pretend and imagination-focused, and it could be sensory-based, motor, social, or all of them. The playground includes different types of swings to accommodate children's various needs for support, slides, ramps, climbing structures, and more—all of which allow therapists to take it outside and provide therapies in different ways that reflect the "real world." Not surprisingly, the koi pond and music garden are also popular with the clients who receive services at Leg Up Farm. It is all about being focused on providing children and adolescents opportunities to do what they need to do, to "be children" or to practice and develop skills needed for the transition to adulthood. Therapy sessions are rarely provided indoors when the weather is nice!

For those looking for some sage advice about taking it outside when the option is to also be inside, Ms. Musselman shared:

> We are a comprehensive therapy center that happens to have a really great playground, pond, and music garden. We use the outdoor spaces as a resource—they are not our full-time primary spaces, but we use them when it's a good fit for the client and practitioner. If it is a good fit, do go outside! What kid [no matter their age] doesn't like a playground? We find that taking clients outside can be intrinsically motivating.

Families primarily find out about Leg Up Farm's services through referrals, social media, and fundraising and community events. While there are many stories to share, two stand out as examples of how Leg Up Farm has positively impacted children, adolescents, and their families and why their referral base is strong. One family shared that "to be able to find a place where [our son is] happy and can play, improve, and progress, that is also family-friendly, warm, and inviting, has been one of the most amazing blessings for us." Another family said:

> There will never be a way for us to repay the incredible staff at Leg Up Farm for the incredible gift of life that they have given to our little girl. Her quality of life has significantly improved since starting there and for that we will be forever grateful.

It is work like this that has led to a fairly long wait list, which means that Leg Up Farm does little marketing. Leg Up Farm's annual operating budget is $3.9 million. Pediatric therapy programs provided by Leg Up Farm are primarily billed through insurance as well as through grant funding; however, the therapeutic riding program is funded through a fee-for-service model. Financial aid is also available for families. Please visit www.legupfarm.org to learn more about the programs and services they provide to clients and their families.

Widening the net to include out-of-school learning, Widmer, Duerden, and Taniguchi (2014) identified a link between participation in a two-week residential summer outdoor-adventure program (including rafting and hiking) with a positive attitude towards learning and motivation and a way to minimize summer "learning loss" (p.168). An important take-home statement from the researchers was: "this research might also inform the use of outdoor adventure beyond individuals to guide work with families or even organizations" (p.170).

Get Moving

While it may still seem counterintuitive, as adolescents seek out more autonomy and time with peers, being with caregivers remains incredibly important (Arnett and Jensen 2019). Who adolescents spend time with in nature—by themselves, with family, or friends—matters (Wang, Wu, and Wu 2013). How this time with caregivers happens also matters, so let's spin back to family-based nature activity (FBNA). More time spent participating in FBNAs, such as hikes, camping, family trips, and sports, particularly in middle adolescence, is associated with greater time spent engaged in outdoor activities in early adulthood (Izenstark and Ebata 2016; Izenstark and Middaugh 2022; Lovelock *et al.* 2016). Like in childhood, more time in nature within the structure of the family also increases the likelihood that it will continue into adulthood (Izenstark and Ebata 2016). For example, results of a self-reflection study asking adults to recall nature experiences in adolescence also found that engagement in outdoor leisure activities involving friends or family members was the impetus to continue their nature engagement as adults (Wang *et al.* 2013). The concept of FBNA seamlessly applies to therapeutic intervention with adolescents. Further, engaging in outdoor activities, FBNA or otherwise, equates to more physical activity (Shanahan, Franco *et al.* 2016).

Engaging in preferred physical activity outdoors can be a perfect way to achieve the recommended activity allotment of 60 minutes a day for adolescents (CDC 2022a; Frömel *et al.* 2020). Despite the need to meet this daily recommendation, children and adolescents with developmental disabilities tend to have lower rates of moderate to vigorous physical activity (MVPA) as compared to typically developing peers. This finding clearly points to the need for client-centered physical activity-focused interventions that meet the needs of all adolescents (Yu *et al.* 2021). One example of a structured physical activity program is the Get Outside: After School Activity Program (GO-ASAP). Barfield *et al.* (2021) found that adolescent participation in this program led to increased physical activity, improved sleep, decreased perception of stress, changes in dietary choices, reduced electronic use, and increased social relatedness and confidence. Outdoor physical activity programs need to be structured within a framework to meet adolescents where they are.

CASE NARRATIVE: Promise Ranch Therapies & Recreation

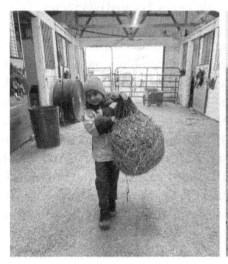

CHILDREN AND ADOLESCENTS HELP WITH BARN CHORES

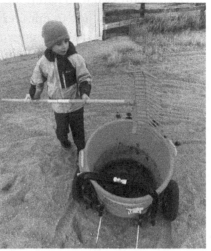

KEEPING THE ARENA CLEAN IS HEAVY WORK

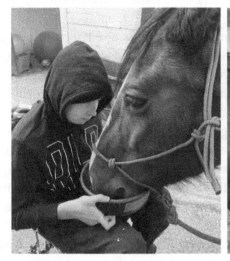

TRUST AND CONNECTION

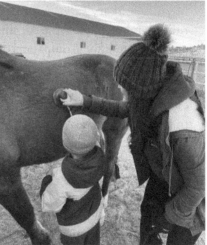

HORSE GROOMING IS THERAPEUTIC FOR BOTH RIDER AND HORSE

Photo credits: Promise Ranch

Thank you to Danielle Braman, MSOT, OTR/L, C/NDT, the Therapy Manager at Promise Ranch Therapies and Recreation, for her help to prepare this case narrative.

With its mission to "enrich our community through connection and inclusion,"

Promise Ranch represents the best of how the holistic needs of a community can be addressed with nature-based therapies. Located on 17 acres in Castle Rock, Colorado, just 30 minutes south of Denver and easily accessible via highway, Promise Ranch is growing their programming. In 2010, they began providing equine-assisted activities (EAA) for children and adults with disabilities and conditions such as cerebral palsy, autism spectrum disorder, developmental delay, traumatic experiences, emotional health issues, rare genetic disorders, and stroke. Promise Ranch uses EAA, which includes hippotherapy, or house-mounted therapy, and ranch-based activities as the primary interventions. Hippotherapy is an evidence-based intervention for treating neurological, sensory, and developmental conditions because it has been found that a horse's gait mimics the natural gait of a person. Tapping into this movement pattern while astride the horse helps people achieve functional independence through motor control (Maresca *et al.* 2020; Murphy, Kahn-D'Angelo, and Gleason 2008). Increasing evidence also supports the broader social-emotional-cognitive benefits of EAA, resulting in an increased demand for these services.

In response to their community's needs, Promise Ranch started offering interdisciplinary services in 2020. In addition to hippotherapy, adaptive riding, and horsemanship for military veterans, Promise Ranch also began providing traditional outpatient occupational, physical, speech and language, and mental health therapies. Furthermore, to meet the community's ongoing needs for health promotion and life skills training, Promise Ranch has expanded programming to include inclusive recreation, vocational skills training, cooking classes, gardening, arts and crafts, exercise, and meditation.

Promise Ranch works with clients of all abilities from as young as two years old to those in their 60s. Therapy services are offered as small groups, one-on-one sessions, and periodic specialized camps. All programming (equine therapy, occupational therapy, physical, speech and language therapy, and mental health counseling) is offered weekly for an hour each session, and groups typically run for nine weeks. Therapy takes place year-round in the indoor and outdoor riding arenas, therapy offices, and the outdoor spaces around the ranch, such as the garden. In addition to the eight full-time therapy staff, Promise Ranch is supported by a facility manager, an equine manager, ten barn staff, and 100 hours of volunteer assistance a week.

The Promise Ranch staff are an interdisciplinary team consisting of an occupational therapist (Ms. Danielle Braman), three occupational therapy assistants, a licensed mental health counselor, a social worker, a speech and language pathologist, a physical therapist, a veteran's program coordinator, and 15 horses. Clients are primarily referred by local community case managers from the local health department. Clients (or caregivers of clients) also self-refer after learning about Promise Ranch by way of social media, the website, or meeting staff at local events such as community festivals, where they host a booth, or holiday events promoted at Promise Ranch, including their winter holiday meet-and-greet with the horses.

When doing hippotherapy sessions, the therapists use the horse's movement to help achieve functional outcomes such as attention to task, executive functioning skills including sequencing and planning, posture, and motor planning. Based on the client's needs, the staff are trained to adapt the therapeutic challenge of an activity by encouraging a client to perform positional changes, changing the horse's pace, modifying the equipment used, or having a client complete work on the ground rather than on the horse. A typical session with the horse includes preparing the horse for riding, which consists of identifying and carrying tack to the hitching posts or arena, brushing the horse, putting tack on the horse, mounting the horse, riding the horse, untacking the horse, and assisting with leading the horse back to its turnout area. Depending on a client's abilities, some or all of these activities are incorporated into the session. Just as in "traditional" therapy, the staff are constantly using task analysis and modifying their therapeutic interventions to provide the "just right" challenge to their clients. A typical therapy session without the horse may involve completing barn chores, such as sweeping, feeding animals, or grounds maintenance. Clients also can interact with small animals at the ranch, including guinea pigs and rabbits. In the therapy rooms, clients engage in activities they would complete in a "traditional" therapy setting. Clients can also garden or cook as part of their therapy program.

Promise Ranch has an annual operating budget of $310,000. The resources needed to keep Promise Ranch running are obtained through fee for service, insurance, grants, and government funding. Therapy equipment, such as toys, games, and crafting and art supplies, are organized and cleaned by the therapists, while the horse tack (such as saddles, pads, reins, and grooming tools) is maintained by the equine manager, who is also an occupational therapy assistant.

Although Promise Ranch have not yet published any of their outcome data, which they have collected via the Bruininks-Oseretsky Test of Motor Proficiency, 2nd edition (BOT-2), and the Sensory Processing Measure (SPM), they are considering doing so. While the quantitative data has not yet been published, they have plenty of qualitative data to support their programming through client stories, such as this one. A ten-year-old girl said:

I like [coming to Promise Ranch] because of the horses and the teachers, and how the teachers help you through stuff and how they talk to you and make you feel calm and get through your feelings. I like it because I get to play games and if I don't want to talk to my parents, I can talk to one of my teachers here and feel comfortable and get help with something I am struggling with. I like that the horses can also help you stay calm sometimes. If you like horses, it might be good to come here. I've learned about the horses, how to tell how they feel sometimes—when they are feeling something, you can tell mostly by their ears, and their facial expressions.

And another client shared: "I like coming to Promise Ranch because the people are so nice. They play fun games, and it doesn't even seem like work. I get stronger and get to practice conversation. I like horseback riding!" Reading these stories reminds us how nature-based therapy can make the work of getting stronger and more resilient feel like fun.

The parents of young clients also have stories that illustrate the benefits. One parent shared:

Our son has a rare seizure syndrome. Because of this, he is globally delayed and has several physical limitations. You can imagine our delight when we found out that he would be able to have weekly hippotherapy sessions to address some of his challenges. Each week he can work on his bilateral control, range of motion, balance, and core strength. He also gets to feel confident, loved, and has time to feel like a real person. What is also powerful to watch is my son's connection to the horses he rides. He is fortunate to have made two new horse friends—Kola and Poncho! They are patient with him. They listen to what his body is telling them. And he can pet them and give them a kiss at the end of each ride. It would make anyone watching be filled with gratitude for these horses. The staff at the Promise Ranch have been wonderful!

The grandparents of a 12-year-old with Down syndrome shared:

We came to Promise Ranch with high hopes of [our grandson] increasing his large motor activity, and he has benefitted so far beyond our initial hopes. He was hesitant at first, but the staff was encouraging and patient and now he can't wait to be at the ranch and to see the horses. We have seen great strides in many areas. While his balance is greatly improved in class, we see how that has helped him in general with running, playing, climbing stairs, and much more. We also see the improvement in his core strength, which has helped his posture and general activities. He has even improved his speech as he has learned to communicate effectively with the horse and therapist. Finally, he has built tremendous confidence on the horse, which is displayed in other settings. We are grateful to Promise Ranch and their tremendous programs!

As Promise Ranch works to connect their community and create an inclusive place for healing and growing, they are creating a beautiful place to be. Ms. Braman, the therapy manager, shared her personal reflection of working at Promise Ranch:

The smell of fresh hay. The sounds of a horse whinnying. Watching a beautiful creature do what they were born to do. When I walk onto the ranch, I feel calm. I feel inspired. The sensations that welcome me to work are familiar yet exciting every time I am here. Nature-based therapy has changed the way I think as a therapist. I used to go to work with an "agenda" of activities for my clients to do. Whether it was completing a certain task or lifting a weight x number of times. But being a clinician in a natural setting, I realized that there is no need for an agenda. Brushing a rabbit, watering flowers, planting seeds, or snuggling against the whiskers of a horse provide tons of therapeutic benefit. Yes, I facilitate this magical experience our clients can engage in and ensure that while they are brushing this magnificent beast, we are working on a range of motion and gross motor coordination. But our clients don't even know they are doing therapy most of the time. The refreshing gulp of nature re-energizes our clients and offers a space for huge therapeutic gains. Our clients achieve amazing things in our program, and it is so inspiring.

Exposure to nature not only helps heal clients; it can also make therapists better clinicians!

Although Ms. Braman finds nature-based therapies to be effective, energizing, and refreshing, she recognizes that there are challenges. The two major challenges the staff face when providing therapy at the ranch are the weather and animals. To address these challenges Ms. Braman recommended to "always have a plan B." She shared that she may have planned for a session outside exploring nature or planting flowers, but then when a huge thunderstorm rolls in, it is not an ideal situation, and she has a backup plan for working in the barn. Also, she made clear that animals have needs of their own. If they cannot be incorporated in the session due to illness or behavior, the therapist must respect that and find an alternative. When a situation like this arises, it becomes a spontaneous opportunity for therapist and client to discuss the importance of respecting the animal's needs and boundaries, and how showing this same level of respect for themselves and for other people is equally important.

According to Ms. Braman, the benefits of providing therapy services at Promise Ranch far outweigh the challenges. For many clients, the benefits of receiving their therapies in an outdoor, experiential setting include unique opportunities for quality-of-life improvements. Interacting with animals and engaging in nurturing and purposeful activities at Promise Ranch is motivating in a way that therapy in a clinical setting may not be. To this end, Ms. Braman shared, "I feel re-energized after I go for a short walk outside. Imagine being a client who has typically only done clinic-based interventions. The experience is uplifting and inviting."

Ms. Braman's lessons learned about "taking it outside" included being flexible to expanding services to best meet the community's needs and keeping an open mind when looking for outcomes. For instance, the staff at Promise Ranch found that a natural fit between the ranch environment and individuals with disabilities has been the opportunity for life and vocational skills training and purposeful work. Building on that natural fit, Promise Ranch diversified their services to include inclusive recreation and employment training to provide more social, leisure, and work opportunities for their adolescent and young adult clients with developmental disabilities. Through equine-assisted therapies, ranch-based recreation, and work skills training, clients with developmental disabilities have forged connections with animal partners. These connections with the animal partners have provided opportunities to practice care for others, instead of always being "cared for," which has helped to build their executive functioning skills and has improved the clients' communication skills. The expansion of services led to improvements beyond what they had initially imagined!

The beauty and healing nature of Promise Ranch is obvious while working with the horses, when spending time outside, and in the moments when they are truly serving their community and providing the programming unique to each client's needs. You can learn more about Promise Ranch at www.prtr.org.

References

Maresca, G., Portaro, S., Naro, A., Crisafulli, R. *et al.* (2020) 'Hippotherapy in neurodevelopmental disorders: A narrative review focusing on cognitive and behavioral outcomes.' *Applied Neuropsychology: Child 11*, 3, 553–560.

Murphy, D., Kahn-D'Angelo, L. and Gleason, J. (2008) 'The effect of hippotherapy on functional outcomes for children with disabilities: A pilot study.' *Pediatric Physical Therapy 20*, 3, 264–270.

As discussed in Williams *et al.* (2018) and developed by Ian Williams in 2009, the ChANGeS framework contains five key factors for enhancing planning, implementation, and participant outcomes in outdoor programs. While not overtly intended for a therapeutic program, there is great synergy to be had when considering a therapy-outside model of practice. The five factors are below.

- Challenge: experiences in which participants are extended and have their abilities and personal resources stretched in tasks that may appear at first to lie beyond their reach.
- Activity: being actively engaged in a learning environment requiring physical, emotional, cognitive, and psychological involvement.
- Nature: immersion in natural environments characterized by green space, fresh air, freedom from distraction, and simple living.
- Guided experience: making meaning from experiences through leader guidance and reflection, goal setting, metaphor, and debriefing.
- Social milieu: being part of a functional community involving small-group living, social modeling, giving and receiving feedback, and negotiating new relationships.

(Williams et al. 2018, p.23)

Using the ChANGeS framework, outdoor adventure programs such as Get Outside After School Activity Program (GO-ASAP), Fit2Lead, Crossing the Alps, and The Journey (Barfield *et al.* 2021; D'Agostino *et al.* 2019; Mutz and Müller 2016; Opper *et al.* 2014) could potentially be adapted to meet the needs of adolescents with developmental and other disabilities.

What matters is that adolescents need to be outside, every day, engaged in physical activity in safe and inclusive spaces. This can include park programs, going to camps, and school trips, which are examples of health-promoting ways to increase MVPA (Zarr, Cottrell, and Merrill 2017). For now, and for the sake of their healthy development, we need to "run" with this knowledge and develop viable strategies to ensure that adolescent clients are given safe and barrier-free opportunities (Piccininni *et al.* 2018) to participate in therapy outside.

CASE NARRATIVE: Yellowstone Boys and Girls Ranch (Rocky Mountain College OT)

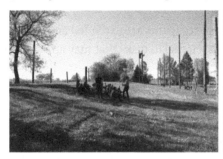

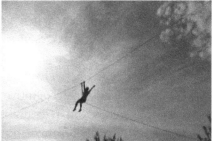

GATHERING TO TALK ABOUT
THE ROPES COURSE

SOARING TO THE HIGHEST POTENTIAL

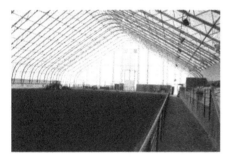

THE SCALE OF THIS INDOOR ARENA IS BREATH-TAKING
Photo credits: Yellowstone Boys and Girls Ranch

Thank you to Taylor Clark, OTD, OTR/L, for her help to prepare this case narrative. Please note that at the time of writing this case narrative, Dr. Clark was a student in the Rocky Mountain College OTD Program class of 2022 and provider of occupational therapy services. Dr. Clark is now the first occupational therapist hired by Yellowstone Boys and Girls Ranch! Kudos to her and the staff for recognizing the value of occupational therapy. Dr. Clark was also instrumental in championing and starting the on-campus Serenity Garden and programming at the college. This case narrative is featured in Chapter 6.

Located in Billings, Montana, the Yellowstone Boys and Girls Ranch (YBGR) is a residential mental health facility for youth, aged 11–18. The mission of YBGR is "Caring people preparing youth for life." The website is www.ybgr. org. The YBGR currently has facilities for equine and aquatic modalities, as well as massive gardens, greenhouses, and animal husbandry programs.

All participants in the YBGR program are living with mental health diagnoses and working towards goals developed by the therapy team. The youth participate in monthly treatment reviews during which they read their goals and weigh in on their progress. Diagnoses range from autism to oppositional defiant disorder to substance abuse. Many of the participants are diagnosed for the first time at YBGR, while others come to the facility with a diagnosis having utilized other mental health facilities across the country for most of their lives. The primary goals for most youth at YBGR are learning and developing coping and self-regulation skills. While many of these youth return home, some will be required to live in group homes or independently upon discharge, so learning communication skills and self-help skills that enable them to care for themselves are also common goals for all the youth.

Beginning in April of 2021, the Rocky Mountain College Occupational Therapy Doctorate (OTD) program partnered with the staff at YBGR to implement occupational therapy on campus using the facilities already available to youth and staff. Recognizing an unmet need, the YBGR occupational therapy program was developed according to the theory that occupation-based mental health services would provide preventative and restorative measures for the youth in Montana. April 2021 was the first time YBGR offered occupational therapy on campus, although they had contracted for outpatient services in the past.

Occupational therapy practitioners at YBGR have opportunities to utilize equine, aquatic, low- and high-ropes courses, gardens, and off-campus outings such as hiking to provide occupation-based mental health services in real time for youth in their current environment. Having occupational therapy available on campus increases the frequency with which clients and staff can access the services and allows practitioners to utilize the clients' natural environment. The relationship between the occupational therapy program at Rocky Mountain College and YBGR further increases the access these youth have to therapeutic activity-based services.

Occupational therapy services are provided indoors and outdoors onsite at the private facility as well as off-campus for therapeutic excursions. Occupational therapy is designed to address mental health and sensory integration vulnerabilities. While the entirety of the 410 acres of the Yellowstone Boys and Girls Ranch (with 240 acres used for the on-campus ranching operation) is available for use by staff and youth, the current site for occupational therapy is housed in a building on campus that was previously used as a lodge for youth and then as the medical clinic. Being located in the center of campus allows for easier access to all outdoor and active recreation facilities and equipment. The YBGR has both maintenance staff and youth at the facility who are paid to participate in "work crew" vocational training. Together, both staff and youth are responsible for the maintenance of campus facilities.

Occupational therapy services are offered as small groups or one-on-one, depending on the youth's needs. In alignment with the facility staffing, the largest therapy group contains eight youth and two staff as the campus ratio is four youth to one staff member. The program participants will flow in and out of groups as their needs dictate. Most group sessions are 45 minutes, though some sessions can last for 75 minutes depending on the activity. Currently, all youth enrolled for occupational therapy receive one group or individual session per week unless there is an unexpected absence. Below are just some of the therapeutic outdoor activities facilitated by occupational therapists that participants engage in as part of intervention services (they are easily graded by offering varied levels of support and individualized to meet the specific needs of each youth):

- outdoors ropes course
- gardening and greenhouse work
- riding bikes
- taking care of pheasants
- water balloon activities
- sports, such as basketball
- equine activities
- off-campus opportunities: hiking, biking, kayaking.

The occupational therapy program is designed to run year-round. Activities vary based on weather, but the facility has many options for and supports indoor, outdoor, and off-campus activities. There is minimal marketing of the occupational therapy program as it is currently available only to those who already use the residential-based services. Currently, youth at YGBR are the sole users of occupational therapy services.

Truly reflective of an academic–community partnership, the Rocky Mountain College OTD students provide services under the supervision of a licensed occupational therapist. The students can also, if they choose to, complete both of their level I and II fieldwork rotations as well as class assignments such as running therapeutic groups at YBGR. Initial training and continuing education opportunities are provided by the facility. Research has been conducted that examines the benefit of sensory-based approaches from admission to discharge from occupational therapy services. Many of the sensory-based approaches being studied use outdoor spaces and include nature-based activities.

The occupational therapy program is supported by an interdisciplinary team composed of the director and executive director of residential services, therapists, mental health workers, a physician assistant, and medical directors (physicians), who are all part of the treatment team. The occupational therapists meet or communicate with the treatment team to ensure optimal outcomes for the youth. At a minimum the occupational therapists attend monthly treatment-plan reviews for youth on their caseload, but depending on the youth and their needs, this might be daily.

The Rocky Mountain College occupational therapy program was the recipient of a substantial grant that was used to buy all the initial supplies for the program that were not already available on the YBGR campus. This funding has hugely supported the program. Ongoing funding for the program happens through grants, billing for services through insurance, and local, state, and federal funding. The occupational therapy program requires a minimum budget of $15,000 per year to cover the cost of supplies and equipment. Donors and practitioners who run the groups acquire all resources needed to complete the group. The campus itself has a plethora of supplies collected throughout its years of operation, which can be creatively used during therapy sessions. The occupational therapist is expected to plan all groups and take into consideration what is needed and what is already available, and to get everything organized and ready for therapy. The Rocky Mountain College OTD Program and YBGR, within the span of its inaugural year, have hired a full-time occupational therapist (Dr. Clark), who also supports the continued interactions of occupational therapy students on the YBGR campus. This is innovation at its finest!

Both youth and staff alike have expressed their interest and connection with the program. Two youth who received occupational therapy services shared their thoughts about their experiences:

- "I feel better when I am out in nature."
- "Being outside is what helps me manage my anger."

The staff at YBGR have been incredibly welcoming and continually communicate their gratitude. In one such instance, the lead psychologist told Dr. Clark a story about a group he had run in a lodge on campus where quite a few of the youth on her caseload lived at the time. Dr. Clark shared that she had been feeling a little down because two of four youth who were needed to work with her for initial assessments refused services immediately. She said, "It's disheartening, but it's their choice. The lead psychologist went into the lodge to do a group session, and one of the youths who refused made it general knowledge that they weren't going to be doing occupational therapy—that they had really stuck it to the therapist who tried." Well, not just one, but all of the children on her caseload who lived in that lodge told the other youth that decision was a huge mistake, and if they had the choice, they should try to get into occupational therapy because it was so fun and there was so much great work being done. What a resounding endorsement from those who are the recipient of services!

Dr. Clark also shared that most of the referrals are for sensory issues. One of the youth on her caseload was scored very high on the sensitivity and scales, this was leading to some serious outcomes. He had been refusing school because the input was just too overwhelming and resulted in a lot of engagement in self-harm behavior. Dr. Clark went to his on-campus residence before school for an occupational therapy session and found the youth visibly miserable: physically and emotionally defeated. Dr. Clark and the boy decided to walk to the horse barn, about a ten-minute walk. As they walked, Dr. Clark reported that she could see him loosen up with each step they took. By the time they got into the turnout (a large, open space where horses spend most of their time grazing) and started doing some serious work focused on sensory integration and Mahler's interoception curriculum (2018), the boy was a whole new kid. He began speaking up and talking about what leads to feeling hopeless. The walk back after therapy was just as beneficial. As they walked back together, he was starting to feel anxious, but Dr. Clark and the boy were able to talk about a plan to stay engaged and in the present, and they were able to discuss his goal to work in a mental health field. Being outside and working with the horses created the opportunity: skilled occupational therapy expanded on it and solidified the lesson.

There are, as Dr. Clark suggests, benefits and challenges to taking it outside, but the benefits outweigh the challenges. On the benefits side are the opportunities to reconnect with oneself, with nature, and with adaptive hobbies that support the needs of those in the mental health community. Nature provides an endless source of therapeutic opportunity depending on the practitioner's creativity and reduces the level of expectations on a child during a session. The mood-enhancing benefits of sunshine are subtle but an important part of addressing mental health issues. The challenges that Dr. Clark identified are that in Billings, during the winter months, snow and ice can be a limitation. Many of the youth are not provided with the proper clothing or footwear to be doing extensive activities outside. There is also inherent risk in the outdoor environment and engagement in activity outside, issues addressed in Chapter 2.

This is Dr. Clark's advice for those considering outdoor practice: "Let the clients take the lead. Incorporating assessment tools such as the Occupational Profile and/or the Canadian Occupational Performance Measure into the evaluation process will often prompt clients (in general) to share their perspective and interest in being outdoors." And—voilà!—the opportunity to take it outside is ready and waiting.

Wrapping It Up

Although it is important to promote time outdoors for adolescents (and for everyone), understanding the environments where they live, play, socialize, and learn is also important. Perceived safety is a factor for participating in outdoor play; lower perceived safety is associated with lower rates of outdoor play (Kepper *et al.* 2020). Additionally, air pollution can impact the safety and quality and amount of time spent outdoors (Dong *et al.* 2018), important considerations for any outdoor therapy program to take seriously when site planning.

Nature enhances spaces for adolescents to support engagement in recreation, to move their bodies, to experience restoration, and to socialize. These places include nature preserves, forests, beaches, gardens, parks, and backyards. As therapists, starting with creating a mindset that these existing spaces can be used for therapy with adolescents marks a critical first step toward taking it outside.

NUGGET OF NATURE: CHOOSE YOUR OWN ENDING—LOOSE PARTS FORAGING

This highly adaptable activity will facilitate movement outdoors and promote creativity, and can be easily tailored to meet the interests of any client. After foraging for loose parts outside, encourage the forager to make an obstacle course (or you as the therapist can set the course), string the objects to make a mobile, or make a collage and take a photo. The materials listed below cover all three activity options. If choosing just one ending, you would not need all the materials listed.

Materials you will need

- Stopwatch (or timer on a mobile device)
- Checklist and pencil or pen
- Pedometer or smartwatch
- Small container, bag, or basket for collecting the found materials
- Chalk
- String (at least a 5' length)
- Scissors

- Ruler, chopstick, or something rigid from which to hang the found objects
- Sheet of solid colored construction paper
- Camera

Steps to facilitating the foraging

1. Explain the project to your client, provide them directions for foraging, and give them a small container or bag to hold the object while they are foraging. Consider choosing one of the three instructions below. We encourage you to think about what you are working on with your client and tailor the instructions to meet their needs. For example, if you are working on following instructions, give them a checklist; if you are working on increasing physical endurance, give them a set number of steps to take or a time parameter. Additionally, discourage clients from touching trash unless you provide requisite protective equipment (e.g., gloves and hand sanitizer).

2. Provide a specific time (e.g., seven minutes) and encourage them to find (within the time frame) as many small objects outside as possible such as sticks, small rocks, flowers, seeds, or leaves.

3. Provide a checklist that specifies how many or what objects need to be found. If working on fine motor skills or writing, ensure the writing utensil you provide is appropriate for your client. Examples include: a set number such as four unique objects and five objects that are the same, a checklist of colors (e.g., something green, brown, yellow, tan, red, orange), or a checklist of characteristics such as something soft, hard, smaller than a grape, larger than an apple, heavy, light.

4. Provide a minimum number of steps or a certain distance they must walk. To count the steps, use a pedometer or smartwatch, and to establish the distance we recommend choosing a known route that has an established distance.

5. Once the found objects are collected, give your forager instructions for what to create. This is the "choose your own ending" portion of the activity.

6. Move it! Either direct the forager to create an obstacle course using the found objects or you as the therapist can set up an obstacle course and have the forager run through the course. If on pavement or a sidewalk, use chalk to enhance and add more structure to the course. Place the objects on the ground and far enough apart that your client will have to move to participate. Examples of directions and movement to consider are: twist and turn, run, jump, skip, tiptoe, hop, bend and touch, crawl, and walk around.

7. String it! Provide string and a ruler or stick (or other rigid object to hang the string from) and encourage the client to make a mobile. The mobile could

consist of a single long string connecting all the objects or multiple strings connecting a few of the objects on each piece. Foragers can wrap the string around objects such as a small rock or thread the string through objects like a leaf or flower petal. If you have an indoor therapy space, consider displaying the mobile as a way to bring some nature inside!

8. Photo it! Provide your client with a piece of construction paper to use as the background and then encourage them to create a collage or display with the found objects. Once the art piece is complete, take a photo of the creation. If you complete this activity multiple times, the photos can be a fun way to compare the different foraging experiences.

How to make the activity easier

- If providing a checklist, provide more concrete instructions on the checklist. Instead of listing "4 unique objects and 5 objects that are the same," list "1 rock, 1 seed, 1 flower, 1 stick, and 5 leaves."
- If creating an obstacle course, reduce the number of obstacles and distance required to move.
- If stringing the found object, consider helping with wrapping and tying the objects onto the string.
- If displaying it, consider simplifying the instructions to "find one object on our walk."

How to make the activity more challenging

- Modify the instructions to increase the distance or step-count required.
- Modify the instructions to make the checklist longer or more specific, such as "find a white rock, an oak leaf, and a dandelion flower."
- Modify the obstacle course to increase the number of obstacles and the complexity of the course, such as adding more paths to choose within the course.

CHAPTER 6

Young Adulthood

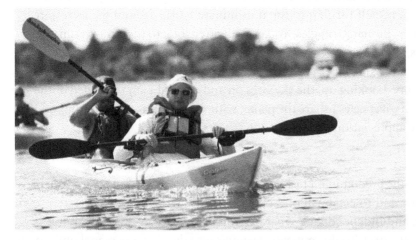

WATER ACTING AS A GREAT EQUALIZER FOR THOSE LIVING WITH A SPINAL CORD INJURY
Photo credit: Empower SCI

Introduction

Spanning from ages 18 to 25–30 years, young adulthood is also referred to as emerging adulthood (Arnett 2000; Simpson 2018). It is the transition period between adolescence and adulthood and, like all other periods of development, has its unique tasks and challenges. As young adults transition into adulthood at about age 25, the prefrontal cortex of the brain has matured, so that executive functions and emotional stability are better established and, accordingly, better decision making is possible. Physiologically, bone mineral density continues to increase, while physical growth concludes in young adulthood (Hochberg and Konner 2020).

THIS MUCH I KNOW—MADELYN

I never had an extravagant experience with nature where I instantaneously understood its profound role in my wellbeing. Rather, I noticed fleeting moments of peace when walking past blooming flowers or feeling a graceful breeze on my cheeks. For a second, my attention shifted to something other than the grinding minutiae of day-to-day life. I became a part of a world beyond my spheres of work, school, and relationships, something beyond my social identities. As someone who has struggled with mental health problems, this release was deeply freeing. Over time, I found myself turning to the non-human world around me as respite from my human struggles. Today I will often look to the sky—in times of stress, gratitude, anger, and sadness. The size, variability, reactions, unity, provisions, and sheer power of the sky washes me clean with profound humility. Looking up, the sky goes on and on, and I am reminded of the millions of species I share the planet with, of the release of letting go, and of the appreciation for the healing aspects of nature.

Several of the predominant tasks of young adulthood include working to achieve autonomy and to establish oneself as a person with their own lifestyle, own identity, and independence separate from their caregivers (Havighurst 1972; Pusch *et al.* 2019). To do so means beginning to develop a personal philosophy that comprises opinions, goals, preferences, likes, and dislikes.

NUGGET OF NATURE: GARDEN MOOD-BOARD COLLAGES

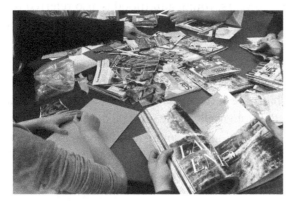

Using magazines and other media to create mood boards
Photo credit: Amy Wagenfeld

Designing a dream outdoor space is highly preferential and involves making choices. This activity is best done in a group to promote social-emotional skills as clients will need to share and negotiate for materials. Working in a group presents clients with an opportunity to engage in spontaneous conversation as well as sharing when the collages are complete. If working one-on-one with a client, this activity provides choice making and opportunities to practice fine motor skills, such as cutting and gluing.

Materials you will need

Adapt the following materials as appropriate for your client group:

- Illustration or poster board (at least 11" x 17")
- Glue or another adhesive
- Scissors
- Magazines, advertisements, photos, and catalogs
- Various colored papers (e.g., construction paper, origami paper, wrapping paper, and sketch pad paper)
- Markers, crayons, and/or colored pencils
- Small items such as buttons, paper clips, ribbon, string, sea glass, shells, flower pods
- Work tables

Steps to facilitating mood-board collage activity

1. Place materials in the center of the table.
2. Provide each client with a piece of illustration or poster board.
3. Ask clients to close their eyes and imagine what their dream outside space could look like.
4. Allow clients time to use the materials to create a visual of this imagined space on their mood board. If an image of something specific is not available, encourage clients to draw it or to write about it. For example, if there is no image of a swing, a client could draw one or write "large tree swing" on the mood board.
5. Encourage each client to share their mood board with the others at the end of the therapy session. Discussion prompts can ask, for instance, about where the space is, what inspired it, what makes it special, and how it makes you feel to think about it.

How to make the activity easier

- Tear pictures from magazines instead of cutting.
- Assist clients with placing items on their mood board.

How to make the activity more challenging

- Stand to complete the activity.
- Work in teams to create a dream outdoor-space mood-collage board.

Making social connections and finding one's community typically takes place in young adulthood, which may lead to developing long-term intimate relationships. During this stage of development, young adults typically foster a sense of political awareness, and pre-existing and new friends are increasingly important as they transition away from dependence on their families of origin. Some young adults will marry or be in committed relationships and may begin to start a family. Joining the military, in the United States, is normally something that only young adults can do. Becoming involved with social and civic groups that are of interest such as in sports, music, religious, non-profit, and advocacy often occurs during young adulthood.

THIS MUCH I KNOW—PHELAN

At the current moment, nature to me means having to shovel my driveway during a winter in Michigan. While shoveling, I usually wonder why I decided to move somewhere that the weather hurts my face. But when I'm done, I look up at the sky, take a big breath of the cold air, and realize, though Mother Nature forced me outside, it's all worth it. Being outside gives me an opportunity to clear my head from work and life. When I see the still neighborhood lit up in the bright snow, I'm thankful I get to be outside...even if I still wish I had a snowblower instead of the shovel.

An initial career or career trajectory is typically established during young adulthood. Along with a career and autonomy comes fiscal responsibility. Learning to manage a budget and maintain a household are tasks that are associated with young adulthood. All these higher-level milestones or tasks are possible because, cognitively, young adults have reached a high peak of intellectual development, particularly with working memory and processing speed (Hochberg and Konner 2020). Never again during the lifespan is the brain so sharp and well tuned.

We do want to acknowledge the non-universal nature of young adulthood. Not all 18- to 30-year-olds can experience a period of development where they gradually assume responsibility and discover their personal philosophies. Without education and wealth, many people in this time of life assume all the tasks and full responsibilities of adulthood (Abrego 2019; Galambos and Martínez 2007).

THIS MUCH I KNOW—AUDI

I was lucky to have grown up in the Pacific Northwest on a forested piece of property. I've always had a deep respect for nature; my favorite activities were climbing trees and exploring in the woods. As a young adult, recreating out in nature became my number-one form of self-care. From walking in local parks and outdoor spaces, to riding my bike along a scenic byway, to hiking in the mountains, nature is my place of inner stillness.

For me, the tranquility and solitude of the mountains is the best place to fully engage in mindfulness meditation. The rich sensory experience of hiking solo through a forest alongside a creek or lake, the smells of pine and wild rose, sunlight streaming through the trees, the sounds of water and birdsong filling the ears, and the crunch of pine needles and snow underfoot bring me into a state of presence I simply can't access in my everyday life. The minutiae of my day, my worries, my to-do lists, and the endless stream of chatter in my mind all seem to melt away as I become fully immersed in my surroundings. The ego meets true humility in the magnificent presence of mountains.

Therapeutic Benefits of Nature: Young Adults

Research looking at the therapeutic benefits of nature specific to young adults reveals that exposure to nature positively impacts all aspects of development: physical, social-emotional, and cognitive. Additionally, gratifying nature-based experiences in young adulthood are important for future positive engagement with nature in adulthood. For young adults to feel comfortable in nature and appreciate being outdoors, the process of experiencing the joys and wonders of nature actually begins in childhood (Sugiyama *et al.* 2021). This means children need access to safe outdoor spaces and caregivers must support outside play because early experiences in nature impact future impressions of it. Young adults who grew up playing in wild outdoor environments and developed positive feelings about nature and outdoor activities are more likely to look for employment in outdoor sectors than young adults who lack these experiences. Furthermore, young adults with positive feelings about nature are then more likely to share their love and care of nature with future generations (Broom 2017; Sugiyama *et al.* 2021). The time children and adolescents spend outdoors can shape future leisure and vocational opportunities and also help nurture the planet by supporting environmental sustainability. Being outdoors really can open doors on multiple levels!

CASE NARRATIVE: Serenity Garden (Rocky Mountain College OTD)

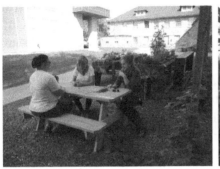

SEATING IN THE GARDEN PROVIDES A SOCIAL SPACE AND COULD BE USED FOR TABLETOP ACTIVITIES

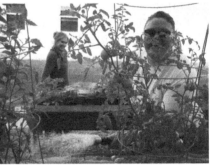

HAVING A LITTLE FUN IN THE GARDEN

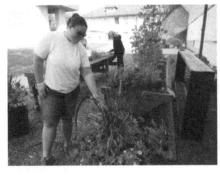

THIS SMALL GARDEN IS TUCKED IN BETWEEN TWO BUSY ACADEMIC BUILDINGS, BEAUTIFYING AND MAKING GOOD USE OF A PREVIOUSLY UNATTRACTIVE SPACE ON CAMPUS
Photo credits: Emily Schaff

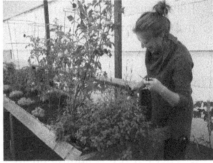

THE GRATIFYING JOY OF HARVESTING HERBS

Thank you to Twylla Kirchen, PhD, OTR/L, Founding Program Director, and Emily Schaff, Administrative Assistant, for their help to prepare this case narrative.

An innovative example of how an educational program can take it outside is the relatively new Rocky Mountain College (RMC) OTD program located in Billings, Montana. With a mission to "prepare clinicians, educators, researchers and future leaders in the profession through engaged, experiential and evidence-based educational opportunities to expand knowledge about the health benefits of occupation," their nature-focused, occupation-based activities are making a positive impact on the health and wellbeing of the campus population. Educators and students, take note: you too can transform your campuses into health-promoting learning spaces, such as the 100' × 550' serenity garden installed by the students adjacent to the OTD building.

Rocky Mountain College's OTD program was developed to meet the unique needs of people in Montana. The OTD program focuses on engaged learning, community-based practice, entrepreneurship, mental health, rural health, and culture. Students begin identifying community-based, rural-focused programming needs during the first semester of the program. Many of the programs that students choose to support are located outdoors and promote the health benefits of engaging with nature and natural environments. One of the projects that was initiated by their inaugural class and sustained and enhanced by following classes is the on-campus serenity garden.

In their first semester, the RMC OTD students are required to select a project that addresses a need in the community. Students noticed a vacant and unattractive area in between the OTD building and the science building, and decided to meet with facilities management and the Dean of Students to obtain permission to create a serene sensory garden that would benefit students, faculty, staff, and visitors. Recognizing it is a matter of social justice, the first group of students built wheelchair-accessible garden beds and planted vegetables and grape vines. It took approximately $1000 to start the program; the costs were mainly for wood and materials to build the planters, soil, and plants.

The second cohort of students applied for and received a $2500 college grant and added more planters, a bench, and a water feature, and repaired an outside wall where community-based murals are now hung. The students also collaborated with the undergraduate Botany faculty to submit and obtain a grant to install a heated and cooled greenhouse that was built in fall of 2021. The program is now fully grant-funded and supported by the RMC OTD program. While no formal onsite research has been conducted, it is eagerly anticipated.

Most of the participants who engage in the serenity-garden program offerings are students, faculty, and staff of RMC. It makes a difference in students' lives, with one saying this about the garden: "I feel as if I am transported out of the drudgery of class. I can clear my head and go back in the building in a better place than I left it." The garden has also been used with children and their families, and all ranges of adults who are participating in projects with the RMC OTD students. People have learned about the serenity garden program through the RMC newspaper, word of mouth, and an article about the program published in the *Yellowstone Valley Woman* magazine in September 2021.

The site is large enough to accommodate 24–30 people at the same time, and participation is open enrollment. With an addition of a heated greenhouse, the program is open year-round. Ten students, overseen by Dr. Kirchen, run the program, and volunteers also help tend the garden with tasks such as watering. No formal training has been provided as the program is an "all hands on deck" and learning-together effort. About tending the garden, one student shared, "It is therapeutic to be able to care for the plants and watch them grow."

Knowing full well that a garden is never done, students are continuing to add to the serenity garden. Some of the recent additions have included a walkway to promote accessibility, a water feature, and a greenhouse. Students have facilitated community-based groups with children and older adults in which they picked vegetables and herbs from the garden and used the OT kitchen to prepare a variety of fresh and delicious dishes.

The materials needed to run the serenity garden program include:

- planters
- vegetable plants
- flowers
- herbs
- soil
- bark ground covering
- bench
- water feature
- grape vines
- poles and wire (for grape vines)
- putty and paint for wall murals
- hoses and watering source
- greenhouse and supplies.

When asked to provide some advice to anyone thinking about a college campus serenity garden, Dr. Kirchen shared the following: "Think outside of the box. Explore grant funding to cover cost. Collaborate with the other programs, facilities management, and leadership at your college or university. Empower students and let them create something beautiful." While on the topic of students, Dr. Kirchen was quick to recognize the contribution of the RMC OTD students who planned, initiated, and sustain the serenity garden.

And as we wrap up this case narrative, we share a few of Dr. Kirchen's final thoughts about the benefits of taking it outside. She said:

> There is nothing more powerful than the experience of fresh air and sunshine. Students are often confined indoors for hours at a time. This can cause fatigue, frustration, and at times depression. Creating a therapeutic outdoor space for students, faculty, and staff to explore can greatly enhance mood, attention, and overall educational outcomes.

She is so right!

Nature-Based Outdoor Adventure Programs for Young Adults

Research conducted with young adults shows that nature experiences such as hiking, biking, running, and outdoor exercise improve cognition and attention as well as self-awareness (Mayer *et al.* 2009). For college students, engagement in intentional outdoor nature-based programs reduces stress (Sharma *et al.* 2020). There are also well-identified, wide-ranging benefits associated with an immersive nature experience that include relaxation, reduced stress, enhanced emotional health, and spiritual connections (Roberts *et al.* 2016; Warber *et al.* 2015). In fact, much of the research related to the impact of nature on young adults centers on participation in outdoor wilderness programs. For example, the Norwegian grounded concept of *friluftsliv* (pronounced free-loofs-leaf), translated as open-air life, is a means of experiencing wild nature either alone or with others (Mutz and Müller 2016; Taylor 2010). Applying the concept of *friluftsliv* to a group of undergraduate students at a German university who spent eight days in the wild with no access to comfort amenities, including mobile phones, was the focus of an interesting research study. During their time in nature, the students engaged in ten-mile daily hikes, rock climbing, camping, fishing, foraging, and swimming. Pre- and post-testing of the *friluftsliv* experience revealed that the students felt their mental health had improved. They were less stressed, felt a greater sense of self-efficacy, were more mindful and happier, and felt a greater sense of life satisfaction (Mutz and Müller 2016). As therapists and practitioners, these immersive outdoor experiences have the capacity to heighten the meaningfulness and impact of our services. And although we may not be leading an eight-day wilderness camp with our young adult clients, we can provide smaller doses of concentrated nature to achieve similar goals.

NUGGET OF NATURE: NATURE IMMERSION ON A SMALL SCALE

The activity can be facilitated outside or indoors. It engages multiple senses and can be facilitated with all clients, regardless of mobility or cognitive level. Adapt it as needed to engage your clients in a way that is meaningful for them.

Materials you will need (for one client)

- Three 5-gallon-sized bags, each filled with stalks of either fresh or dried aromatic herbs like mint (including myriad varieties such as peppermint, apple, and chocolate), thyme (generic, lemon, orange, juniper), lemon verbena, lemon balm, lavender, rosemary, and scented geraniums. An alternative to dried herbs is to gather a basin full of soft and pliable fresh pine needles.
- A large bowl or basin
- Tray or tabletop workspace

Steps to facilitate the sensory immersion experience

1. Encourage your client to strip the leaves off the stalks of herbs and place them in the bowl or basin.
2. Invite them to plunge hands or feet into the basin of herbs.
3. Encourage your client to crunch or tear the herbs between their fingers or toes.
4. Have them scoop and pour handfuls of herbs over their forearms and rub them into their skin.
5. Discuss with your client how it feels and smells and what their emotional state is after immersing themselves in their herbal "bathing" experience.

How to make the activity easier

- Strip the leaves off their stalks in advance and place only leaves in the bags.
- For clients with limited extremity function, place the herbs in the bowl and bring the bowl to them.

How to make the activity more challenging

- Prior to telling your client the names of the herbs, encourage them to guess what they are, based on smell alone.
- Encourage them to use their non-dominant hand to strip leaves, inviting them to think very deliberately about what they are doing.
- Have your client keep their eyes closed while stripping leaves off the stalks.

Established in 1941 by founder Kurt Hahn, Outward Bound is one of the most widely recognized programs of its type. The Outward Bound Trust is based on the principles of "physical fitness, craftmanship, self-discipline, and compassion" (Hickman-Dunne 2019, p.282). Outward Bound started in Scotland (U.K.) and over the past 80 years programs have been established throughout the world. Outward Bound came to the U.S. in 1962. The Outward Bound USA mission is "to change lives through challenge and discovery...predicated on the belief that we seek, embrace and value adventure and the lifelong adventure of learning" (Outward Bound 2021, para.1). Typical Outward Bound programs are geared towards neurotypical young adults and include extended kayaking trips and/or long-distance hiking trips with backpacks. Like other immersive wilderness experience programs, with modification and adaptation, you may find the Outward Bound model useful when developing therapeutic outdoor adventure programs for clients with physical and mental health issues.

CASE NARRATIVE: Empower Spinal Cord Injury

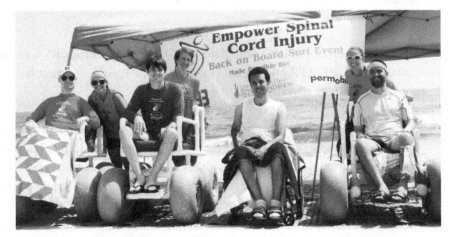

EMPOWER FOUNDERS AND PARTICIPANTS AT BEACH
EVENT USING AN ADAPTED MOBILITY OPTION

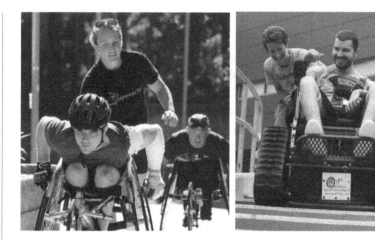

ADAPTED CYCLING

TRIALING AN ALL-TERRAIN CHAIR ON STEPS

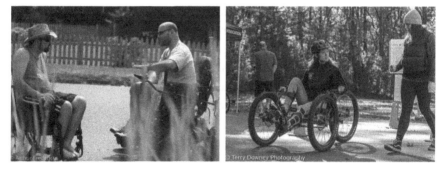

MENTORING IS AN IMPORTANT
COMPONENT OF THE EMPOWER
PROGRAM

Photo credits: Empower SCI

KNOBBY CYCLING PROVIDES A UNIQUE
OPPORTUNITY FOR OFF-ROAD BIKING

Thank you to Elizabeth Lima Remillard MS, OTR/L, LSVT BIG, CRS, Carinne Callahan, MS, PT, ATP, and Jessica Goodine, MS, PT, NCS, for their help in preparing this case narrative.

Founded in 2012, by physical and occupational therapist co-founders Carinne Callahan, Jessica Goodine, and Liz Remillard, Empower SCI, Inc., is a non-profit corporation that enables individuals with spinal cord injuries (SCIs) to lead happier, more meaningful, and more independent lives. Empower SCI. seeks to fill the gap in the current rehabilitation process created by decreased lengths of stay at rehabilitation hospitals, reduced outpatient services, and a shortage of specialized client-centered care during recovery from a spinal cord injury.

Often, there is also a disconnect between when an individual is ready for community-based rehabilitation and when they are deemed eligible for these rehabilitation services. The time following a spinal cord injury can be complicated by grieving, orthopedic restrictions, pain, and the healing of broken bones. It can take up to a year, if not more, to work through the gravity of the situation following this type of injury. Ms. Callahan, Ms. Goodine, and Ms. Remillard wanted to create a rehabilitation springboard to launch people beyond simply surviving, and into living their best lives. Thus, the focus of Empower SCI is to provide individuals with SCIs the opportunity to participate in further rehabilitation, beyond the basics of activities of daily living, at a time in their lives when they are mentally motivated, physically healed, cleared by their healthcare provider to participate, and have a longer-term focus beyond the initial shock of experiencing a spinal cord injury. The goals of the program are to help clients work toward improved physical and mental health, independence, and overall quality of life.

Empower SCI provides holistic one-to two-week-long intensive residential programing. The program integrates structured skilled rehabilitative services such as physical therapy, occupational therapy, and recreational therapy, with social-emotional services such as peer mentoring, rehabilitation counseling, education, and informal knowledge sharing between individuals who are going through similar experiences and challenges. To participate, clients must have a spinal cord injury and are typically over 18 years old. Most clients are in their 20s or 30s, but Empower SCI has served clients as young as 16 and as old as 65 years old. Each year the intensive residential program is offered in New York and in Montana, to accommodate clients from both coasts of the United States. The program consists of a combination of individual and group therapy sessions and adaptive recreation such as yoga, painting, cycling, kayaking, surfing, and dance. Before every program, each client establishes a set of unique goals and programming. The programming is then tailored to meet those goals and intended to maximize their ability to lead a happier, more meaningful, and independent life.

In addition to intensive residential programs, Empower SCI supports adults living with spinal cord injuries by running day-long wheelchair skills courses at various sites across the United States, hosting monthly virtual "Empower Hour" sessions to provide social connection for people with SCIs, and facilitating a yearly mountain bike fundraising event (the Knobby Tire fundraiser event, which raises both awareness of adapted mountain biking and funds to support Empower SCI programming throughout the rest of the year). Data on client goal attainment, independence, and quality-of-life measures has been collected with plans to analyze and publish the results.

The intensive residential programming happens in Missoula, Montana, and Stony Brook, New York, in outdoor spaces such as the quads on college campuses that Empower SCI partners with, as well as local beaches, harbors, rivers, and bike trails. The programs are offered as one- or two-week sessions offered twice a year in June and July. These programs are completely run by volunteers. The team includes physical therapists, occupational therapists, certified recreational therapists, massage therapists, rehabilitation counselors, nurses, personal care assistants, assistive technology professionals, and peer mentors. Professionals such as occupational and physical therapists, rehabilitation counselors, and nurses are licensed in either Montana or New York. Therapists provide one-on-one and group sessions. All staff assist with recreational activities. Volunteers arrive on campus prior to the clients for a two-day training on spinal cord injury, physical and psychological complications, transfer techniques, use of specialized recreational equipment, and program schedules. The therapeutic activities are provided in large and small groups and one-on-one; hence, it takes about 60–70 staff to run the programs. Noteworthy is that during the COVID-19 pandemic, although the intensive residential programs were not held in person, they were delivered virtually. All aspects of the intensive programs were included, but there was a greater focus on peer mentoring, group work, and education due to the online platform.

In its inaugural launch in 2012, staff ran their pilot program completely with volunteers on a budget of $18,000 to pay for room and board at the colleges and obtain liability insurance. Over time, Ms. Callahan, Ms. Goodine, and Ms. Remillard have acquired equipment, which can be costly. Cycles and custom adaptive surf boards can cost more than $4000 each. The list of equipment needed to run the program is also extensive. It includes sports wheelchairs, handcycles, helmets, grip adaptations, kayaks, paddle adaptations, seating supports, Mobi-mats, foam, personal flotation devices, beach wheelchairs, surf boards or stand-up paddle boards, tents, drums, tri-fold mats, plinths, sewing machines, splitting material, lockline, Velcro®, cooking materials, shower chairs, commodes, personal protective equipment, cleaning supplies, and arts and crafts materials. Some of this equipment, which is stored in a storage unit, was purchased through grants. The staff try not to acquire too much equipment because storage facility costs can exceed $2000 a year, and therefore they rent what they do not own from vendors such as Spaulding Adaptive Sports in Boston or DREAM Adaptive in Montana.

To set up recreational activities, the Empower SCI team readies equipment such as Mobi-mats (rigid mats that allow beach access for wheelchair or other mobility users) or plywood to allow wheelchairs to more easily roll over sand or other less wheelchair-accessible terrains, and they set up pop-up tents to offer shade. While the availability of paved boardwalks, accessible bathrooms, and parking is ideal, staff have a propensity for further adapting to whatever the local environment offers. In addition, staff have found that participants prefer to be outdoors when given the option. When programming on the college grounds, the preference is to facilitate non-outdoor-based activities outdoors in areas that have a building overhang, or other shelter that offers shade to help facilitate improved thermoregulation (Price and Trbovich 2018). To create a best fit between the clients' level of function and the activity, adaptation is a key component of the Empower SCI program. For instance, when kayaking for someone with paraplegia, the staff may use a single-person kayak with pontoons to prevent tipping, foam padding to reduce pressure points on bony prominences inside the cockpit of the boat, and a regular paddle; but the staff use a tandem kayak that has lateral supports and wrist grips for the paddle for an individual with tetraplegia.

Empower SCI is funded through a combination of grants, fee for service, federal, state, and local funding, private donors, corporate sponsorship, fundraising, and foundation support. Their yearly budget covers insurance, licensure, housing, food, purchasing equipment, equipment rentals, storage, marketing, travel, and accounting. Word about the program is shared via social media such as Facebook, Instagram, and through the Network for Good email-based newsletters.

There is an abundance of positive feedback about the Empower SCI experience that we are honored to share. They include:

I think there's an idea that there's more possibility for me to live an adventurous and explorative life and I hadn't thought that before.

—Emmett

There is so much adaptive stuff out there that I didn't even know about, and I can't wait to try it all. Every day was a highlight—you know, trying new things, walking more, the sports—everything was great. Everyone made me feel so empowered every day, but I guess getting back into the water was probably my favorite: you know, the surfing and the kayaking, it was definitely awesome.

—Denny

There was such a sense of community, family, and fellowship here that I found nowhere else. It was two weeks of incredible fellowship and activities provided by people who all volunteer their time and do it as a labor of love.

When I returned home last year, people could see the change in me. I was more alive. I felt like I was more back in the human race again: so many things I could do that I didn't think I could do. To someone who hasn't experienced it, it's indescribable. I am at a loss for words because it is just so amazing. This will be the most amazing two weeks of your life.

—Joe

There is life before Empower and there is life after Empower. And life after Empower is amazing...

—Andrew

They give you so many opportunities to be okay and be comfortable in your own skin and be comfortable in your own chair. And it shows you're not different, that this chair is not you, you know—it's just how you get around—and everyone has made that so concrete in my life at least that I don't feel different, and I feel comfortable going home and rolling the streets and not worrying like about what people are saying about me, because we're not different.

—Tara

While there are significant challenges associated with running Empower SCI the staff remain undaunted and share the following advice for those considering an interprofessional outdoor therapy program. The weather can and will be unpredictable, and you need to understand complications that can arise from the clients you work with. The staff at Empower SCI always consider psychological as well as physical safety. For instance, they think about past trauma related to being outdoors, as many clients were injured in the water. Their clients may have poor temperature regulation and sensation below the level of the spinal cord injury, which is a serious problem in summer months in terms of the risk of sunburn and overheating outdoors. Without the right equipment and forethought, terrain can be a barrier to accessibility. This could lead to getting stuck in sand or the corrosiveness of saltwater irritating sensitive skin. Always thinking and being aware of what could go wrong and being prepared to deal with physical and psychological issues are critically important.

Here's a wonderful endorsement for taking it outside: "Do it! Mediums like water can be great equalizers and a welcomed break from sitting in the same chair, all day, day after day. Fresh air and being in green and blue spaces are therapeutic interventions of their own." Please check out an inspiring video, https://youtu.be/x6veZszAZtA, and visit Empower SCI's website at www.empowersci.org.

Reference
Price, M.J. and Trbovich, M. (2018) 'Thermoregulation Following Spinal Cord Injury.' In A. Romanovsky (ed.) *Handbook of Clinical Neurology*. Amsterdam: Elsevier.

For young adults with cancer, group-based outdoor adventure interventions such as rock climbing and hiking experiences improve coping skills, self-confidence, and autonomy as the programs are goal-directed and intended to challenge each participant and encourage a proactive group mentality (Rosenberg *et al.* 2014). For example, results of one study found that young adults with cancer who participated in a week-long outdoor adventure program reported decreased levels of stress and improved self-efficacy and experienced a greater sense of social support (Zebrack, Kwak, and Sundstrom 2017). An additional study showed that young adult cancer survivors who participated in a six-day outdoor adventure program demonstrated improved body image, greater self-esteem, and reduced depression (Rosenberg *et al.* 2014). As part of a holistic body-and-mind intervention approach for young adults with cancer, engagement in outdoor adventure programming leads to increased physical activity, which in turn may improve self-image, confidence, and rehabilitation (Gill *et al.* 2016).

CASE NARRATIVE: Ocean Therapy

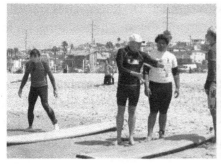
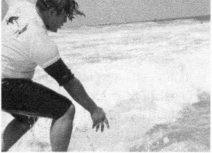

PREPPING TO CATCH A WAVE

WORKING HARD TO FIND A BALANCE IN THE BODY AND MIND TO STAY UPRIGHT ON A SURFBOARD

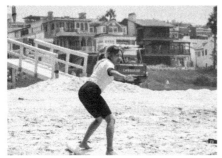
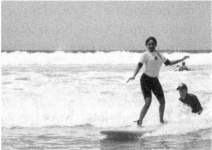

LAND PRACTICE IN ADVANCE
OF A SURFING EXPERIENCE
Photo credits: CraigBlankPhoto.com

SUCCESS ON THE WATER
AND IT FEELS SO SWEET!

Thank you to Carly M. Rogers, OTD, OTR/L, past Director of Programs of the Jimmy Miller Memorial Foundation, and Ms. Nancy Miller, Co-founder of the Jimmy Miller Memorial Foundation, for helping to prepare this case narrative.

When we think of "outside," we often think of forests and greenery. We think about therapy in gardens and climbing trees. What about the beach? That is exactly where Dr. Carly Rogers went to support veterans and at-promise youth (youth from difficult and challenging backgrounds). Prior to becoming an occupational therapist, Dr. Rogers was a Los Angeles County Ocean Life-guard who worked as a Water Awareness, Training, Education & Recreation (WATER) Program Instructor. One day, she saw a child with cerebral palsy excited to get out of his wheelchair and into the ocean water. She thought to herself, "We need to get these kids surfing!" Dr. Rogers later started her occupational therapy journey and wrote the Ocean Therapy program for a class project.

In 2004 Dr. Rogers' friend and colleague, Jimmy Miller, died. One of Jimmy's gifts was instructing Dr. Rogers in how to teach surfing, which was foundational to creating Ocean Therapy. After Jimmy's death, the Jimmy Miller Memorial Foundation (JMMF) was started, and Dr. Rogers was recruited to implement the surf therapy program she had conceived. The JMMF is:

> a non-profit 501(c)(3) Foundation dedicated to honoring Jimmy Miller by supporting the healing of mental and physical illness through surfing and ocean-related activities. Through recreational, educational, and mentoring programs, the Jimmy Miller Memorial Foundation...bring[s] together surfers, educators, therapists, lifeguards, and friends to help people affected by mental and physical illness feel the joy and healing power of the ocean and surfing.

Dr. Rogers served as the Director of Programs for 12 years.

Ocean Therapy is a community-based occupational therapy program that combines surfing, group processing, and social participation. The program is designed to provide an inclusive and supportive social setting where participants can gain self-efficacy through experiencing the ocean and acquire new surfing skills in a safe but unpredictable environment. Please take some time to watch a TED Talk about Ocean Therapy that Dr. Rogers presented at: www.youtube.com/watch?v=Wfb8tHn8Xv4.

The program serves at-promise youth and adolescents aged 6–19 years old who have histories of trauma, behavioral or emotional problems, or learning or educational disabilities. Ocean Therapy also has contracts with the military to provide services to both active-duty military personnel as well as U.S. military veterans and their families. Participants are recruited through participating organizations with the JMMF. Some participating organizations include clients from the Greater Los Angeles Veterans Affairs Healthcare System, USMC Wounded Warrior Battalion, Uplift Family Services, Richstone Family Center, Just Keep Livin Foundation, and Didi Hirsch Mental Health Services. Ocean Therapy is held in Manhattan Beach, California, and also bi-monthly at Marine Corps Base Camp Pendleton in Del Mar Beach, California. Along with these services, the JMMF continues to expand its treatment population, which now includes first responders and children and their families affected by cancer. Along with increased treatment populations, locations have also expanded.

Ocean Therapy is inclusive! Participation in Ocean Therapy does not require any previous surfing experience or to be able to swim, as the program takes place in shallow water with close supervision. Some clients come with advanced surfing skills and others have never put their feet in the sand. Youth participate in distinct cohorts that are coordinated through their participating agency and typically engage in a one-day surf experience. Active-duty U.S. military service members participate on an open-enrollment basis and can join at any time for bi-monthly sessions. Each group contains 10–12 participants. Sessions are held between January and November with a break for the holidays and challenging winter conditions. Sessions are four hours long and are supported by volunteers, professional surf instructors, a beach coordinator, safety coordinator, and a licensed therapist with surfing competency as the session facilitator. Each session begins with a check-in and discussion circle on an overview of the program, schedule for the day, safety, a discussion theme, and a group response. Then, on-land surf instruction begins, followed by surfing in the water with a surf instructor and water volunteer. As program coordinator, Dr. Rogers used her occupational therapy lens to help grade surfing through a backward chaining model. A midday discussion is held with debriefing on the experience in the water, affirmations, and strategies for a second session. The second surfing session is held and is followed by lunch and a final discussion. Participants may choose to engage in research, which is directed by a JMMF research coordinator. Funding for Ocean Therapy is provided by private foundation and government grants, government funding, client benefits, and donations.

Ocean Therapy was first implemented in 2005 and several research articles have been published outlining and discussing the evidence-based impacts of the program. Research on the program showed that Ocean Therapy provided hope for participating youth. The research also noted that participation in Ocean Therapy was supportive for combat veterans with PTSD and reduced their symptoms of depression (see references below). In addition to standardized questionnaires, participants have shared their personal reflections. The impacts of Ocean Therapy that have been experienced by the participants and their support networks are evidenced in the research. For example, one youth participant reported:

> There was a person who went to Ocean Therapy who felt nervous at first but excited to try something new. They went there knowing how to describe themselves, all their worries and their thoughts. But when they tried surfing, and got up there on the wave, they didn't know who they were anymore because all of their thoughts went away. Riding a wave, who they thought they were as a person went away for those split seconds and then they reached the shore, and every step became a mystery. They didn't know who they were before—without their eating disorder—but up there on the wave, that person with the eating disorder went away. They got a chance to see who they might be. They didn't know who they were when they reached the shore, but it gave them a sense of possibility.

A Marine participant said:

> In combat, you wait, and you wait, and then you engage in an intense firefight fighting for your life. In surfing, you wait, and you wait, and then you engage in a pure natural adrenaline rush. I never knew how beautiful Mother Nature could be.

A Wounded Warrior Battalion commanding officer reported:

> When the Marines come back from running or cycling, they're tired and

feeling a bit better, but when the Marines come back from Jimmy Miller, the change in the barracks is visceral; you can feel that something in them has changed.

Dr. Rogers recalled this poignant Ocean Therapy moment with us, which we share verbatim:

Joe arrived at the beach for an Ocean Therapy session wearing his PT [physical training] gear, camo green shirt, shorts, socks, and boots. As he put his pack down, I asked, "You going to take off your boots?" Laughing, Joe remarked, "I don't know, I'm from Georgia, I've never put my feet in the sand." As we all watched, Joe removed his boots and slowly maneuvered his feet into the sand and replied, "Alright, alright...I got this. I'm feeling you...now where's that surfboard?" Joe was a Marine who had served in Iraq. He shared that he had been diagnosed with both PTSD and a TBI [traumatic brain injury]. Shortly after his feet touched the sand, Joe was up and riding a wave wearing a helmet—a natural athlete, ecstatic about his experience, exclaiming with his hands held high.

Two weeks later, we returned for another Ocean Therapy session on base at Camp Pendleton. As a therapist, I was discouraged to find that Joe was not in attendance as the program is self-referred (or occasionally "voluntold" to attend when staff feel the Marine would benefit). I asked where Joe was and one of the other Marines said he had an appointment. The session moved forward, and we were in the water, Marines standing up here and wiping out there. As I pushed a Marine into a wave, I looked up and Joe had grabbed a board and was paddling past me. I exclaimed, "Joe, you're here! Where are you going?" "I need my waves!" he replied.

Later we came back to the Marine-deemed "kumbaya circle." I asked a question to the group, "How does this make you feel?" Joe, pacing side to side, digging his feet into the sand, replied, "I'll tell you how this feels. I was just at my mental health appointment, and they said I need to talk about the past. But here, I don't want to talk about the past, I don't want to talk about Iraq, I want to live, I want to look forward, I want to SURF!"

There are a multitude of challenges to "taking it outside" such as access to the ocean, cultural awareness of ocean-related sports, and traditional medical model approaches to therapy and funding, as noted by Dr. Rogers. As is evidenced through all that Dr. Rogers has shared, the benefits are endless. Although a beach is not accessible to all, Dr. Rogers advises practitioners who are thinking about taking it outside to "expand the limits of what currently exists." Practitioners can provide an opportunity for participants to experience nature by engaging in nature-based interventions. She suggests that nature-based recreation entities such as kayak instruction, surf instruction, or rock-climbing instruction companies already exist and can provide a medium through which a therapist can develop programming. When consulting with nature-based entrepreneurs, Dr. Rogers has a three-step plan she recommends:

1. Find a company or organization that is instructing the nature-based activity of interest.
2. Find a population in need and an agency to coordinate with.
3. Connect with a university to conduct research to determine the program's effectiveness and share the results with the greater community.

Dr. Rogers has provided actionable steps we can all take to connect our local clients and communities to nature! For more information about Ocean Therapy, please visit https://jimmymillerfoundation.org.

References

Marshall, J., Ferrier, B., Ward, P.B., and Martindale, R. (2020) '"When I was surfing with those guys I was surfing with family." A grounded exploration of program theory within the Jimmy Miller Memorial Foundation.' *Global Journal of Community Psychology Practice 11*, 2, 1–19.

Rogers, C.M., Mallinson, T., and Peppers, D. (2014) 'High-intensity sports for posttraumatic stress disorder and depression: Feasibility study of ocean therapy with veterans of Operation Enduring Freedom and Operation Iraqi Freedom.' *American Journal of Occupational Therapy 68*, 4, 395–404.

Sarkisian, G.V., Curtis, C., and Rogers, C.M. (2020) 'Emerging hope: Outcomes of a one-day surf therapy program with youth at-promise.' *Global Journal of Community Psychology Practice 11*, 2, 1–16.

Promising results have been identified with nature-based therapeutic programs for young adults with mental health conditions. A recent study examined the impact of providing green care or green work on farms for young adults receiving care at a specialized interdisciplinary psychiatric treatment facility in Norway (Steigen *et al.* 2018). The green care or green work intervention involved outdoor activities such as tending to plants and animals as well as cooking. All participants had treatment-resistant mental health diagnoses such as trauma, anxiety, depression, and eating disorders (Steigen *et al.* 2018). Following their green care or green work farming intervention, participants, even those with low expectations at the outset, reported being either pleased or very pleased with the intervention, and more likely to engage in therapy. Despite reservations, nature appears to have the uncanny ability to engage even those who are skeptical or may not think it possible to participate in therapy. Like their counterpart wilderness programs, outdoor-therapy farming programs for young adults with mental health challenges are a potential alternative or supplement for traditional mental health programming.

CASE NARRATIVE: Pacific Quest

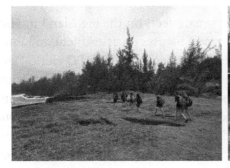

SOCIAL HIKING IN NATURE IS
HEALTH PROMOTING

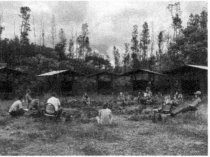

GROUP MEETINGS TAKE ON A NEW AND
POSITIVE MEANING WHEN FACILITATED
OUTSIDE—TALK COMES EASIER

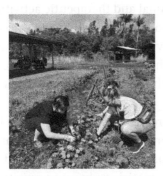

GARDENING IS AN EVIDENCE-BASED
INTERVENTION TO IMPROVE PHYSICAL
AND SOCIAL-EMOTIONAL HEALTH
Photo credits: Pacific Quest

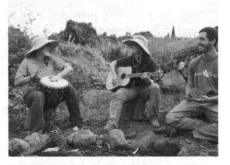

MUSIC MAKING INVITES PARTICIPATION
AND CONNECTIVITY

Thank you to Suzanne McKinney, MA, Owner and Outreach Director, for helping to prepare this case narrative.

Launched in 2004, Pacific Quest (PQ) redefines behavioral therapy by utilizing a neurodevelopmental and experiential approach to treatment. This approach, which includes therapeutic sandplay therapy, horticulture, integrated psychiatry, yoga therapy, physical activity, and mindfulness, integrates evidence-based therapeutic methods and whole-person wellness to motivate personal change and sustain a healthy community. Noteworthy about PQ is that it is home to one of the only outdoor sandplay structures in the world. Sandplay is an evidence-based, hands-on therapeutic method that, through the use of symbols such as sand, water, and small objects that represent a person's inner psyche, the client is better able to express their inner psyche, thus allowing for deeper self-understanding and healing beyond talk therapy.

Located on 35 acres (1,524,600 square feet) on the big island in Hilo, Hawaii, the fee-for-service PQ program focuses on assessment and intervention during an 8–12-week residential experience. The PQ clinical staff includes a psychiatrist who provides telehealth and integrated health services, a naturopathic physician who serves as the medical director, a pediatric neuropsychologist who serves as the clinical director, a psychologist, four additional licensed primary mental health therapists who are trained master's-level therapists seeking an innovative work experience, and two trained field therapists enrolled in graduate therapy programs. Residents, adolescents (aged 13–17), and young adults (aged 18–24) throughout the United States (and internationally) enroll in PQ where they engage in activities that increase emotional health and wellbeing. All educational and therapeutic activities and interventions provided at PQ are individualized to meet individual needs and abilities. PQ is accredited by Cognia (www.cognia.org). Their program curriculum provides up to five credits for all high school students. Resident IEPs are requested upon admission so the PQ therapists can incorporate these interventions into treatment as needed.

Individualized treatment programs are created and updated weekly by the therapy team and include specific plans for field activities and accommodations. For example, a resident may have specific anxiety or trauma related to water, which would determine if and how they participate in ocean activities. Therapists communicate with the field teams several strategies to facilitate guided activities for safe and optimal treatment. Through this client-centered treatment model, PQ continues to pioneer a cutting-edge approach to outdoor therapy, providing multiple opportunities to address brain development and enhance social, cognitive, and physiological functioning necessary for sustainable growth. In alignment with a nature-based neurodevelopmental and experiential approach to treatment, PQ's mission is to "cultivate sustainable growth in our residents, in our families, in our communities, and in ourselves."

The founders of PQ, Mike McKinney and Chris Kaiser, began as guides in a traditional "survival-based" wilderness program. There they realized the importance of outdoor programming, but also saw the need to treat adolescents and young adults who have more internalized behaviors and distress. Through their previous work as guides, the founders recognized that the adolescents and young adults would benefit from a more gentle, nurturing environment and process to facilitate change. Also, the founders recognized the importance of providing a physically and psychologically safe environment, which now entails incorporating relevant cultural and ecological factors such as a curriculum that integrates Hawaiian history and celebrations, cultural norms, and environmental education into treatment. With an entrepreneurial spirit and a desire to help adolescents and young adults reach their potential through therapeutic and educational program-ming outdoors, Pacific Quest was founded.

A typical resident at the PQ program is usually struggling with internalized distress. Often residents both experience anxiety, depression, trauma, grief, and loss, and are dealing with complicated family systems and relationships. Residents typically come to PQ after trying many other modes of treatment. They come seeking an alternative way to understand themselves and gain strength and confidence to move forward in a positive way. Programming is delivered year-round, indoors, and outdoors, either one-on-one or in small groups that address physical and mental health, and sensory and educational needs. Throughout the treatment process, residents and families complete the Youth Outcome Questionnaire (Y-OQ). Results are gathered at admission, discharge, and specific points post-discharge. At the individual level, this data better equips the treatment team to craft interventions/treatment approaches to meet a resident's needs. The meta-data empowers the PQ development team to evaluate treatment efficacy long-term and enhance programming. The capacity for PQ is 16 adolescents and six young adults at any given time. During the COVID-19 pandemic, the PQ team delivered the family portion of the program virtually. This included once-weekly calls with a primary therapist and a two-day intensive program with families and the resident. Post-pandemic, the family program includes single and group family and parent group therapy sessions. Families also join their child for horticulture and experiential activities described below.

The outdoor spaces on the 35-acre campus were chosen for their accessible qualities, garden possibilities, access to residences and staff, and to provide ample space for individual and group treatment. Onsite staff maintain the outdoor spaces. Most of the ongoing necessary materials to run the program are for the garden and other experiential activities such as swimming, paddle-boarding, hiking and exploring national and local parks, yoga, gardening, and music. The materials needed to facilitate the experiential activities include gardening tools and supplies, paddleboards, kayaks, yoga mats, and outdoor shelters known as "hales." Hales are wooden open-air shelters that the PQ founders designed to provide shelter from the elements and for individual space and time for refuge and reflection. Additional materials are clothing, which includes swimming and weatherproof gear and shoes. Equipment needs are determined by the treatment team and purchased/managed by the PQ logistics and facilities departments. Startup costs for PQ included land purchase and gear. The annual and monthly costs include salaries for the 100 staff involved with the program, the building lease, land maintenance, property rental, utilities, and general use costs.

PQ markets through their website (www.pacificquest.org), affiliations such as the Association for Experiential Education (AEE) and the National Association of Therapeutic Schools and Programs (NATSAP), alumni referrals, and therapeutic consultants. PQ is nationally recognized as a Gold Status–designated research program by the NATSAP and the University of New Hampshire. To date, well over 1000 PQ residents and families have been a part of this study. Staff at PQ are deeply committed to this research and remain dedicated to utilizing the outcome data to deliver the most comprehensive and evidence-based treatment for every resident and their family.

We are grateful to share two meaningful stories that exemplify the worth and value of PQ's programs and staff through the voices of a former resident and a parent of a child who was in the program. First, the former resident:

> I attended Pacific Quest for 99 days beginning in April of 2010. What I once believed to be a punishment, I now clearly understand to be a privilege. Today, I am grounded through the seeds that were first planted at Pacific Quest. The roots grow deeper, the stalks stand taller, and the fruit tastes sweeter still—nearly a dozen years later. With time came perspective, progression, and appreciation, and my journey on the Big Island is now one I remember fondly.
>
> Initially, I held resentment, even hatred, for the program that seemingly held a spotlight on my darkest moments and deepest insecurities. I was embarrassed to accept, trust, or forgive myself; to love myself felt beyond the realm of possibility. Acknowledgment of suffering and trauma meant there was work to be done. In this sense, standing among dead crops and overgrown weeds was easier than tilling, planting, and tending the garden. Pacific Quest, however, provided the environment for me to do the work: to start the work, really, as the work continues today. Any hostility toward the Pacific Quest program was, in many ways, a reflection of my own self-worth and not of the program itself. Now, as I continue to evolve, reflecting on my time at Pacific Quest can only be seen as beautiful. This is not to say my

passage was without suffering, no; but it was certainly beautiful, nonetheless. Pacific Quest provided the foundation—a nursery and fertile soil—for growth.

I remain deeply grateful for the opportunity that Pacific Quest provided. I often long for the simplicity of the day in the life at the program. External pressure, distraction, and expectation fell away, and I found permission to be honest with myself. Being in the program provided the chance to touch moments of peace that, before arriving on Hawaii, I was unaware existed. I stay connected to this feeling of peace and solace, knowing I can return to that same state of mind at any time. With each new day, I challenge myself to strip away trappings surrounding me and ground back to the love and lessons learned from Pacific Quest.

A parent shared:

The Pacific Quest program was a life-transforming experience for our 15-year-old son who was depressed and going down a very dark, dangerous path after being diagnosed with a learning disability in his freshman year of high school. Pacific Quest helped our son to self-reflect and understand himself, and taught him coping mechanisms and how to self-advocate. They helped him and our family learn to communicate together in a thoughtful productive way. Pacific Quest's team is incredibly talented, and their program is powerful, effective, and enduring. Where school was once a daily dose of torture pre-Pacific Quest, our son just graduated high school with honors, won an award for Achievement in Learning, and was cited as having the best live presentation to the faculty and senior class. My husband and I are grateful every day and will never forget the team at PQ.

What advice did Ms. McKinney share? She told us, in no uncertain terms, "Do it now! Don't hesitate! Just taking a client outside for a walk or into a garden space for a session can change the way the client sees and feels things." In terms of the benefits of taking it outside, Ms. McKinney told us that "the outdoors provides new and real access to address challenges, desires, goals, and hope. Getting outside fully integrates health."

Realities of Programming

Longitudinal studies of wilderness and green care/green work programs are needed to determine the duration of effects and their long-term changes, be it for young adults at university, those living with or after cancer, people with developmental delays, or those with mental health issues. But research should also extend beyond effect duration and impact, to understand how young adults can and do access care. For instance, one of the realities is that for many young adults, engaging in wilderness outdoor-adventure programs is not within their financial means or is not covered by insurance. Hence, while its benefits are recognized, access to such life-affirming programs is not equitable. In an increasingly urbanized society, it is imperative that nature experiences be provided to all young adults, or, better still, to everyone regardless of situation or circumstance, as nature heals. Perhaps best said as: "Nature is vital to us, as it satisfies human physical needs, and aesthetic and spiritual needs" (Broom 2017, p.35). We all need it.

CASE NARRATIVE: Triform Camphill Community

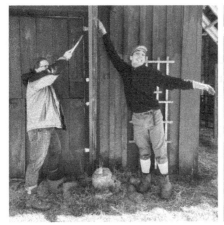

PRIDE IN ACCOMPLISHING OUTDOOR CHORES

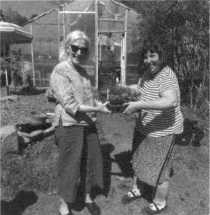

INTERGENERATIONAL PROGRAMMING AT THE GREENHOUSE

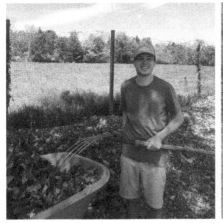

GARDEN MANAGEMENT

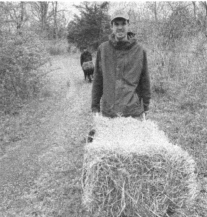

WORKING AS A TEAM TO MOVE HAY

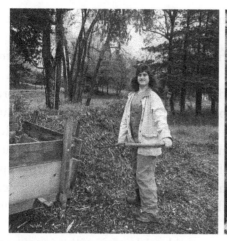 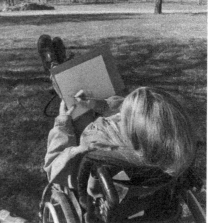

THERAPY OUTDOORS CAN EASILY
LEAD TO A SENSE OF PRIDE
Photo credits: Triform

AN ARTISTIC CONNECTION WITH NATURE

Thank you to Carol Fernandez, JD, Vice Chair of the Board of Directors for the Triform Camphill Community, for her assistance with preparing this case narrative.

Located in picturesque Hudson, New York, Triform Camphill Community (Triform) is one of 15 Camphill communities located in North America and is a member of the Camphill Association of North America (www.camphill. org). The first Camphill school community was established in Scotland in 1939. The aim of Camphill, from its outset, was to create an environment in which individuals with special needs could receive the care and support they need to live full and meaningful lives.

Triform was created in 1979 by a small but dedicated group of experienced Camphill co-workers. Its original mission was to provide work training to underserved individuals living in the local community. Forty years later, the mission has changed and expanded into being a youth guidance intentional community where residents and co-workers live and work. It is one of only two Camphill communities in the U.S. specifically dedicated to supporting young adults with special needs to transition to adulthood, as they each assume their unique place within their adult world.

As a Camphill community, Triform bases its work on the recognition of the spiritual integrity of the individual regardless of ability, and aims to provide residents with dignified and meaningful work, a healthy social atmosphere, and a vibrant cultural, artistic, and spiritual life. Triform is dedicated to building a vibrant community life for young adults with special needs that is a supportive environment offering the possibility for healing, growth, and self-development.

Triform is a transitional youth guidance program designed for young adults aged 18–30 years old. The Triform residents all have some sort of developmental and/or intellectual disability diagnosis. They come to Triform when they have finished their public-school programs to build their adult lives, learning to live in an integrated community, sharing responsibilities, and building friendships. They learn to take care of themselves and others and learn what it means to take care of a home. The day-to-day living, therapy, and activities at Triform happen all the time, because householders there share their homes with those who live and work at Triform. It is their home that they share with residents.

What makes Triform unique among residential communities or programs for those with special needs—and why it is featured in this book—is that it is a biodynamic farming and gardening campus. Biodynamics refers to "a holistic, ecological, and ethical approach to farming, gardening, food, and nutrition" (www.biodynamics.com). The program integrates home and community life with work skills development, classroom activities, therapies, and a rich variety of social/cultural experiences, all while being on a beautiful 500-acre property with easy access to the great outdoors. The rural character of the community, beautiful buildings, and peaceful, verdant landscape creates a sense of peace and wellbeing that supports this unique and effective approach to working with individuals with special needs. The entire Triform campus is fully utilized by various parts of the program and community members. There are indoor activities such as ceramics and fabric arts, which are done in fully accessible indoor studios; there is a full commercial bakery, also indoors. Additionally the programming includes farming, landscaping, and animal husbandry, which all take place outdoors. As a self-contained, inclusive program, the community is made up of young adult participants (referred to as residents), short-term co-workers, and householders and their families. The community is responsible for the maintenance of the campus. Other staff include office personnel, a nurse, and various therapists and instructors who come to the campus periodically (such as therapy group providers and yoga instructors).

There can be up to 40 participants on the campus, with the majority being residential. Tuition for residents is generally private pay, with some residents receiving support from their home states. Participants in the day rehabilitation (dayhab), non-residential program receive Centers for Medicare and Medicaid's Home and Community-Based Services (HCBS) funding. New residents generally begin the program in September and dayhab participants may begin at different times during the year.

There are eight homes where the staff, who are called householders, reside with participants and co-workers. The householders live on Triform's campus with their families, and are people who have chosen to live in a community dedicated to helping young people with special needs. There are also volunteers, called co-workers, who come for a few months to a year, with many staying for additional years. Triform and other nearby Camphill communities provide training for both householders and short-term co-workers. As a mainly residential program, the bulk of Triform's expenses are ongoing and related to programming, maintaining houses and other campus facilities, and for paid staff. Marketing for all the Camphill communities occurs through social media, the specific community's website, and personal outreach. For more information about Triform Camphill Community, please visit www.triform.org.

Wrapping It Up

In this chapter, we looked at the developmental tasks associated with young adulthood and how research evidence supports that nature-based experiences positively impacts them. In this stage, when brain development is reaching its peak, nature can mediate and buffer the challenges of navigating through young adulthood. Sometime between the ages of 25 and 30, young adults become adults, and nature continues to matter, just perhaps in different ways.

NUGGET OF NATURE: SEED BOMBING

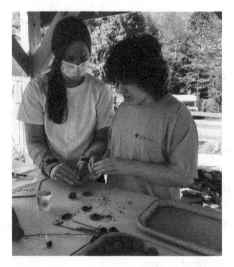

MAKING SEED BOMBS
Photo credit: Monarch School of New England

Wildflowers and plants that attract pollinators are great for our ecosystem and can be beautiful additions to our landscape. When considering where to drop your seed bombs, consider a plant pot, a flowerbed, or a meadow. Making the seed bombs is fun for all ages; tossing or crushing and then sprinkling the "seed bombs" can be exciting; and the anticipation of watching the flowers bloom can be inspiring. Drop seed bombs in spring or summer, or whenever your prime growing season is, to optimize growth. Consider making seed bombs with bird food for dropping in the winter. While you will not see any flowers grow, you will get to watch birds eat! The instructions show how to make the seed bombs and offer a few conversation starters if you decide to make the activity social or even intergenerational. Bombs away!

Materials needed to make approximately 20 large golf-ball-sized balls

- Mixing bowl
- 2 tablespoons of seeds: either purchased flower seeds or seeds collected from the garden (when possible, use native plants that will benefit your community)
- 1 cup of peat-free compost (found at a local garden center)
- ½ cup of powdered clay (found in craft shops)
- ¼ cup of water
- Baking sheet
- Optional: paprika or chili powder (to discourage birds or rodents from eating the seed bombs)

Steps to make seed bombs

1. In the mixing bowl, add 2 tablespoons of seeds, 1 cup of compost, and ½ cup of powdered clay.
2. Slowly add in ¼ cup of water, mixing with your hands until all ingredients are combined.
3. Take golf-ball-sized (1½") clumps and roll them into balls.
4. Place the balls on the baking sheet and leave them to dry in a sunny spot.
5. Once dry, plant your seed bombs within a few days.
6. Sow them before or shortly after the seeds germinate by dropping them on soil—in pots, in bare spots of a flower bed, or, with permission, in meadows or lawns.
7. Get excited and check back to see what grows.

Conversation starters to use while making seed bombs

These questions are open-ended and can be used to spark conversation:

- What is the best surprise you ever had?
- What is your favorite flower?
- What kind of landscapes do you like?
- What is something special about where you live?

How to make the activity easier

- Instead of making balls, allow clients to make whatever shape they can.
- Have ingredients pre-measured and in the bowl already mixed, so that clients only need to add water.

How to make the activity more challenging

- As an alternative to rolling seed bombs into balls, encourage clients to make more elaborate shapes such as cubes or hearts.

Instructions adapted from "How to make a seed bomb" (The Wildlife Trusts n.d.)

CHAPTER 7

Adulthood

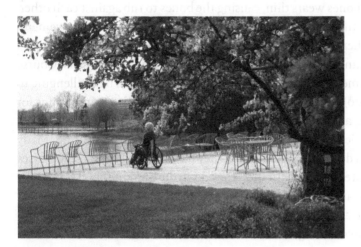

A PEACEFUL SPOT OF REPOSE
Photo credit: Amy Wagenfeld

Introduction

Adulthood follows young or emerging adulthood and precedes older adulthood. This developmental period extends from age 30 to 65. For our purposes, we will refer generically to this period (the longest in human development) as adulthood, unless otherwise specified when we are referring directly to the middle years of adulthood. This 35-year age span is often a time when the aging process starts to speed up (Lumen Learning 2022). Age-related declines in some areas of function may emerge toward the end of this period, but for most people they occur gradually and are adapted to easily (Cronin and Mandich 2016).

Adulthood is for most people a period of "good" physical and mental performance, but how we age is multifactorial. The uncontrollable factors that impact aging, such as biological and genetic, are called primary factors. Secondary aging factors refer to elements such as diet, physical activity, and drug and alcohol consumption, which are within our control. Regardless of primary or secondary aging factors, our bodies typically show signs of aging toward the end of adulthood. Skin becomes drier and less supple, and wrinkles appear. Gray hairs appear and hair loss or thinning is common. Weight gain during adulthood is not uncommon (Amarya, Singh, and Sabharwal 2018). Men tend to put on weight in the abdominal region and women in their hips and thighs. For women, fertility declines and, typically during their 50s, menopause occurs (Lumen Learning 2022).

Some common physical conditions that are associated with adulthood are the onset of osteoporosis, the loss of bone density, and arthritis, which may affect the hands, spine, hips, and knees (Cronin and Mandich 2016). As we age, the cartilage between bones wears thin, causing the bones to rub against each other, which can lead to stiffness, reduced flexibility, pain, and loss of joint movement, regardless of whether there is a diagnosis of arthritis (Cronin and Mandich 2016). Additionally, immune function is not as strong as it was in earlier years (Course Hero 2023). For some adults, the loss of physical function can be challenging to accept (Glover 2000). Nonetheless, moving and staying active is important for physical, cognitive, and mental health.

Adults may notice sensory changes, especially in vision and hearing. Many adults experience a decline in vision, and if they have not yet begun using glasses for reading, computer use, and distance, they do so during adulthood (American Optometric Association n.d.). Some may begin to use hearing aids. For most adults, these visual and auditory changes are small and gradual, and therefore easily accommodated through corrective lenses or hearing aids.

NUGGETS OF NATURE: 20/20 RULE

You can use the 20/20 rule to relieve eye strain and enjoy a bit of nature. Relieving eye strain is part of good self-care, especially while spending extended periods of time working on a computer. Set a timer for 20 minutes and when it goes off, softy refocus your gaze out of a window or at a house plant that is 20 feet away, for 20 seconds.

During adulthood, typical age-related changes of the brain and nervous system are minor and do not affect overall function, and cognition remains relatively intact (Cronin and Mandich 2016; Lumen Learning 2022). Although there are subtle changes in cognitive function, most people do not experience noticeable changes in performance until late adulthood. In fact, middle adulthood is a period of peak performance in the mental abilities of inductive reasoning, spatial orientation, vocabulary, and verbal memory (Cronin and Mandich 2016). Interestingly, crystallized intelligence grows and fluid intelligence declines during middle adulthood. Crystallized intelligence is the accumulation of knowledge, skills, and strategies we amass over our lifetimes. Fluid intelligence refers to information-processing skills, which decline in middle adulthood, as adults do not problem-solve as quickly as young adults (Course Hero 2023). But practical intelligence—our problem-solving skills, and a component of fluid intelligence— tends to increase, which is important because it helps adults solve real-world issues and supports goal-directed behaviors (Blanchard-Fields 2007; Lumen Learning 2022). All in all, as the types of intelligences may shift, adults may come to the end of adulthood with slower problem-solving capabilities. But with the amassed knowledge and improved practical problem-solving skills that come with more years of life, there is little observed change in intelligence. Adults who maintain a physically active lifestyle and challenge themselves mentally tend to experience less cognitive decline as they age than those who are not active or mentally engaged (Graf, Long, and Patrick 2017).

NUGGET OF NATURE: CARING FOR MIND AND BODY— A SIMPLE WAY TO ADAPT A GARDEN HAND TOOL

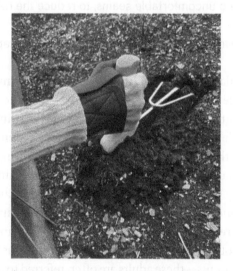

ALTERNATE USING AN ADAPTIVE GARDEN TOOL TO INCREASE COMFORT AND MINIMIZE STRUCTURAL DAMAGE TO THE HAND
Photo credit: Ryan Durkin

This modification can turn a standard hand garden tool into one that is more comfortable and ergonomic for a client or yourself. There are ergonomically designed garden tools on the market, which you may find helpful and worthy of purchase for a therapeutic gardening program.

Trial them before purchasing, if possible.

Materials you will need

- Plumber's foam pipe insulation, approximately 1.5" diameter
- 18" duct tape
- 18" compression wrap (also known as athletic wrap or Coban)
- Scissors

Steps to create a modified hand garden tool

1. Cut a piece of foam the length of the garden tool handle.
2. Cut a vertical slit to open the foam.
3. Place foam over the handle of the garden tool.
4. Secure in place by wrapping the duct tape around the foam.
5. Make certain there are no uncomfortable seams, to reduce the risk of blisters.
6. Using the same procedure as in step 4, cover the tape with athletic web wrap to allow for better grip surface.
7. Again, make certain there are no uncomfortable seams, to reduce the risk of blisters.
8. When the wrap gets dirty, remove it, and replace with a clean piece of wrap.

For adults, this period of life, particularly middle adulthood, is typically a time when they demonstrate competence in a diverse array of activity demands, occupations, and roles. Tasks associated with adulthood may include settling into a comfortable rhythm with a life partner, being financially independent, progressing in a career, adjusting to the demands of aging parents, parenting, and grandparenting, identifying and participating in meaningful leisure pursuits, and contributing to one's community (Glover 2000; Havighurst 1952; Merriam and Mullins 1981, pp.136–137). A decline in function in any of these areas during middle adulthood would be considered a non-normative pattern (Cronin and Mandich 2016). A common social-emotional task of adulthood is simultaneously raising children and caring for aging parents—these adults are often referred to as the sandwich generation—while balancing the demands of maintaining a healthy lifestyle to advance to older adulthood most successfully. Personal attitudes and beliefs can influence aging (Hertzog *et al.* 2008). As such, lifestyle and personal expectations often define adults' levels of satisfaction with physical and mental performance (Cronin and Mandich 2016).

THIS MUCH I KNOW—ROSE

After many years of working as an occupational therapist, I went on to pursue a doctoral degree. I enrolled in a fully online program that came with its own set of newness and challenges. As a full-time staff therapist, private practice owner, wife, and mom of twin boys, achieving life balance was challenging. I trialed various ways to achieve balance but was unsuccessful. I was later inspired by one of my instructors who encouraged me to spend time in nature. I began to take walks outdoors during my breaks. I even walked on rainy days. Recently, I discovered and adopted a new way to work. I have been spending time in nature at a local park near my home. I call this place my *park office*. Previously, I would leave work, head straight home to take care of my family, then complete schoolwork. This routine contributed to feelings of stress and burnout. Currently, I head to my park office after work to unwind and study. This practice has enabled me to feel better and be fully present with my family. My family notices the changes and I feel good about it. I cannot say that I've found a perfect recipe for balance but stopping at my park office has changed the way in which I balance. My park office has been restorative. I hope that you also find a place in nature where you can experience balance and restoration. Where's your park office?

NUGGET OF NATURE: HERBAL DREAM PILLOWS

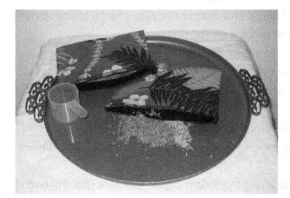

Dream pillow
Photo credit: Amy Wagenfeld

No matter how old we are, sleep is important! While this activity is appropriate for most anyone over the age of five, inviting adults to make herbal dream pillows offers a positive diversion and can be a great activity for someone rehabilitating their upper extremities. It is a way to connect with nature while not necessarily being outside, although working outside always provides added benefits for the mind and body. The activity can be social or completed as a one-on-one activity with a client, and perhaps provide a pathway to a relaxing night's sleep.

Materials you will need

- Table covers (optional)
- Dried lavender flowers
- Dried fennel seeds
- Dried dill seeds
- Dried lemon balm leaves
- Four large plastic bowls
- Cookie sheets or trays with lip (1 per client)
- Four small 1–2-tablespoon scoops
- Dream pillow bag (4" x 6" cotton bags with Velcro closure)
- Lavender essential oil (optional)
- Glue or glue gun

Steps to make a dream pillow

1. Cover the workspace.
2. Place the dry herbs in bowls.
3. Set out a tray and dream pillow bag for each client.
4. Pass around bowls of herbs and encourage your clients to scoop out one scoop of each herb and place it on the tray.
5. Using fingers, clients can gently mix the herbs together.
6. Open the dream pillow bag.
7. Using pincer fingers, ask clients to place the herbs in the bag, filling it about three-quarters full.
8. Place 2–3 drops of lavender essential oil in bag (optional).
9. Tightly close the bag, making certain the hook and pile of the Velcro are securely connected.
10. Run a bead of hot glue along the Velcro seam to ensure that the bag stays closed.
11. Gently shake the bag to mix the herbs and oil together.
12. Clients can now place the dream pillow bag inside their pillowcase.
13. Sweet dreams!

How to make the activity easier

- Use a whole-hand grasp to scoop and place herbs in bag.

How to make the activity more challenging

- Instead of leaves and seeds, provide clients with stalks of dried herbs and have them strip leaves from their stems.
- Add tool use by encouraging clients to spoon herbs into bags.

Emotional regulation becomes more adaptive and situationally specific based on prior life experiences during adulthood (Zimmermann and Iwanski 2014). It also represents a time of reflection and wonder about one's contribution to the world and a finite realization that life is not eternal (Glover 2000). Long-term partner or spousal, familial, and close friend relationships can be very important during adulthood. A task associated with adulthood is determining what makes life meaningful. Adults may ask themselves, "Am I helping to shape the future generation? Am I being the most creative and productive person I want to be? Am I helping to contribute to society in small or larger ways? Am I proud of what I have done and continue to do?" Contrary to popular belief, concepts of a midlife crisis being inevitable or that adulthood is a more stressful period of life than others are not supported by research (Cronin and Mandich 2016). As stated by Graf and colleagues (2017), "successful aging is not merely an end point": rather, it is a journey (p.222).

Therapeutic Benefits of Nature: Adults

For several millennia and "across many cultures of the world, influential traditions in science, philosophy, poetry, and religion have emphasized the role that nature plays in providing feelings of wellbeing" (Bratman, Hamilton, and Daily 2012, p.118). But how much exposure to nature is "enough"? While we believe that there is never enough nature in our lives, this is our biased opinion because we love it so much. That said, a large-scale study of adults in the U.K. found that a cumulative total of 120 minutes per week spent outdoors and, in some capacity connecting with nature, yielded benefits such as perceived good health and wellbeing (White *et al.* 2019). The two hours of nature contact could be experienced in one go or distributed throughout the week. This dose response was consistent whether the participant had nearby access to nature or had to travel to be in nature. The bottom line is: if a person spent 120 minutes a week connecting with nature, the results were positive. Beyond the good health and wellbeing benefits a person derives from spending time in nature, there is the very real power that nature has to amplify the effects of therapy when it is provided outside because being in nature makes people feel healthier and well.

NUGGET OF NATURE: SOUNDS OF NATURE

While outside or near an open window, at regular intervals that are appropriate for your client's mobility status, invite them to stop, take an audible breath in and out, close their eyes (if it is safe for them to do so), and then listen for ten seconds. Cues could be "What do you hear?", "What do you not hear?", and "Are there sounds you have never heard before?" Be creative and spontaneous, as sounds are never static. As a therapist/client team, continue the "move, stop, and listen" pattern, traveling in different directions, turning your heads to the right and left, up and down, and listening and observing.

Being surrounded by nature and interacting with natural materials has the capacity to improve multiple health outcomes, including mental and physical health, wellbeing, and cognition (Bratman *et al.* 2012; Fieldhouse 2003; Pearson and Craig 2014; Wilkie and Davinson 2021). In fact, experimental and cross-sectional studies with adults find that engagement with outdoor physical activity appears to be more beneficial for mental health status than indoor physical activity (Bailey *et al.* 2018). How do you feel after taking a walk in a park, in the woods, or on the beach?

CASE NARRATIVE: Walk with a Doc

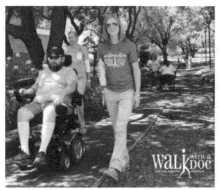 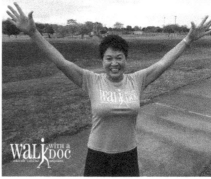

No matter how it happens, outdoor exercise is healthful here

Celebrate!

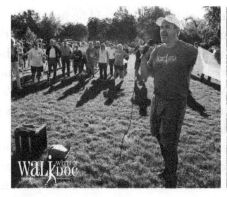

DOCTOR TALK

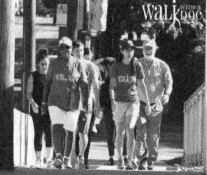

IT IS HARD TO RESIST SMILES WHEN THE WALKING IS GOOD

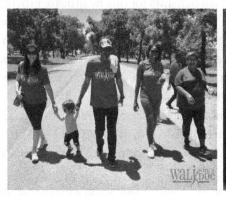

IT TAKES A TEAM

WALKING IN AN URBAN SETTING

Photo credits: Walk with a Doc

Thank you to Rachael Habash, MA, Chief Operating Officer, and David Sabgir, MD, FACC, Chief Executive Officer, from Walk with a Doc, for helping to prepare this case narrative.

How often have you gone to the doctor and been told to exercise more, eat healthier, and get more sleep? How often have you taken this advice to heart? We know and have heard, time and again, the tenets of good health, but following through can be difficult. Dr. David Sabgir also knew this when he was completing his cardiology fellowship in 2005 in Columbus, Ohio. He found that people were not listening to his exercise advice, and he felt that he was limited by what he could do in a clinical setting. So he invited his patients to take a walk with him in a local park on a Saturday morning. To his surprise, over 100 people showed up, energized and ready to move.

When Dr. Sabgir suggested this practice to other physicians, many were appreciative of the idea but did not believe it would be sustainable or achievable on a large-scale platform. Dr. Sabgir was undeterred. In 2009, the practice of physicians walking with patients began to branch out to other communities. In 2015, CNN featured a story about Walk with a Doc, which spurred national interest to start Walk chapters. As of 2021, there are Walk with a Doc programs in 600 communities around the globe, in 48 states in the U.S., and 37 countries worldwide.

Walk with a Doc programs are open to people of all ages and abilities. Anyone can join and there is no cap on the number of participants. Each walk is facilitated by volunteers and a current or future healthcare provider, who may be a doctor, a medical student, or a dietitian. Healthcare providers and volunteers commit to hosting 12 events per year, approximately once monthly. On average, there are 22 participants for one healthcare provider.

The 60-minute walks are held in local parks or other safe walking loca-tions. Walk chapters are encouraged to use accessible locations as much as possible to ensure as many people who are interested can attend and par-ticipate. Each free event starts with a brief health discussion, followed by a walk with a healthcare provider. Discussions while on walks may cover more general topics such as conversations about exercise and healthy eating. They may also be more pertinent to current issues such as with the COVID-19 pandemic when talks focused on the importance of vaccines and wearing masks.

Each community participating in Walk with a Doc starts with an onboard-ing process. Initial costs are $650 to establish the program and then there are limited ongoing costs such as liability insurance. Walk with a Doc events are advertised through physician invitations, social media, marketing, press releases, and word of mouth. For people who may not have a nearby Walk with a Doc program, are unable to access one near them, or who were not ready to attend an in-person event due to the COVID-19 pandemic, there are opportunities to attend a virtual Walk with a Doc. An alternative option for participation is viewing a video on a specific health topic from a health professional sent via email, and walking in nature safely with a friend or family member.

Walk with a Doc has conducted research to determine the impacts of the program. According to results of the most recent annual qualitative survey, being in a Walk with a Doc program increases participants' physical activ-ity and helps them feel more in control of their health. Specifically, 92% of walkers feel they are more educated and empowered about their health since starting Walk with a Doc, 79% report getting more exercise, 79% feel more confident in their interactions with healthcare providers, and 98% enjoy the refreshing concept of pairing healthcare providers with communities outside the traditional clinic setting. Additionally, 70% of physicians feel the program helps them educate their communities. In 2017, a pilot study conducted in partnership with the Robert Wood Johnson Foundation and Limetree Research demonstrated increased physical activity, social connectedness, and knowledge of healthcare issues among Walk with a Doc participants. In this study, it was found that 63% of participants increased their physical activity since joining Walk with a Doc. Anecdotally, walkers and program facilitators alike shared that being part of the program increased their energy level, improved their mood, and broke down perceived barriers between walkers and healthcare providers.

Walkers and healthcare providers alike shared their inspirational stories. Participant Sherman Transou joined a heart support group after receiving a heart transplant. The doctor running the group invited him to participate in a Walk with a Doc in his community. Mr. Transou said, "I started to build my strength again and was eventually able to complete a half-marathon. I use my story to help inspire others." Denee Killion, RN, BSN, a Walk Leader from the U.S. Department of Veterans Affairs in Omaha, Nebraska, shared that she observed two Vietnam War veterans confide in one another in a way they had not with others while they were walking. Dr. Kansra shared that "Walk with a Doc is an opportunity to get fitter; it is a way for patients to meet others looking for company to walk with; it is education; it is laughter; it is camaraderie; it is group therapy." Dr. Ghiloni told us that he "loves the opportunity to motivate people to change their lifestyle to improve their health without the red tape involved in an office visit. I love the fact that participants have nothing to fear." We can see that walkers and healthcare providers equally benefit from this program.

Dr. Francis Peabody said, "The secret in caring for the patient is in *caring* for the patient." Walk with a Doc lives up to this. There's no better way to show someone you care about them than showing up outside the office to listen and walk with them. There is no other corporation, non-profit or for-profit, combining physical activity, social connection, and education with physicians and their communities on a year-round basis. This linkage between clinic and community fills a void in healthcare and is making preventative medicine a viable solution. While Walk with a Doc was started to address the sedentary epidemic, it has since evolved to include health education, social connection, and nature. For more information on Walk with a Doc, please see https://walkwithadoc.org.

Research shows that nature contact improves mental health (Pearson and Craig

2014). A study related to the mental health of inpatient hospital nurses comparing indoor to outdoor work-breaks found promising results. After 13 weeks, the nurses who took daily breaks from work outdoors in a garden were significantly less burned-out than the nurses who took their breaks indoors (Cordoza *et al.* 2018). If we extrapolate these results to inpatients in healthcare facilities, how might patients (and therapists) feel if they could have therapy outside? Would they feel less burned-out? Would they feel more willing to engage in therapy? Would they return home healthier? What important research studies these could be! If your "take it outside" model is healthcare-based, think of what we could all learn from results of such a study.

CASE NARRATIVE: Positive Strides

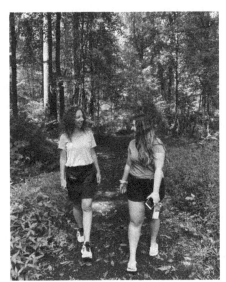

MENTAL HEALTH THERAPY FOR MIND AND BODY
Photo credit: Positive Strides

Thanks to Jennifer Udler, LCSW-C, Founder and Director of Positive Strides Therapy, for her help in preparing this case narrative.

Positive Strides is a private, fee-for-service psychotherapy practice located in Montgomery County, Maryland, that incorporates the power of walking and nature to help in the healing process. The inspiration for Positive Strides is a wonderful example of personal experiences being the catalyst to start something new and innovative. In 2012, Ms. Udler spent five months training with the Montgomery County Road Runners Club. She was in the First-Time

Marathon training program with a group of other aspiring marathoners. As they ran, they got to know each other, and started talking about their lives—sometimes even working through various personal problems. During this time, Ms. Udler felt inspired that, yes, this was the perfect model for therapy. It felt very natural for people to open up while in a state of motion—a way to move forward both physically and mentally. She decided to take the steps to move forward with the idea for a walking-therapy private practice, which she would soon name Positive Strides Therapy, launching in 2013. Since then, Ms. Udler learned that there is a great deal of research supporting this method of practicing therapy and explaining why it is a powerful way to conduct a therapy session. Positive Strides is a perfect example of putting research into practice.

Through the practice of walking outdoors in a safe and serene outdoor environment, Positive Strides–licensed counselors mainly provide individual, one-to-one mental health therapy to clients who are experiencing depression, anxiety, grief, loss, and other life transitions and stressors. Therapists facilitate services with a holistic approach that includes understanding the person in their environment. Finding meaning in movement and a verdant outdoor setting, clients are able to move through their difficult situations with the warmth, care, and professionalism of well-trained therapists. The 50-minute walk-and-talk sessions take place outside year-round in local parks that provide a variety of natural and paved trails. That said, when weather interferes, they provide telehealth counseling as a backup option. Ms. Udler said that this looks more like a traditional therapy visit, although the therapists may still try to incorporate some references to nature.

Typically, Positive Strides therapists see children, teens, and adults with some form of anxiety disorder, mood disorder, or adjustment disorder. Some clients do not have a clinical diagnosis and are seeking counseling due to a stressful situation, such as divorce, loss, or relationship concerns. Their goals are often to decrease their anxiety, improve their mood, and learn coping skills for managing the stress that is occurring in their lives.

This is what a therapy session might look like. Therapists will walk with their clients during the 50-minute session. Ms. Udler shared that sometimes these walks are pretty straightforward—just a paved path through a well-maintained park. Other times, the walks are more challenging, including hilly terrain or excursions off the path. Clients who are adventurous may want to wade through water in a creek or climb a hill that has no path. Children often take advantage of the playfulness of the environment, and will spend time picking flowers, identifying insects, or trying to catch a frog.

Initial costs to start Positive Strides included licensing fees, bank fees, LLC registration fees, and website development. Ongoing costs include website, marketing, administrative overhead, licensing fees, and malpractice insurance. Staffing wise, the counselors in the Positive Strides Therapy practice are responsible for their clients, and an administrative staff supports the organization virtually. While Ms. Udler uses social media platforms such as LinkedIn, Facebook, and Instagram to market the program, most of their clients are referred by a fellow professional, a graduated client, or a friend. Keeping it simple, the only materials needed for facilitating Positive Strides are for clients and counselors to wear comfortable walking shoes, dress for the weather, and carry a water bottle.

There are several wonderful comments that clients have shared about their therapy experiences and one from a Positive Strides therapist that we share below. A teen client said:

> Working with my therapist at Positive Strides has helped me gain the skills to better cope with my anxiety. When I walked during therapy, I was able to generate new ideas for handling difficult situations. These ideas helped me feel as though I have more control and will be really helpful in the future when I am far from home. I think it was easier to make progress in a nature type setting as opposed to an office because I was able to think and talk more freely.

Another client reported that "Nature, fresh air, sunshine, and exercise make me feel better. However, I rarely carve time out for myself to walk. Walking during therapy is a way to improve my body and my mind."

Jennifer Firestone, LCSW-C, a walk-and-talk therapist with Positive Strides, shared that her most memorable outdoor-walking therapy moment took place in the snow:

> While walking for the first time with a client while it was snowing, we marveled at the beauty and were able to discuss how things in life can change, much like the weather. Sometimes we can see things changing in our lives like being able to look at the weather forecast...and sometimes we get caught in a surprise rain or snow shower. How do we cope? By learning how to be flexible and adjust...jump in the puddles, dance in the rain, make a snow angel, throw a snowball, make a snow person, and have a big cup of hot chocolate, tea, or coffee.

Ms. Udler's take on therapy outside is invaluable and, frankly, quite realistic. She feels that the benefits of being outdoors during therapy are countless. Clients are comfortable in the natural environment where they walk. The physical act of walking engenders a sense of freedom to relax, nurtures increased creative thinking, and enhances positive mental and physical function. Clients are less worried about eye contact and are free to discuss their worries in a judgment-free zone. Walk and talk is great for people who love to exercise, and enjoy the outdoors, as well as for those who are looking to try to increase their level of exercise by adding more movement into their routine.

Confidentiality is something to be cognizant of. Although the therapist would not disclose to anyone they encounter during walk-and-talk sessions that they are with a client, and are sure to walk in a quiet and less-populated path, one challenge does include maintaining confidentiality: by the nature of walk and talk, a person may be recognized by a fellow park pedestrian. Another challenge is to be able to predict and prepare any issues or concerns that day regarding the client's emotional state. If the client is very upset, what is the best way to handle their emotions? Professionalism is important, and being aware of who and what is going on around the park can play into the therapy. Ms. Udler always advises therapists to be aware of where the client is emotionally, and be flexible to take breaks for sitting, or maybe staying close to the entrance of the park/parking lot, in case help is needed.

When asked to share some sage advice for those considering "taking it outside," Ms. Udler shared:

> Do your homework and think critically. There are classes, tutorials, articles, and books on the subject. This is not just a session outside; consider all the factors involved. In addition to learning more about walk-and-talk therapy, the number-one thing is to maintain your professional self, and that the client's needs come first. As a therapist, you need to maintain your boundaries just as in the office, and be flexible with things like clothing, walking side by side, and welcoming a client to a shared space.

A final and fascinating thought that Ms. Udler leaves us with is that while walk-and-talk therapy may sound new, it has been around for a long time. Freud walked with the composer Gustav Mahler on a four-hour walk-and-talk session (Sasso 2020). She reports that the field is growing, and therapists are learning that creative therapies allow clients to access counseling in a way that a traditional office setting does not. People need choices, and we as professionals need to be flexible, adapt, and be available to new and different options for providing therapy. We could not agree more. For further information about Positive Strides, please see their website at www. PositiveStridesTherapy.com.

Reference

Sasso, D.A. (2020) 'The walking cure.' *Psychiatric Times*, August 3. Accessed on 12/3/2023 at www.psychiatrictimes.com/view/walking-cure.

A common intervention for supporting wellbeing is called mindfulness-based stress reduction (MBSR). A study with college faculty, staff, and students compared the outcomes of a six-week MBSR intervention that was facilitated in three different environments: a natural environment (a local public park), a built outdoor environment (a courtyard on the college campus), and an indoor environment (a seminar room). Wellbeing and nature connectedness were assessed at the outset of the study, during the intervention, a week after the intervention ended, and then one month later (Choe, Jorgensen, and Sheffield 2020). Those adults who participated in the natural outdoor condition demonstrated the most improved mental health status and strongest connection with nature. Most exciting was that these outcomes were sustained a month following the intervention (Choe *et al.* 2020). Mindfulness in nature appears to have lasting impact, which gives further support and rationale to conducting therapy outdoors.

Experiencing nature while walking, gardening, or exercising makes people feel better and have a more positive outlook; it helps with focusing and remembering details; and it enhances strength and physical fitness (Hall and Knuth 2019; Soga, Gaston, and Yamaura 2017). While people benefit from being in nature even if they must travel to get to it (White *et al.* 2019), not everyone is afforded this opportunity. Lacking easy and nearby access to natural outdoor environments, adults living in urban environments experience increased rates of attentional fatigue and limited chances to restore mental capacity. The result of such deprivation and loss of mental capacity can lead to stress, impulsivity, anger, and poor decision making (Zijlema *et al.* 2017). Experimental research comparing the impact of 50-minute walks in a natural environment, such as a park, with an urban cityscape environment found effective benefits for those who walked in nature. In this study, participants completed an extensive battery of psychological and cognitive assessments before and after the walk. Those who walked in nature showed decreased anxiety, rumination, and negativity as well as improved working memory, compared to the participants who walked in the urban environment (Bratman *et al.* 2015).

THIS MUCH I KNOW—SUSAN

It's just instead of taking a nap, I take a walk outside. I don't know what it is, but I just feel more awake and alive. You know, you're out there and your mind refocuses and you're able to feel more present and energized.

If you are providing care in an urban environment, consider looking for a site with trees and natural bodies of water when taking your practice outside, if it is feasible. To further illustrate the power of nature itself, a study of momentary subjective wellbeing and environmental conditions found that adults reported being happier when they were in any type of natural green environment as compared to urban environments (MacKerron and Mourato 2013). And remember, if you are limited to the urban cityscape, it is still worth it to spend time outside with your clients, as you can (at minimum) experience daylight! Think about this. If we are happier when outside and in nature, how might this impact goal attainment in therapy if it were facilitated outside?

CASE NARRATIVE: Central Oregon Veterans Ranch

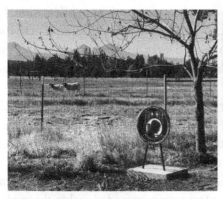

A SPECIAL PLACE FOR VETERANS

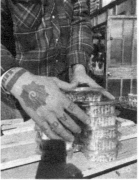

LOVE MICROGREENS

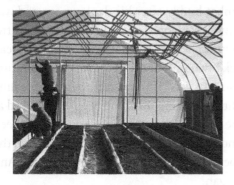

WORKING IN THE HOOP HOUSE
Photo credits: Central Oregon Veterans Ranch

Thank you to Alison Perry, MS, LPC, Founder and Executive Director, for her help in preparing this narrative.

The Central Oregon Veterans Ranch (COVR) is located between Central Oregon's two largest cities, Bend and Redmond; it is a 19-acre farm that provides agriculture-related learning, volunteer opportunities, and peer-support services for veterans. COVR's services are specifically tailored to meet the needs of veterans who have experienced trauma, particularly combat veterans. The original vision of the program stipulated that the property on which COVR is situated should provide adequate outdoor space, farm/agricultural qualities/structures, and breath-taking mountain views. "The Ranch," as COVR is often referred to, harnesses the beauty of the natural environment—the geographical setting, active agricultural operations, animals, and other natural features—to create a welcoming and non-stigmatizing environment for veterans. As an alternative to the medical model, the Ranch offers a holistic model of intervention that focuses on community building and support rather than symptom management or alleviation. It is a self-paced environment that offers veterans an array of outdoor activities, a sense of belonging, and opportunities to learn and grow organically. Aptly stated as its mission, the COVR is "a working ranch that restores purpose and spirit to veterans of all ages."

Ms. Perry shared that she worked as a licensed professional counselor (LPC) and trauma therapist in the traditional medical model of the Department of Veterans Affairs (VA) for six years. She worked in both hospital and rural outpatient clinic settings. In 2007, while working at the Portland VA Medical Center, she had a case that illuminated the limitations and sometimes retraumatizing effects of the interventions provided within the medical model. Her client was a 22-year-old Iraq War veteran who had been drugged and sexually assaulted by his combat buddy after his deployment and was exhibiting new symptoms of paranoid schizophrenia. He was viewed by the system as a "high needs" or "complex client." One day, Ms. Perry got a call that he was in the psychiatric lockdown unit at the VA, throwing furniture and threatening staff. Her first thought was "If I'd been through everything that vet had been through, I might be reacting the same way." She looked at a colleague who also cared for the veteran and said, "I wish we had a sheep ranch out east where we could send these vets, where they could work on the land, sleep under the stars, and be in a community of other veterans." And so, with that quick exchange, it began!

In 2012, Perry attended a 40-hour Contracting Officer Representative (COR) training course in Long Beach, California, for her new VA position in a housing program, followed by a personal retreat in Albuquerque, New Mexico, with Bill Plotkin (author of *Nature and the Human Soul*) and Richard Rohr. It was the juxtaposition of these two experiences so close together that inspired Ms. Perry to make the decision that she would leave the VA to pursue her vision of an alternative model of healing for traumatized veterans. Her plan was to take a couple of different steps professionally to diversify her skill set to help equip her for this new journey. Her COR training, work on a Department of Labor grant for a community college, and a brief stint as executive director of another veterans' non-profit in Central Oregon gave her enough confidence and community connections to get started.

In 2013 she formed an advisory board of veterans, veteran family members, and healthcare providers. Over the course of the next two years, the group was able to obtain its 501(c)(3) non-profit status and secure enough funding to partner with an investor to secure the current 19-acre Ranch property. Operations began with Ms. Perry and a small group of veteran volunteers in April of 2015.

The majority of veterans engaged in the Ranch community are combat veterans and have served in Iraq, Afghanistan, or Vietnam. The community also includes veterans who have survived other types of military trauma, such as life-altering physical injuries or sexual assault. Most have a diagnosis of PTSD, and many have service-connected disabilities. As there are far fewer females than males in the military, and even fewer who have served in combat roles, most participants are male. The Ranch was intentionally designed as an alternative to therapeutic models that evolved out of traditional settings where women were the primary recipients of services (see Winerman 2005). Ms. Perry calls COVR's model a "backdoor approach" to engaging veterans (male and female) who may shy away from or reject therapy models where therapist and client sit face to face, eye to eye, to talk about feelings, thoughts, and traumatic memories directly and explicitly. The Ranch is more of a "shoulder to shoulder" approach that honors the autonomy and agency of veterans, allowing them to share and process at their own pace.

While participants are primarily male, outreach is not gender-specific, but focused on levels of psychological and moral injury, typically related to wartime experiences. The Ranch does not provide housing or transportation, but current services include daily agricultural activities, volunteer opportunities, and a general social environment that veterans typically access anywhere from one to four times a week. Veteran participants include those who are employed, unemployed because of disability, pursuing education, or retired.

The overarching goals and outcomes for COVR participants are primarily psychosocial and spiritual health, and secondarily education. To that end, services are provided in multiple ways: large and small peer-support groups, one-on-one counseling with a licensed counselor, one-on-one peer support, agricultural workshops and classes, and veterans-only Alcoholics Anonymous

(AA) meetings. COVR also offers various volunteer opportunities for veterans—team projects and/or tasks that can be done independently, such as feeding animals and operating farm equipment.

Groups meet weekly, year-round, for about 60–90 minutes, and volunteer activities are available weekly. Individual counseling and peer support happens in structured and unstructured formats, and the length of time varies according to each veteran's needs. Often veterans participate in a combination of the above services, which contributes to the sense of community and camaraderie that is so often missing post-military.

Services are offered on an open-enrollment basis. Group size is rarely limited, except for when there is limited physical capacity for an educational course or the nature of the training dictates smaller group sizes (such as suicide prevention or special topic workshops). Services are primarily provided outdoors or under a general-purpose medium-sized military tent. Feeling wind drafts connects being in the tent with nature, and in cold months, the pellet stove facilitates warmth and contributes to a sense of coziness. In inclement weather, the Ranch house may be used. Not only have veterans reported that they prefer meeting in the tent, as compared to the Ranch house, but they also find it reminiscent of their time serving in the military.

The activities performed in the agriculture programs involve either receiving or sharing knowledge and include classes in how to grow lettuce hydroponically, regenerative farming and ranching techniques, animal care, how to operate farm equipment, and gardening and growing food. Almost all activities involve group projects where relational bonds are forged between veterans and shared physical work mimics the experience of teamwork, purpose, and pride of military service. Additionally, participation in the natural environment—sun, soil, wind, animals, and plants—facilitates a sense of peace, joy, and increased wellbeing.

The main commodity necessary to run COVR is people! Staff, veteran volunteers, and certified peer-support specialists comprise the team. As of 2022, there were a total of eight paid staff at COVR. All staff are either veterans or veteran family members, which helps support the veteran-specific culture of the organization, and COVR seeks to provide ongoing training in service of maintaining a trauma-informed environment. An operations and program manager manages the day-to-day operations and oversees management of the property and service delivery to veterans, including a staff composed of ranch manager, greenhouse manager, veteran outreach and education coordinator, and peer support specialist. Another staff member directly involved in day-to-day operations and program delivery is a veteran behavioral health peer-support specialist, a position made possible through a contract award from the Oregon Health Authority (OHA). This position requires a state certification for peer support. There is a requirement for this position/program to have supervision from a licensed mental health professional, such as Ms. Perry, who is a licensed professional counselor, which can be inside or outside the organization.

In addition to staffing, the other materials necessary to keep the Ranch operational include farm and agricultural equipment, greenhouse infrastructure and supplies, animals, and feed. The executive director, board of directors, and development staff are responsible for raising funds, networking, and bringing resources into the organization. The executive director works closely with all staff to maintain regular communication and outreach to community partners, particularly providers who serve veterans such as the local VA Clinic, Vet Center, Veterans Service Office, and other veterans' groups. The entire COVR staff are adept at outreach on behalf of the Ranch for materials, supplies, equipment rental, and other types of donations.

The ongoing maintenance needed to keep COVR running is organized into different program budgets such as greenhouse/hydroponics, pasture management, education/training, and peer support. COVR and its programs are funded through grants, private donations, fundraising, and community events. Events range from onsite fundraisers that welcome the general population onto the property, such as the Annual Armed Forces Day Plant Sale, to larger more formal events such as a Hollywood-style Gala that kicked off in 2022.

As you will soon read, the tireless efforts of the staff make a huge impact and change participants' lives for the better. Ms. Perry was generous in providing several standout stories about the immense value that COVR has had on its participants. Below we share three of them, all different but all transformative.

A combat veteran of the Iraq war (OIF or Operation Iraqi Freedom) came to COVR in 2017, later describing the Ranch as his "last stop" before planning his suicide. Referred by a veterans' housing non-profit, he had dropped out of VA care and exhausted all viable options. The first person the veteran was greeted by at COVR was a Vietnam veteran, who escorted him into Ms. Perry's office, where he proceeded to break down and share his history of trauma. A fit young man in his 30s, he was interested in the non-clinical opportunity to connect with fellow combat veterans in a natural setting and through shared physical volunteer work. Soon this veteran was coming out several times weekly, receiving support from peers and working on the Ranch, including helping wrangle wily sheep for shearing. The veteran found the vigorous work rewarding, and the support of peers (and an environment where he was understood) to be life-saving. Later he would say, "the Ranch saved my life."

A veteran of the Afghanistan war (OEF or Operation Enduring Freedom) came to the Ranch with his mother, a fellow Army veteran. He had dropped out of college because of high levels of anxiety related to PTSD, inability to focus, and inability to relate to peers. He and his mother began coming out weekly, assisting in the COVR greenhouse with planting, harvesting, and preparing lettuce for market. They also participated in other volunteer activities, including support for events on site (annual plant sale) and off site (such as festivals and fundraisers). The mother and son veteran pair participated at the Ranch for over a year, until one day Ms. Perry realized she was not seeing them anymore. At breakfast one morning with a veteran community partner who was friends with the young man, he shared:

> You know why we're not seeing so-and-so at the Ranch anymore, right? He was finally able to go back to school. It was the act of getting out of isolation, working with peers, and working in the greenhouse that gave him the confidence to go back.

A male Army veteran, who had sustained a lifelong back injury while serving in the military and was marginalized, repeatedly beaten up, and sexually assaulted by his unit for being "useless," arrived at the Ranch after having struggled for years with chemical dependency, relationship issues, and multiple suicide attempts. The Ranch staff discovered that the veteran had been raised on farms and ranches in northern California. Upon coming to COVR, the veteran felt an immediate sense of safety, trust, and comfort. He also felt right at home in the farm environment and began picking up volunteer tasks and jobs until he was hired as a ranch supervisor. Bringing his knowledge and expertise to COVR's agricultural environment gave this veteran a renewed sense of purpose and self-worth. Acceptance by veteran peers contributed to a profound sense of belonging—a stark contrast to his treatment in the military after being injured and considered "useless." The veteran's mental outlook, relationships, and progress in recovery began to improve. In a video testimonial, he spoke about the welcome he received, and the purpose he found at COVR; his concluding words were priceless: "The Ranch has a way of bringing your soul back."

Like all therapeutic programs, Ms. Perry was able to articulate both its benefits and challenges. For her, the benefits of working outside of the traditional clinical or medical environment include a shift in how "therapy" or healing happens:

Participants get to experience a more organic, natural way of relating and communicating as human beings on a journey of healing. Nature and the natural environment provide the "third thing" that can help support and mediate the healing relationship in a more organic fashion, different from the provider/client dualistic split of the modern medical model. Clients/participants often feel more at ease, "at home," and less stigmatized in a natural setting.

And realistically speaking, the challenges include "navigating safety, privacy, and the changing landscape of boundaries outside of the medical/clinical setting."

For all who might be considering a similar model, Ms. Perry offered this advice:

Consider privacy, safety, liability, and corresponding insurance policies and disclosure statements. Ask yourself, is your intervention using a nature-based activity, or is it about the environment, or both? What is the intended outcome of your activity or use of a nature-based setting? Consider whether and how boundaries or boundary issues might present themselves outside of a traditional clinical or medical setting.

In other words, take the time to carefully consider what you want your therapy outside program to be and how to make it work best for your intended client base. For this particular model, funding and organizational structure (non-profit) are also critical. More information about COVR's innovative programming can be found at www.covranch.org.

Reference
Winerman, L. (2005) 'Helping men to help themselves.' *Monitor on Psychology 36*, 7, 57.

It is important to consider our clients' preferences and collaborate with them to ensure nature-based interventions and recommendations are appropriate. We are eager to support the notion that everyone should experience nature on a regular basis owing to the evidence base supporting its health-promoting effects. Nevertheless, something important to consider is the intrinsic motivation of our clients. In a study of adults with common mental health disorders (CMD), which include depression and anxiety, Tester-Jones *et al.* (2020) determined that the benefits of a "green prescription," which is a physician's recommendation to be in nature for a specific amount of time per week, came at the cost of reducing the participant's motivation to be outside. While adults with CMD derive the same health-promoting effects that the general population does, when given a "green prescription," they are also likely to experience a reduction in intrinsic motivation to be outside (Tester-Jones *et al.* 2020). The take-home message is that we must be thoughtful in the ways that we recommend nature contact outside of therapy, whether a client has an identified mental health condition or not. In fact, the choice of being outside for therapy must also be respected. Remember that nature can happen inside as well.

CASE NARRATIVE: Destination Rehab

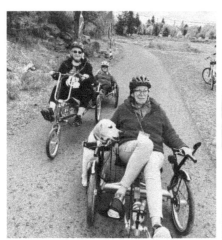

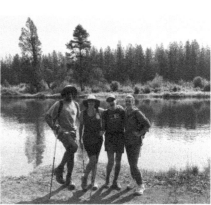

GETTING OUT AND RIDING BIKES WITH FRIENDS

HIKING TO UNEXPECTED PLACES

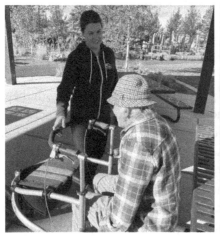

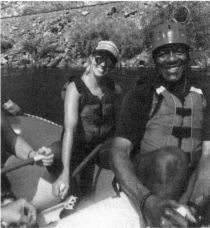

'SIT TO STANDS' ON DIFFERENT PARK SEATS   SMILES COME EASY WHILE OUTSIDE AND RAFTING

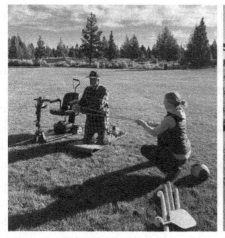 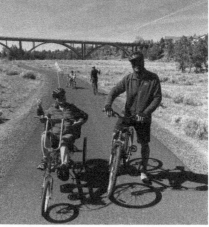

STRENGTH TRAINING IN THE PARK   THE DESTINATION IS ADVENTURE
                                 AND REHAB

Photo credits: Destination Rehab

Thank you to Carol-Ann Nelson, PT, DPT, NCS, MSCS, Founder and Director, for her help preparing this case narrative.

Located in Bend, Oregon, Destination Rehab's mission is "Empowering adults with neurologic conditions to experience outdoor adventure through individual physical therapy and group wellness programs!" Their goal is to empower adults with neurologic conditions to experience outdoor adventure and enjoy their time outside. Destination Rehab provides an array of services including one-on-one physical therapy, outdoor-based group support programs, weekly fitness classes, and other services to promote health, independence, and community reintegration.

   Started in 2016 as a physical therapy practice, Destination Rehab is organized as a non-profit in the State of Oregon, recognized as a 501(c)(3), and is the only outdoor non-profit physical therapy practice for adults with neurologic conditions in Oregon. The organization is staffed by three physical therapists, one donor journey coordinator (employed to raise money for the organization), and two part-time administrative staff, and is supported by five board members and over 20 volunteers. Destination Rehab now serves over 150 individuals annually with neurologic conditions, including 25+ caregivers and support team members. Destination Rehab recognizes the need for integrated and closely coordinated services for this vulnerable population. To address this need, it has active partnerships with Oregon Adaptive Sports and the Bend (Oregon) Parks and Recreation Department. Destination Rehab is also partnered with more than ten regional medical professionals and organizations that provide services such as adaptive sports, cycling and paddling gear, orthotic creation, neurologic testing, recreational centers, regional support groups, and health education. As part of their outreach and partnership, Destination Rehab hosts an annual event (with Oregon Adaptive Sports and other community organizations) that includes outdoor sports, wellness, and fun activities, and showcases all Central Oregon has to offer.

Dr. Nelson worked in outpatient neurological rehab for many years before starting Destination Rehab. Her motivation to create Destination Rehab was based on reality. She was shocked to see that although patients made gains in the clinic setting, they were not able to bridge the gap to greater involvement in the outdoors and local community. As someone who loves the outdoors and sunshine, Dr. Nelson could not imagine how it would feel to be homebound and not know how to get back to the outdoor community activities that make life fun and meaningful. She recognized a gap in the rehabilitation process: practitioners were successfully getting people home, but then there was little follow-on care, resource provision, or training to get people back to full community participation, which left them unable to access the activities and adventures that create memories with loved ones and add more significance to life. Dr. Nelson recognized that when someone was stuck at home, their world became smaller and smaller, and breaking out of that cycle was very challenging. She was (and remains!) keenly aware that beyond physical rehab, people also required emotional and cognitive rehab, and they could thrive with exposure to a wide array of environments beyond the home environment. Destination Rehab was created to fill those gaps and provide the missing follow-on care resources to broaden people's worlds and get them back outside and re-engaged in the community.

Participants come to Destination Rehab because they do not want to "live out the rest of [their] days on the couch," and they realize that they want their lives to be filled with experiences beyond the inside of their homes. Many participants have been backpackers, long-distance cyclers, rock climbers, skiers, and kayakers. Engaging in past outdoor recreation provides incredible memory-making experiences for their participants, who want to continue to participate, despite now needing a modified approach. Dr. Nelson has noted that many participants have lost friends because they can no longer keep up with their former lifestyle and are looking for a new community of positive people who understand the challenges of a neurologic condition and are determined to experience life at its fullest. The drive to connect with a community of people who are drawn to nature prevails.

The majority of Destination Rehab participants have diagnoses such as multiple sclerosis, Parkinson's disease, brain injury, spinal cord injury, stroke, or cerebral palsy. Programming includes individualized one-to-one sessions, and both large and small wellness-oriented groups. For example, visits for physical therapy are facilitated one to one for ten weekly sessions; the Adventure Group meets weekly for six months starting in the summer and is a cohort of 12–20 people; and there is an ongoing twice-weekly fitness program for about 12 people called Peak Fitness. The holistic goals that Destination Rehab addresses with their young adult, adult, and older adult clients encompass physical and mental health, sensory integration, and education. Summed up, the goals are all about building confidence to participate more fully in the best part of life—what matters to the client.

Services are provided indoors and outdoors in both built and non-built environments. The staff sometimes rents a local gym space, taking care of the clean-up after use. They also offer drop-in days at the local rock-climbing gym and recreation center where they use the workout areas and pool. The majority of days are spent meeting participants at local parks and trails, and taking advantage of grassy surfaces, natural trail obstacle courses, pickleball courts, water for kayaking, and picnic benches that facilitate practice with various functional transfers. Bigger picture: there are no physical limits to the Destination Rehab program—the entire outdoors is their space! With that said, the Destination Rehab team is realistic and always selects sites with an accessible bathroom, shade, and somewhere to take a seated break, which could be on a walker with a built-in seat or a chair that the staff brings along to every session.

It takes people, gear, time, and creativity to run Destination Rehab. The staff includes three full-time physical therapists, one full-time donor journey coordinator, a full-time clinic program assistant, and one part-time occupational therapist. All three physical therapists are passionate about spending time outdoors and are Board Certified Specialists in Neurologic Physical Therapy. The donor journey coordinator is responsible for networking, fundraising, and marketing. The clinic administrative staff work from home and in the field and are responsible for scheduling, participant contacts, participant forms and referrals, and assisting with physical therapy and group sessions. In addition to paid staff, Destination Rehab is supported by over 20 high-quality volunteers. The volunteers are current or retired medical professionals, kinesiology students, and physical-therapy doctorate students who are supervised onsite by a staff member. The equipment needed to run Destination Rehab's programs includes a vehicle to haul and store rehab equipment gear, such as functional electrical stimulation equipment, orthotics, overground walkers, walking sticks, data collection tools (i.e., Blaze-Pods—www.blazepod.com), and Kinesio tape; and outdoor sports equipment such as recumbent trikes, kayaks, stand-up paddleboards, and snowshoes. The amount of time dedicated to providing direct services changes with the seasons. In the summer, there is more programming, while in the winter months, the focus is on education, the staff's professional development, and team strategic planning. The staff are creative in facilitating the programs to run without a dedicated office space and by utilizing several community locations that can be swapped out depending on the weather.

Dr. Nelson shared that their strongest marketing platform is word of mouth. They also connect with clients via referrals from local neurologists, support groups, speech and language therapists, and occupational therapists. In addition, they actively promote the programs through their website and on social media platforms.

When discussing financial requirements and startup costs, Dr. Nelson offers newcomers a bit of advice. She recommends "starting with two staff members—a director/clinician and a second clinician—then hiring a fundraiser as soon as possible." To start Destination Rehab, Dr. Nelson used her personal vehicle and $2000 of her own money to purchase equipment. The current programs, now six years in, are funded by grants, fees for services, billed to insurance, donations, and fundraising. Their operating budget is close to $400,000 a year and 80% is dedicated to staffing. In addition to providing creative care outdoors and managing a business, Dr. Nelson is working with Oregon State University to complete research projects. She regularly presents at national conferences and on webinars: her recent American Physical Therapy Association (APTA) presentation had over 600 attendees, a testament to the rising interest in taking therapy outside!

Destination Rehab participants often have goals related to improving independence, community participation, confidence, and quality of life. They achieve these goals through the facilitated experiences of new adventures that challenge them to push beyond what they thought was possible, to rediscover favorite activities, and to join Destination Rehab's community of mentorship and support. Another beautiful feature of the programs is how destigmatizing the interventions and activities are; the participants are often working out in a park or on a lake, which to any passer-by would look like another high-intensity workout or leisure activity. Beyond the qualitative and observed improvements, Destination Rehab's three physical therapists perform a range of tests during one-on-one physical therapy sessions including the six-minute walk test, the Berg Balance scale, the Mini-BESTest, TUG, the Walking Impact Scale (Walk-12), Modified Fatigue Impact Scale, and participant confidence rating scales. This testing provides impressive data to show that they are making big impacts! In 2020 the team provided 1019 direct service hours which increased in 2021 to 2100 direct service hours. On average, they have found that over the course of ten weeks, participants improve their six-minute walk test scores by 40.27%. Dr. Nelson generously shared some specific intervention plans, which you can find at the end of this case narrative.

She finds that the challenges associated with running innovative outdoor-based programs are wide-ranging, but certainly not insurmountable. The first challenge is often related to selecting a location that has sufficient parking, accessible restrooms, benches with shade, van access to unload the equipment, varied terrain, shelter from inclement weather, is easily found on a map, and is not too crowded. Once the location is settled, there are further challenges related to the weather (e.g., rain, heat, smoke), getting the participant's family to understand and support the programs, protecting the participant's privacy, and addressing their fears. This is a novel program, and many participants fear the unknown.

Despite the challenges, Dr. Nelson and her team have created innovative solutions. They discuss the issue of participant privacy (or potential lack thereof when working in a public park) with the participants and their families during initial screening calls. They carry their equipment in and carry it out; just like conscientious hikers, they "pack it in and pack it out." They dress in layers for the weather and are constantly mindful of offering shade and hydration. The team carries extra water and packs extra food. Equipment and structures can be sanitized on site. They are mindful of scheduled children's camps and reschedule to a less crowded park. And the team members have liability insurance coverage that is portable, meaning it extends wherever services are being rendered.

Furthermore, there are outstanding challenges that more traditional indoor-based practices face as well. Sometimes it is challenging to locate new participants who do not find the right meeting spot or show up at the wrong time, and there are efficiency losses related to transporting and loading equipment. Despite these frustrations, Dr. Nelson shared sound advice that can apply to any practice, indoors or out:

> Be willing to start simple and grow based on your local clients' needs. Be creative and always have your problem-solving hat on. When participants see you approach challenges with positivity and confidence, they will begin to feel the same way!

Destination Rehab's programs are helping people get outside, live more active lives, and make positive memories. Dr. Nelson offered some feedback from a few participants who were eager to share their experience. A participant living with multiple sclerosis wrote:

> I have issues with walking due to my left side being weak. Before starting with Destination Rehab, I was unable to walk far distances and often stayed inside, sitting in a chair, because my knee collapsed with weight on it. Now, after six months of working with the team at Destination Rehab, I feel confident walking, swimming, and getting outside. The physical therapists are professional and caring, they are right there watching you and helping you, and most importantly giving you the confidence to try new things. Destination Rehab reintroduced me to outdoor activities and changed my mindset on what I can do. Knowing I cannot stay in PT forever, they recommended I start the Destination Rehab Peak Fitness program where I can attend the weekly exercise class and try things on my own. This program, along with the others Destination Rehab offers, provides a community for me and my peers living with neurologic conditions and helps me meet people that I can do things with. I have tried new things like pickleball and kayaking and feel confident to go outside with my husband and play horseshoes and other activities that I would not have tried in the past.

Another participant who is recovering from a stroke shared:

> I love that it is outdoors and keeps me physical. I feel I have a say in what we are doing, and I am able to provide input for what we are doing. Most PTs in the past that I worked with—I just had to do what they told me, so it's so nice to give feedback and be heard. It really is just so different than anything I could have experienced at a traditional PT office. The PTs are so thorough: they ask questions, listen, encourage you to do your best, and are so positive. Adventure Group has been great! My wife and I love meeting new people and seeing new places we would not have seen. It is fun to be with the group and have people there to cheer you on. It reminds you that you are not alone. There is always laughter, positive feedback, and they show you it is okay.

And his wife said:

> We love the kayaking and being out on the water. We have enjoyed it so much we purchased kayaks for ourselves and look forward to going! We love seeing new things, and at first this sounded scary...the unknown...but now we get excited to try new things and don't hesitate when asked to. Every experience we had so far has been great. I like that they involve me and welcome me

during the activities. I had to take over everything—driving, taking care of the house—I didn't realize how much my husband did before his health issues, and now all the responsibilities are on me, so it's nice that the PTs recognize and acknowledge that. Not only did my husband's life change but mine did as well.

To learn more about Destination Rehab, please visit, www.destinationrehab. org.

Four Potential Intervention Plans
Functional Strength
The following bullets provide general ideas for how to address functional strength when working outdoors with participants.

- The participant walks on natural stairs or inclines using mobility aids as needed.
- They perform "sit to stand" from varied bench surfaces.
- They pull a weighted sled.

Consider modifying the activities using kettlebells, dumbbells, resistance bands, and a weighted vest.

Balance
The following bullets provide general ideas for how to address balance reactions when working outdoors with participants.

- The participant walks on a soft surface with perturbations (e.g., walking over grass that has natural bumps in the terrain).
- The participant and therapist play pickleball.
- They use stand-up paddleboards.
- They walk a dog on a leash.

Consider modifying the activities using agility ladder, sports equipment, cones/targets on ground, and inclines.

Stand-up paddle boarding (SUP)
The following bullets provide a general protocol when stand-up paddle boarding with a participant.

- Once the participant is familiar with the equipment and has demonstrated requisite safety understanding, start the session in shallow water.

- As the therapist, follow the mantra "Action–Observation" and provide verbal instructions when needed.
- Encourage them to start off in a quadruped or tall kneeling position.
- Take time to go through weight shifting, head turns, and paddling in different patterns, while walking beside them in the shallow water.
- As the session progresses, and if appropriate, encourage the participant to practice standing up, paddle in shallow water, and then move to deeper water.

Bicycling

The following bullets provide a general protocol when bicycling on a recumbent bike with a participant.

- Begin the session by setting the bike up and familiarizing the participant with the equipment and safety protocols.
- Practice transferring on and off the bike with the participant.
- Discuss and demonstrate bike management skills: using the brakes, turning the bike, adjusting the length of the bike, and adjusting the seat on the bike.
- Before heading out on a ride, have them demonstrate how to turn, start/stop, go in reverse, and go fast/slow.
- When planning the ride, it is important to consider the following features:
    - How many hills are on the planned route?
    - How many intervals will you encourage the participant to complete?
    - When targeting power training, encourage them to use a higher-numbered gear.
    - When targeting endurance and speed training, encourage them to use a lower-numbered gear.

When implementing any intervention plan, but especially any outdoor intervention, be sure to consider the following questions and aspects of the activity:

- How much problem solving will the participant be doing?
- Do they present with cognitive or memory challenges?
- How much multitasking will they be doing?
- How will the participant follow or find the intended route?
- Does the environment present high or low distraction levels?

- Has the participant used the equipment before, or will this be novel equipment?

As therapists, we are always working to help our participants get healthier, stronger, faster, more independent, and more confident. As therapy progresses, we may find ourselves in the lucky position of needing to make an activity more challenging! These are a few go-to modifications to increase the challenge of an activity:

- Throw a ball at the participant during the activity for added distraction.
- Add weight to the activity (e.g., they wear a weighted vest).
- Add a metronome to the structure of the activity so they have to keep on beat.

Nature-based interventions also have the capacity to enhance population health and wellbeing (Shanahan *et al.* 2019). Social cohesion is a construct associated with interpersonal connections and factors that impact quality of life. Research has found that access to urban nature such as parks, greenways, and gardens provides the venue for people to meet and connect with others, experience social support, find common ground, and develop community, which leads to improved social engagement as well as physical activity (Jennings and Bamkole 2019). These same benefits can be found through indoor social gardening activities (Wagenfeld, Schefkind, and Hock 2019). Collectively, this leads to improved mental health and wellbeing, enhanced immune function, and general wellbeing (Jennings and Bamkole 2019).

CASE NARRATIVE: Cascade Girl Organization's Bee Heroes America

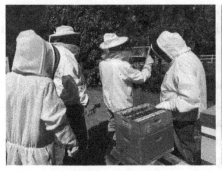 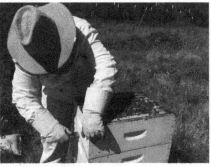

Mission-driven task to inspect the frames

Opening the frames

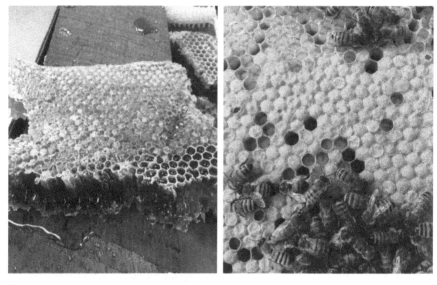

HEALTHY HIVES PRODUCE HEALTHY HONEY   LIKE BEES, HUMANS CAN WORK
                                      BETTER AS TEAMS

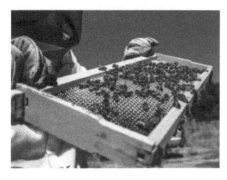

MANAGING THE HIVES
Photo credits: Cascade Girl Organization

Thank you to Sharon Schmidt, PMHNP, Psy.D., Certified Master Beekeeper, Founder and President of Cascade Girl Organization, for her help in the preparation of this case narrative.

Cascade Girl Organization's Bee Heroes America program has a mission that works toward several goals: to aid the survival of bees and all food system pollinators; to educate veterans about bees, agriculture, and beekeeping; and to foster community connection and inclusion. Bee Heroes America is an innovative and unique program offered through the White City VA Rehabilitation Center and Clinics in Southwestern Oregon, which aims to educate veterans and support their social reintegration.

The inception story of Bee Heroes America started when Dr. Schmidt fell in love with bees as a child. Her father grew up on a Wisconsin dairy farm where Dr. Schmidt's grandmother was the beekeeper, and the small insects were often the sole source of dietary sweets during the years of the Great Depression. Dr. Schmidt's father (a WWII veteran) passed along his sense of wonder and curiosity about the tiny creatures' seemingly magical attributes.

Long after completing her master's degree in nursing and her doctoral degree in clinical psychology, to answer her own questions about beekeeping in the apiary (a place where bees are kept), she began seriously working with honeybees and, in 2020, earned a master beekeeper certificate from University of Montana. Over the course of six years, Dr. Schmidt's interest in science and love of bees, combined with her work in mental health, particularly with people with PTSD, culminated in the ideas behind Bee Heroes America.

In the apiary, she noticed the delicate exquisiteness of her bees and how much focus it required to manipulate frames without hurting them. Over the years, Dr. Schmidt resolved many of the questions she harbored about the "best" ways to keep bees. She learned how bees interact with their environment when left to their own devices and how she could partner with them to help them do what they want to do. The bees obliged by being good teachers, stinging her when she was not careful. Their teaching paid off, and she became more willing to do things in ways they could accept. Dr. Schmidt realized that both a sense of wonder and a dose of healthy respect for their stings had their role in keeping beekeepers focused. These were valuable lessons for her work with veterans. Meanwhile, Dr. Schmidt found that keeping bees allowed entry into a variety of experiences with truly wonderful people she would have never otherwise met.

Her then hobby began to inspire others, including a retired veteran friend who had deployed repeatedly and came back with multiple physical and psychological battle scars. Dr. Schmidt realized that beekeeping harbored enough elements of wonder and danger, altruism, and courage to facilitate attention and focus. She began to believe that those factors plus exposure to the outdoors and nature might help individuals with PTSD modulate mood and engage intentionally instead of being caught up in the endless cycle of numbness and re-experiencing that come with PTSD.

Research confirmed what she had perceived: that veterans coming back from active duty could benefit from activities designed to help them reintegrate into their communities and that they tended to form a sense of kinship with other veterans who had experienced similar stressors and challenges (Anderson *et al.* 2019). In her work, Dr. Schmidt had noticed that veterans were mostly disinclined to talk about the experiences of battle during deployment.

However, she saw that they sensed and had empathy for the effects of trauma in others. Further, she observed similarities between veterans and bees; the veterans, having been trained to work together to defend their homes and families, possessed the capacity to work together like a functioning hive. In contrast to the work of war, she shared that working with bees can be a positive and restorative focus, bringing a group of veterans together in the constructive task of helping the bees to protect their home and family.

Bee Heroes America provides an opportunity for veterans to become fully immersed in their own sense of wonder about a society of tiny individuals—a society that makes its own very sophisticated decisions for the good of the hive. The program provides veterans with a structure to integrate into the beekeeping community, which then assists their return to local community life. The program also facilitates exposure to nature, which, according to Dr. Schmidt, has several positive effects. The first is restoration, which, based on the attention restoration theory, is that peaceful experiences involving nature minimize the negative impact of sustained focus on mental health (Kaplan and Kaplan 1989). The second is the idea that the beekeeper is exposed to 30,000–60,000 tiny individuals engaged in highly organized activity and as such she proposes a "mirror neuron effect" (Cook *et al.* 2014), which might also have an organizing effect for the beekeeper. Another effect is improved mood regulation. Dr. Schmidt proposes that the potentially healing outdoor effect of exposure to the beneficial *Mycobacterium vaccae* may, based on studies of rats and mice, potentially inhibit inflammatory responses in the brain and help regulate mood (Foxx *et al.* 2021; Frank *et al.* 2018; Schmidt 2020).

Bee Heroes America offers beekeeping instruction and practice with fellow veterans. As of early 2021, Bee Heroes America had delivered the first education module to their inaugural cohort of veterans. The program is delivered both virtually and in person. The online component consists of six education sessions that are each one-and-a-half hours long. The education modules, which cover introductory topics related to beekeeping, are delivered via an online meeting platform. Dr. Schmidt teaches with the assistance and oversight of the Director of Recreational Therapy at the White City VA Rehabilitation Center and Clinics. At the conclusion of the initial education modules, veterans are familiar with information about honeybees and their care as well as the roles of some of the other pollinators common in agriculture. While online, peer mentorships are also facilitated to connect the veteran to the larger beekeeping community. Following the online portion of the program, two experienced beekeepers will join the team to help take students to the next phase, which is to start beehives and to learn about how to observe and care for the hives.

The in-person sessions are facilitated on the White City VA Rehabilitation Center and Clinics campus at the beehives, where veterans will learn and practice caring for the live beehives and participate in mentorship. To foster community integration, Bee Heroes America encourages veterans to join local beekeeping events and facilitates activities with local farms and local beekeepers. A typical in-person session includes meeting at the hives, caring for the hives as needed, learning activities such as checking for mites or repairing beehive frames, and harvesting wax or honey. Although not mentioned in the previously listed activities, important outcomes include experiencing nature, recognizing a common bond with the hive and its mission of protection and growth, improved focus and awareness in the present moment (bees will correct you if you are not focused and aware of what you are doing!), a sense of harmony with the cycles of nature, a sense of mastery, a common bond with others who care for bees, and a sense of pride in constructively assisting the bees to do what they want to do. Additional sessions are planned for weekends to bring all veterans together for special activities and celebrations.

All participants, thus far, are veterans receiving care through the U.S. Department of Veterans Affairs' domiciliary program. The domiciliary program provides long-term rehabilitation to veterans who are at risk for homelessness, substance abuse, and/or mental illness. The program is offered as recreational therapy in a group setting; any veteran who wishes to join can be referred by their primary care physician. The most recent cohort at Bee Heroes America included 20 veterans. The beehives were donated to the program, as were the bees.

The beehive location on the VA campus was selected based on various criteria: accessibility via a vehicle, sufficient flat space to accommodate the beehives, distance from human activity, and access to water, shade, sunlight, and flowers. The equipment needed to run the program includes protective gear, hive tools, smokers, storage equipment, materials to test and treat bees for parasites and other harmful pests, honey extraction and bottling equipment, and educational materials such as books and computers. Additional expenses include paying for an online meeting platform subscription and covering the cost of travel for some of the volunteer instructors. Some of the equipment was donated, but funding for additional equipment, materials, and expenses are from grants, fundraising, and through the Recreational Therapy budget at the VA.

Because beekeeping is a unique and multifaceted activity, Dr. Schmidt and her team understand that not every veteran will want to become a beekeeper and that the activity can also facilitate interests in other areas. They approach each cohort cycle expecting that some will choose not to work directly with bees. Their passion may be to plant flowers, learn about hive building, maintain equipment, find pollination opportunities, market hive products, or paint, decorate, or clean hives, and still others will enjoy the process of making honey. Some may just want to watch it all happen and that too is OK!

The reason for the multifaceted expectations is that the goal of Bee Heroes America is to provide a space for every veteran to participate at their own pace and interest level—and to express their feelings while connecting with others at whatever level is comfortable—all while outdoors. Even in the startup phase, Bee Heroes America is helping veterans connect. Dr. Schmidt shared some of the feedback she has received from the veterans, which included "being fascinated with bees" and a few who told stories about how they had participated in similar activities in their youth. A female veteran realized that although she had trepidation about meeting the bees, she would be supported by the Bee Heroes America staff and fellow veterans in this new challenge.

Dr. Schmidt shared that the VA staff have also expressed interest in the Bee Heroes America curriculum, and she hopes to incorporate them in learning this novel skill, thus maximizing therapeutic benefits for patients through mutual understanding. Shared experience can spark mutuality in conversations between staff and clients or family and clients. As participants gain experience with beekeeping, they also gain social capital and status, having acquired new skills and an opportunity to share them with others.

Dr. Schmidt left us with a sweet piece of advice (we would expect nothing less from a master beekeeper). Identifying positive effects of *Mycobacterium vaccae* in the soil and the potential for mirror neuron activation as healing factors, she said, "Outdoor activities have so many potential healing benefits including the sounds and smells of nature." We agree so much that we wrote a whole chapter about those healing benefits! To see some of the bees and get a better taste for what is happening at Bee Heroes America, check out the website www.cascadegirl.org.

References

Anderson, L., Campbell-Sills, L., Ursano, R.J., Kessler, R.C. *et al.* (2019) 'Prospective associations of perceived unit cohesion with postdeployment mental health outcomes.' *Depression and Anxiety 36*, 6, 511–521.

Cook, R., Catmur, C., Press, C., and Heyes, C. (2014) 'Mirror neurons: From origin to function.' *Behavioral and Brain Sciences 37*, 2, 177–192.

Foxx, C.L., Heinze, J.D., González, A., Fernando, V. *et al.* (2021) 'Effects of immunization with the soil-derived bacterium *Mycobacterium vaccae* on stress coping behaviors and cognitive performance in a "two hit" stressor model.' *Frontiers in Physiology 11*, 524833.

Frank, M.G., Fonken, L.K., Dolzani, S.D., Annis, J.L. *et al.* (2018) 'Immunization with *Mycobacterium vaccae* induces an anti-inflammatory milieu in the CNS: Attenuation of stress-induced microglial priming, alarmins and anxiety-like behavior.' *Brain, Behavior, and Immunity 73*, 352–363.

Kaplan, R. and Kaplan, S. (1989) *The Experience of Nature: A Psychological Perspective.* Cambridge: Cambridge University Press.

Schmidt, S.N. (2020) 'Beekeeping as a healing intervention: Historical background, recent programs and proposed mechanisms of action.' Accessed on 2/12/22 at www.cascade-girl.org/beekeeping-for-healing-and-therapy

Virtual nature also improves mental health. Adult participants who were randomly assigned to watch a video of wild nature demonstrated significantly increased positive affect, improved sense of restoration, and reduced negative mood after watching the video, compared to participants who watched a non-nature video (McAllister, Bhullar, and Schutte 2017). The implications for studies of virtual nature can inform how indoor spaces are designed and arranged to maximize health and wellness when outdoor nature cannot be or is not available. Alternatives could be providing therapy in a room with a view of nature, bringing in plants, or hanging images of nature on the walls of the therapy space. We need nature, whether it is outside or brought inside, no matter how young or old we are, no matter where we live, but especially so when nature is not right outside our door.

THIS MUCH I KNOW—LEE

Nature guides me home
Back to a whole human being...
BEING...
Before my soul, new time, place, pain, doubt, anxiety and deadlines
When I am in nature
I find the ALL that is Me
The synergy between the infinite/unconditional and
a BEING within the basic simple unequivocal grace of KNOWING
I AM WHO AM

NUGGET OF NATURE: QUIET AND REFLECTIVE NATURE ACTIVITIES

- Gaze at the clouds.
- Listen to the sound of the wind.
- Study the vein pattern of a leaf.

- Smell a flower.
- Pick two blades of grass and think about how they are the same and different.
- Listen to a birdsong and sing back.
- Plant a seed.
- Make a rock structure.
- Write a worry on a stone and toss it into the woods or water.
- Listen to the crunching sound of leaves as you walk over them.
- Watch the waves.
- Rub your fingers over herbs and take in the smell.

Wrapping It Up

Adulthood is the longest period in the human lifespan; accordingly, much happens during this approximately 35-year period. In this chapter, we explored some of the age-related changes that affect adulthood and how a plethora of research that nature positively impacts adults. Access to nature matters and can improve the quality of our lives, no matter where we are in the lifespan. How we integrate nature in our own lives and in a therapeutic capacity with our clients can positively influence the trajectory of our lives.

CHAPTER 8

Older Adulthood

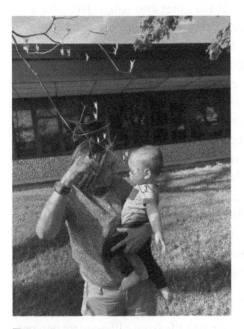

THE NEXT GENERATION BRINGS
A WHOLE NEW PERSPECTIVE
Photo credit: Ben Atchison

Introduction

For the purposes of this book, we consider older adulthood to begin at 65 years old. This number is based on the age most commonly found in the research literature. The U.S. Administration on Aging's 2021 publication reported that there were 54.1 million older adults over the age of 65 living in the U.S., which was 16.5% of the population (Administration on Aging (AoA) 2021). By the year 2060, older adults are predicted to outnumber children and will likely make up 23% of the U.S. population (approximately 94.7 million older adults), while children will only make up 20% (Mather and Kilduff 2020).

THIS MUCH I KNOW—BEN

My morning routine is to pour my first of two cups of coffee and head to my screened-in porch where I am not listening to the news on CNN, I'm not scrolling through my cell phone, nor reading. It's the aroma of the coffee and the morning light that greets me, along with the comforting sounds of the various birds in my trees. I am further comforted by their appearance on my feeders as they fly from the trees, land, and return to their nests. If I move too quickly to stand closer to the screen, they quickly sense the survival instinct of flight. If I'm quiet and still, it feels like a shared experience. They arrive, nibble, return to their nests, and come back to repeat the sequence. They are making themselves at home and doing so without a sense of threat. Sometimes I will sit for an hour before I move on to the daily routine of tending my flower garden. The birds continue their cycle of nest–feeding–nest while filling the air with varied songs. I listen to this while I begin the routine of trimming, pruning, and deadheading every flower in pots, bushes, and trees. It doesn't feel at all like a mundane chore. I drag hoses around to every corner of my ¾ acre of gardens and trees, and while that feels like an annoyance at times, I revel in this participation in nurturing nature. Without pruning, watering, and intermittent fertilization, the hundreds of flowers I'm tending to would cease to thrive. My heart rate is at its best; my mind is not yet swirling in the list of things I need to do. For the next hour or so, I'm enjoying the peace and tranquility of the simple yet powerful blessings of nature.

When thinking about the trajectory of a person's life from a life-course perspective, it can be helpful to reflect on the concept of ageism. Ageism is the prejudice experienced when the estimation of a person's capability is based solely on their chronological age or appearance of age (Applewhite, Backer, and Carpenter 2018). Perspectives and opinions on aging and how older adults are treated are extremely dependent upon culture. Unfavorable stereotypes associated with aging not only affect the thoughts of those younger than 65 years old, but very much affect the perspectives of older adults themselves (Applewhite *et al.* 2018). A recent study found that "82% of older adults reported regularly experiencing at least one form of everyday ageism in their day-to-day lives" and "older adults who regularly experienced more forms of everyday ageism were more likely to [report having] worse physical and mental health" (Malani *et al.* 2020, pp.1–3). How we talk about aging and treat the older adults in our community matters! Here are a few examples of anti-ageist practices that we as individuals can implement in our everyday lives and when interacting with an older adult:

- Do NOT assume an older adult's knowledge of technology (i.e., don't assume they are technology illiterate).
- Do NOT make jokes about older adults or reference being more capable in your youth.
- When someone forgets something, do NOT say they are having a "senior moment."

(Anti-Defamation League 2017; Applewhite et al. 2018)

THIS MUCH I KNOW—ELLEN

We share a conversation with Ellen, a 79-year-old adult woman living with Parkinson's disease and Shannon's grandmother, about nature experiences.

Q: What do you think of nature and being in nature on a day-to-day basis?

A: It's definitely a place I need to go... It helps me, keeps me busy, but it helps me tune out some of the things that are going on in my head. Just sitting on the porch is enough, listening to and watching the birds... I do think nature is good, but when I'm out there, I'm just... I'm right in the dirt. Feeling the different kinds of dirt, determining what the dirt needs, pulling a few weeds, not near enough.

Q: When did you fall in love with gardening and being around nature?

A: Way, way back when I was young, when my dad was working away from home. He'd leave notes for us girls to get out to the garden and weed certain rows, like weed the beets... I was probably in elementary school, 5th or 6th grade.

Q: What made weeding the garden feel special?

A: Well, other than just providing for or producing to help the family have food, it was like, well, this is what we do, we plant beans, and we make cornbread and...ya know, it was a different time.

Q: How is the time you spend in nature special now?

A: Instead of thinking about what I saw on the news or the latest movie or whatever, I don't actually worry about anything when I'm out gardening, other than I don't have enough life left to take care of everything I want. And...well, I think better; well, I don't know about better. But I seem to think much clearer. I find that when we look at things in the long view, we can either become disturbed and disgusted with it or look for the beautiful side of it. In nature it can be easier to find the beautiful side of it.

When thinking about milestones in older adulthood, what comes to mind might be retiring, engaging in more leisure activities, becoming a grandparent, and coping with the growing demands of healthcare management. Each person's experience of older adulthood is unique to them, and if working with an older adult, it is a good idea to ask, "What does a typical day look like for you?" instead of assuming anything. Retirement, though a privilege experienced by roughly 66–82% of older adults, is a milestone that may allow greater time for leisure activities and may lead to a greater need for facilitated or organized social activities (Administration on Aging 2021; Fry 2021). With younger generations, older adults may assume new roles and have more opportunities to engage in or even lead intergenerational programming.

THIS MUCH I KNOW—PEGGY

My personal piece of nature is my garden whether it's in the ground around my house or in pots on my lanai (a kind of veranda/porch). Every morning before I start my day, I like to walk my garden, feel the sun or light rain, and with my cup of coffee or tea, notice all the changes in my plants and plantings. This is my little piece of nature, from the trees in the ground to the herbs in pots in my lanai garden. I derive an immense feeling of personal satisfaction and peace. Rejuvenation! It is amazing to me how a plant can suddenly produce a seed pod or flower that wasn't apparent the day before. I love the little changes and surprises of life from my plants! After that, I can start my day.

The growing demands of healthcare management are often a result of chronic health conditions. Below, we have provided a table with consideration for the most common health challenges faced in older adulthood (Healthy Aging Team 2021).

Table 8.1 General challenges and common chronic conditions faced by older adults: Conditions reported by Healthy Aging Team (2021) by the National Council on Aging

Typical associated diagnosis	Potential modifications for participation
Decreased Endurance or Energy Levels	
Hypertension—experienced by 58% of older adults Heart disease—experienced by 29% of older adults Heart failure—experienced by 14% of older adults Chronic obstructive pulmonary disease—experienced by 11w% of older adults	To address decreased endurance and energy levels (Foster and Powell 1992): • Provide opportunities to sit during all tasks. When working while seated, place materials so that clients do not have to reach up high above their shoulders or bend over (Foster and Powell 1992). • Encourage clients to slide materials across a table, as opposed to lifting them. In addition, use mechanical advantage when available, such as a pulley to lift or a wheeled cart to move materials (Foster and Powell 1992). • Consider setting up workspaces closer together to reduce the amount of walking needed. • Encourage clients to work at their own pace, slowly warming up to start and then increasing the pace if and when they feel comfortable. • Encourage clients to take breaks often and as needed. • When working on large projects or tasks, organize the activity so that it is completed in multiple small steps and incorporate frequent rest periods throughout.
Dizziness and decreased balance	
The cause of dizziness is often complex, but peripheral vestibular dysfunction, positional vertigo, and Meniere's disease are the most common causes of dizziness in older adults—experienced by 24% of older adults (Iwasaki and Yamasoba 2014) Decreased balance is caused by many factors; common causes include low blood pressure and arthritis (Salzman 2010)	To address dizziness, decreased balance, and increased fall risk: • Encourage clients to sit in a chair with armrests to work. • If possible, prior to delivering an intervention or leading a program in an unfamiliar setting, conduct a site evaluation for fall risks and propose needed changes to appropriate leadership. Examples of typical modifications are grab bars near toilets, handrails alongside stairs, and raised toilet seats (Mulry *et al.* 2017; Pynoos, Steinman, and Nguyen 2010). • Consider inspecting workspaces for fall risks (Clemson *et al.* 2019): – remove slippery surfaces and loose mats – remove clutter – visually highlight uneven surfaces – turn on all lights. • When providing therapy outdoors, encourage clients to wear well-fitting, rubber-soled, and closed-toed shoes (Clemson *et al.* 2019). • Provide clients with water to maintain hydration no matter if the activities are facilitated indoors or outside.

cont.

Typical associated diagnosis	Potential modifications for participation
Poor grip strength	
Arthritis—experienced by 31% of older adults	To promote grip strength and tool use: • Add a textured surface via tape or another rubbery material to tool handles (Woy 1997). • Build up tool handles—potential materials to build up the handles include pool noodles, pipe insulation, bike-handle tape, and duct tape. Refer to Chapter 7, Nuggets of Nature: Caring for Mind and Body—A Simple Way to Adapt a Garden Hand Tool. • Use adapted utensil holders on the handles of tools.
Limited range of motion	
Arthritis—experienced by 31% of older adults	To address limited range of motion (Rogers and Powell 1992): • Consider purchasing or making specialty tools. The National AgrAbility website (www.agrability.org) has a virtual toolbox dedicated to assistive technology, prefabricated adapted tools, and ideas for creating your own adapted tools (AgrAbility n.d.). • When working with any type of material, such as artwork, gardening, or journaling, place materials at an appropriate height so that clients can work without having to bend over or reach up.
Low vision	
Low vision in older adulthood is commonly caused by "age-related macular degeneration, glaucoma, cataract and diabetic retinopathy" and is experienced by 33% of older adults (Quillen 1999, p.99)	To address low vision (Foster, Duvall, and Powell 1992): • Turn on all overhead lighting and add extra lighting as needed. • If designing a garden or outdoor space for older adults, keep in mind that garden beds or tabletops should be no wider than three feet to limit unnecessary reaching. • Fragrant plants should be planted apart, to promote distinct areas of smell. • Consider adding wind chimes, a water feature, and other noise-making devices to the outdoor space to promote each client's ability to orient to the space by listening. • Incorporate high visual contrast in the outdoor environment and with tools whenever possible. Examples include painting tool handles, fences, and work surface edges a light color, in contrast to the soil or background. • Store tools and materials in the same spot in a standardized way, such as placing them in a bucket or hanging them on a wall. • When providing written material, ensure it is printed in at least 14-point sans serif font and in a high-contrast color pairing, such as black or deep blue text on a white background.

Decreased sensation in fingers and/or toes	
Diabetes and peripheral neuropathy—experienced by 27% of older adults Peripheral neuropathy is also a consequence of some forms of chemotherapy (Padro-Guzman 2022)	To address decreased sensation: • Provide tools with textured surfaces. • Provide extra supervision when working with sharp equipment. • Encourage clients to use both hands when possible (Loveland 2017). • Encourage clients to wear protective gloves when possible and to check their hands for cuts or other injuries frequently (Loveland 2017). • When engaging in fine motor tasks and if clients are frustrated, encourage them to ask for help and/or use adapted tools. • Consider implementing above precautions related to decreased balance (Padro-Guzman 2022).
Diminished motivation to participate in group activities	
Depression—experienced by 14% of older adults	Accept, without judgment, a client's current level of participation and honor their physical presence as participation. The client's physical presence is a form of "being" and may be exactly what a client experiencing depression needs at that time. If you are worried about meeting your program's initiatives or outcome measures, consider making one of the program's initiatives to provide a space for clients to "be" (Rebeiro 2001, p.82).
Mild memory challenges	
Mild cognitive impairment—experienced by 10–20% of older adults (Langa and Levine 2014)	To address mild cognitive impairment: • Promote each client's ability to use tools correctly, by storing them in containers with clearly marked labels and simple descriptions. For example: "pens—tools to write on paper" and "trowels—tools used for digging dirt." • Promote each client's ability to participate as autonomously as possible in the face of organizational or memory challenges by providing consistent routines and visual cues. Consider posting an agenda for each session. Clients with memory challenges may learn to rely on visual aids instead of having to ask for directions for each task (Giles 2017).

THIS MUCH I KNOW—LORENE

I am going to send you the information you need, but first I am going to take a loop through the park so I can get some more energy.

Therapeutic Benefits of Nature: Older Adults

The benefits of nature-based interventions for older adults have been well documented and include physical and functional health improvements (Demark-Wahnefried *et al.* 2018; Han and Wang 2018; Ng *et al.* 2018; Park *et al.* 2016; Yao and Chen 2017), mood boosts and reduced stress (Han and Wang 2018; Hawkins *et al.* 2013), improved cognition (Park *et al.* 2016), and social inclusion (Hawkins *et al.* 2013; Ng *et al.* 2018; Park *et al.* 2016; Park, Shoemaker, and Haub 2008; Tse 2010). And although there are myriad studies that support the cognitive, physical, and social health benefits of nature, the bulk of evidence supporting nature-based interventions with older adults is often related to improved mental health and framed toward the achievement of wellness or improved life satisfaction (Tse 2010; Wiseman and Sadlo 2015). Regardless of whether goals are related to physical, cognitive, or emotional function, when preparing for therapy outdoors or an indoor nature-based therapy program with older adults, some of the best practices connect both the content of the programming and how the program is facilitated.

CASE NARRATIVE: Mood Walks

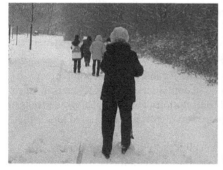

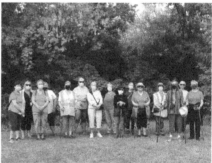

WALKING IS IMPORTANT IN ALL WEATHER AND POSSIBLE WITH THE RIGHT GEAR

THE GROUP GATHERS FOR AN EARLY SUMMER WALK

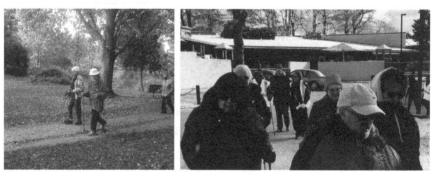

AUTUMNAL WALK

BUNDLED UP AND READY TO WALK

Photo credits: Mood Walks

Thank you to the Canadian Mental Health Association, Ontario Division, for their help in preparing this case narrative.

Mood Walks (www.moodwalks.ca) started in 2008 to increase capacity within the community mental health system to promote physical activities for people with serious mental illness. The program was relaunched as Mood Walks for adults 50+ in 2014. Today, the program is also open to adolescents, adults, and seniors. Mood Walks is a province-wide initiative that promotes physical activity in nature, or "green exercise," to improve both physical and mental health. The program is led by the Canadian Mental Health Association (CMHA) Ontario, with a mission to "work to improve the lives of all Ontarians through leadership, collaboration, and the continual pursuit of excellence in community-based mental health and addiction services." CMHA Ontario works in partnership with Hike Ontario and Conservation Ontario to provide training and support for community mental health agencies, social service organizations, and other community partners to launch educational hiking programs, connect with local resources, find volunteers, and explore nearby trails and green spaces. Mood Walks is funded by various sources, including grants, corporate partnerships, and local funding. Although CMHA Ontario applies for the funding, they ask community agencies to run the program free to their participants; hence, there is no fee to participate in the program.

The inspiration for developing Mood Walks was based on four factors. They are:

1. Evidence shows benefits of engaging in physical activity in green space for people living with mental illness.
2. Mental health services are shifting toward community-based and recovery-oriented frameworks, and physical activity is recognized as an integral part of service provision.
3. Walking is an engaging physical activity, counteracts many of the barriers experienced by people with mental illness, and is accessible and sustainable.
4. Walking in a group lends itself to socializing, spending time in the community at large, and feeling supported.

With the goals of improving physical and mental health, enhancing sensory integration, providing a platform for education, and improving social and communication skill building, the Mood Walks program is delivered outside on public trails, parks, and green spaces, which are managed by whichever entity own the land (whether it is a Canadian province, city, town, or conservation authority). Community organizations need to complete orientation and training before implementing Mood Walks in their community. Safe Hiker and Certified Hike Leader training is required for the people who may be leading Mood Walks. Mood Walks facilitators are encouraged to know local trails and green spaces that are accessible. One of the primary goals is to lead groups that are inclusive and accessible to everyone.

The program is available for anyone living with mental health issues, their family members and friends, or community members at large. Before the COVID-19 pandemic, 8-12 people comprised a typical group, but during COVID-19, its maximum group size was reduced to 5-6 people to maintain physical distancing. During walks, participants are encouraged to wear comfortable clothing and shoes and have a water bottle. Some agencies provide snacks for their participants. The recommended participation is once a week for a minimum of eight weeks, for 45-90 minutes depending on the group's needs. However, the duration depends on the Mood Walks facilitator and the participants. Mood Walks is often structured as a themed program; some of the themes may focus on personal wellness, posture, trail etiquette, a walking meditation, learning about their community, and so on. Although the program has suggested themes, the schedule is flexible.

Participants are encouraged to set SMART (specific, measurable, achievable, relevant, and time-bound) goals throughout the program to give them a sense of direction and help reach realistic goals that they can implement in their life after the program. To keep the program interesting and challenging, Mood Walks leaders can gradually introduce participants to more difficult trails, reduce the number of breaks per session, or increase/decrease the walking speed and duration.

The pandemic reinforced the importance of social connectedness as part of overall health and wellbeing. Due to the COVID-19 restrictions, many partner agencies needed to shift their model for implementing Mood Walks to include virtual components. For example, one agency went online and encouraged participants to walk on their own and then join a virtual meet up with participants to discuss aspects of mental health, self-care, social isolation, stigma, and other topics.

While Mood Walks staff do not ask participants to disclose specific diagnoses, there are exclusive groups designed for people receiving specific clinical intervention. These groups are generally not open to the public. Therefore, there are both open and closed groups. Open groups offer Mood Walks to the general public within their catchment area. Participants join a group on specific dates, and new members do not typically join until the next cohort begins. CMHA Ontario usually recommends one to three trained staff and volunteers to run a Mood Walk and their roles are to lead, ensure safety, and to keep the group together. While therapists, recreationists, schoolteachers, and mental health workers usually run the programs, volunteers and students are always encouraged to participate in the delivery of the program. Accordingly, the interests and availability of time of staffing personnel become integral parts to maintain the program.

Each community agency networks with its partners to generate program materials to run a Mood Walks program such as posters and fillable flyers provided by CMHA Ontario for interested participants. Agencies also get out the word about their Mood Walks program through use of physical and virtual bulletin boards to share updates and information. Another frequently used tool is inviting people to attend an information session on Mood Walks. There are training costs for facilitators by Hike Ontario, which provides Safe Hiker and Certified Hike Leader training, at a cost of $60 per person. In some cases, there are also transportation expenses and additional expenses associated with printing and courier costs for the marketing materials.

CMHA Ontario is building the evidence for this program, but research on the value of exercise for mental health is widespread. CMHA Ontario has seen anecdotal evidence through participant feedback on Mood Walks specifically. Mental health agencies and partners report that Mood Walks improved staff connection to their clients, including those living with serious mental illness, increased community connections, and strengthened a health-promoting culture within agencies. For example, several therapists expressed that the program helped people with common interests bring them together and create a community, helped people build lasting relationships, and helped people to reflect. One recreationist stated that the program allowed part-icipants to connect four domains of health—physical, cognitive, social, and emotional. Here are just a few quotes from participants that clearly speak to the perceived worth of being part of Mood Walks.

- "It is not how far or how fast you can get there; the program is about you and what is good enough for you."
- "Amazing program—gives you a space to reflect, while enjoying nature."
- "I would recommend it to anyone."
- "People built lasting relationships."
- "Mood Walks is a perfect program to focus on mental health and wellbeing of seniors. The program helps us to connect back to the community once you're retired."

Despite challenges—such as ensuring accessible walking or hiking trails for persons living with disabilities, ensuring participants are supported by adequate numbers of volunteers and staff, weather patterns during planned walks, transportation for participants, staff turnover at host agencies, and having participants consistently available for eight weeks in a row to receive the full benefits of participating in Mood Walks—the benefits of being in nature far outweigh any challenges. CMHA Ontario suggested that others interested in establishing a walking program for individuals with mental illness should allow time and space for participants to come together to build social connections. Social interactions and connections are some of the barriers encountered by people living with mental illness. Through Mood Walks, these barriers are reduced and simpler access to mental health services are available for all. You can find more information about Mood Walks at www.moodwalks.ca.

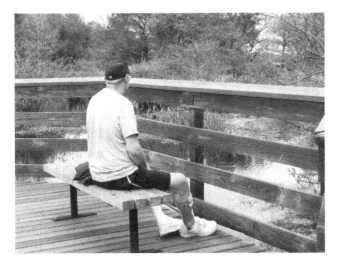

EXPERIENCING SOFT FASCINATION
Photo credit: Amy Wagenfeld

The common factors to interventions that achieved their goals for older adults included physical contact with nature or natural materials, positive interactions with others, and opportunities for responsibility and skill development (Chen and Ji 2015; Detweiler *et al.* 2012; Nicholas, Giang, and Yap 2019; Tse 2010; Yeo *et al.* 2020). A substantial portion of this nature-based literature pertaining to older adults is related to gardening as a modality and intervention. Gardening, an activity based on working with natural materials in synchronicity with nature, is, for some, a very meaningful and familiar activity (Petencin, Diaz, and Kirchen 2016) and should be encouraged. But further consideration is needed for how therapeutic gardening and non-gardening nature-based programs can be developed and introduced to clients to promote more holistic cognitive, physical, social, and mental health outcomes. The body of evidence to support nature-based interventions is rapidly increasing, and we share here just the tip of the iceberg—we hope you feel inspired to dive deeper after reading this book!

CASE NARRATIVE: Rush Oak Park Hospital's Garden Program

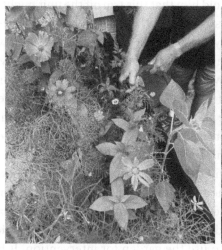

USING A HOSE TO WATER THE RAISED BEDS

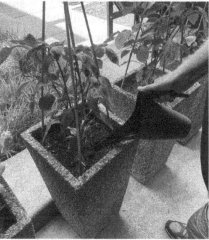

USING A WATERING CAN TO HYDRATE THE VEGETABLES

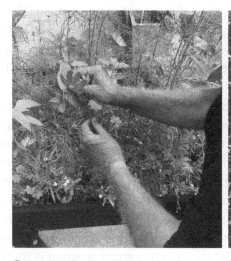

COLLECTING FLOWERS

Photo credits: Ryan Durkin

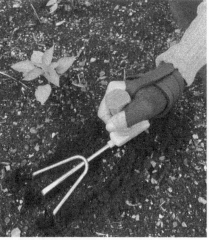

USING AN ADAPTED GARDENING TOOL

Thank you to Ryan Durkin, OTD, OTR/L, MBA, Staff Therapist and Creator of the Rush Oak Park Hospital Garden Program, for his help in preparing this case narrative.

It is often the interesting backstory that explains how the idea for a program germinates. Dr. Durkin shared that when he worked at a different hospital before joining the Rush Oak Park Hospital team, he brought a patient receiving skilled care out to a courtyard in a wheelchair because she told him that she had not been outdoors in several weeks due to her prolonged hospitalization. Once in the courtyard, she told him that this trip off the unit might be the last time she would be outdoors as she knew her health was deteriorating. Dr. Durkin remembers how happy she was to be outside. Her thought was prescient as she passed away during this hospital stay. Her visit outside was, in fact, her last. It was this patient who helped him understand how, for some hospital inpatients, being outdoors is important and meaningful. This patient inspired Dr. Durkin to learn more about and ultimately invest his time and social capital in creating an outdoor treatment experience for this population. At Rush Oak Park Hospital, this inspiration turned to reality.

Therapeutic gardening at Rush Oak Park Hospital in Oak Park, Illinois, started in May 2017 as a supplemental outdoor one-on-one occupational therapy treatment for patients receiving care on the skilled subacute care unit. Over time, disciplines beyond occupational therapy, including physical and recreational therapy, began to use the garden for intervention. It has taken numerous unexpected turns, including closure of the subacute care unit in 2020, but the program prevails. When the program was linked with the skilled subacute care unit, physical therapists brought patients down to the grass portion of the garden to gait train on an uneven surface. The recreational therapist took patients to the garden to join occupational therapy sessions providing they could participate without physical assistance. This linked service enabled group sessions.

Aligning with the Rush Healthcare system mission "to improve the health of the individuals and diverse communities we serve through the integration of outstanding patient care, education, research, and community partnerships," the therapeutic garden program represents a perfect fit for the mission. The intention of the therapeutic garden program is to provide physical and mental health treatment and education for adults and older adults. The program is open enrollment and typically facilitated one-on-one or in groups of no more than three patients and one therapist. During occupational therapy evaluations, information about the therapeutic garden program is shared with patients as an option for where therapy can be provided. Dr. Durkin also presented hospital in-services to other therapists to build awareness of the value of providing therapy outside and the option to do so in the newly installed garden on the hospital campus.

Located on the private grounds of the hospital, the roughly 700-square-foot garden was designed by Dr. Durkin in partnership with the hospital's facilities team who assembled the raised gardening beds, bench, and patio table on the site. The site was selected for numerous reasons. It is located close to a hospital entrance, ideal in case emergencies occur and for inspiration. It had both adequate sunlight for perennial plants to thrive and an existing shade cover for seating, tabletop work, taking rest breaks on warm days, and protection from rain. There were existing, level, concrete walkways to allow patients who use wheelchairs and rolling walkers to safely navigate to the raised gardening beds. The site is also near a water supply, which is a key maintenance factor.

While the major garden care tasks such as mowing and path maintenance are carried out by the facilities team, Dr. Durkin and patients helped with the initial plant installation and continue to assist with ongoing plant maintenance. Shortly before the skilled subacute care unit closed in 2020, a level, grass walking path around native perennial plant beds was installed in a plot of land adjacent to the garden, thus increasing the scope, size, and rehabilitation potential of the garden. Although inpatient-unit patients no longer use the garden, it is now seeing new life with outpatients receiving therapy outside, thereby adapting itself to the ever-changing landscape of healthcare.

Equipment needed for getting the program up and running included hand garden tools such as trowels and cultivators, disposable gloves, a hose and storage box, watering cans, vegetable and flower seeds, pruning shears, bags to gather produce, tomato cages, soil, an off-the-shelf bench, and gardening beds. The smaller items are stored in bags and brought to and from the garden for each session. The hose/storage box and tomato cages are stored inside in a closet in the winter months. The total cost for these items was approximately $1500. Later, a wheelchair-accessible patio table was added to the garden at a cost of $500. Dr. Durkin was responsible for researching and purchasing all items with funding provided by the hospital. Ongoing annual costs are about $150 to purchase soil, organic fertilizer, seeds, and seedlings, and replace tools.

Used in the spring and summer, there are numerous opportunities for therapeutic intervention in the garden. Endurance, fine and gross motor control, strength, balance, use of energy conservation and joint protection principles, and cognition are all addressed by activities such as picking flowers and making floral arrangements, picking vegetables and washing them, pruning, deadheading, and watering plants, planting transplants and seeds, locating plants, and smelling plants. Most of the therapeutic activities at Rush Oak Park Hospital's Garden Program can be done seated versus standing to address energy conservation and joint protection. Watering cans are filled with varying amounts of water to modify challenge. Verbal and visual cueing is upgraded and downgraded during cognitive plant locating tasks. Balance is challenged by placing one hand on the raised gardening bed to working towards no hands while pruning and watering. The garden's location, close to a parking lot for outpatients, has provided an unexpected benefit—a cheering team. Quite often, hospital outpatients going in and out of the hospital offer words of encouragement to patients working on endurance and balance in the garden, telling them, "You can do it" and "You keep going," but Dr. Durkin's favorite was "Now that's great healthcare." Right?

While the subacute program, where the intention of the garden originated, is no longer open, the garden remains standing and is slowly being incorporated into Dr. Durkin's new role as an outpatient therapist with many of the same interventions previously stated, as well as others more applicable to outpatients. They include practicing activity modifications for repetitive stress injuries, trialing stress management and relaxation strategies such as meditation, and practicing visual compensation strategies while tending the vegetables.

Dr. Durkin told us that "taking it outside" requires a high level of flexibility, given that there is reduced ability to control variables in an outdoor environment compared to an indoor environment. In his setting, weather and noise are the two main challenges. Rain and extreme heat can limit the opportunity to safely participate in most activities in the garden, so the decision to take it outside during adverse weather conditions must be carefully considered. Occasional construction projects on the hospital grounds increase noise levels, which makes communication difficult with some patients. These challenges do not outweigh the benefits, and Dr. Durkin and other therapists take every safe opportunity they can to take their patients outside for their therapy sessions.

Dr. Durkin believes that being outdoors has unique healing powers and has encountered few patients who do not appreciate being outside for therapy. He once had a patient ask why hospitals do not have more gardens to do therapy in, given the joy she was experiencing doing her own therapy in the garden. Dr. Durkin told her that hopefully one day all hospitals will. His advice is to explore at least one opportunity to bring your treatment outdoors, to start small and expand the possibilities. Doing so might open the door to many other exciting possibilities to expand the scope of your care. Please see www.rush.edu/locations/rush-oak-park-hospital for general information about Rush Oak Park Hospital.

Evidence Specific to Gardening

Due to the popularity and seemingly ubiquitous quality of gardening literature, we provide a brief synthesis of the research specific to the health benefits of gardening with older adults here. Gardening is a popular leisure activity for many older adults (Ashton-Shaeffer and Constant 2006; Park *et al.* 2016). Interventions that engage older adults in gardening and related activities may result in improved physical, psychosocial, and psychological health as well as overall quality of life, cognitive ability, and socialization (Ng *et al.* 2018; Nicholas *et al.* 2019; Park *et al.* 2016; Spano *et al.* 2020; Wang and MacMillan 2013; Wiseman and Sadlo 2015). Additionally, there is some evidence to support the use of gardening to slow cognitive decline among older adults living with Alzheimer's disease (D'Andrea, Batavia, and Sasson 2008).

NUGGET OF NATURE: PRESSED FLOWERS AND LEAVES

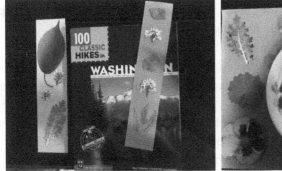 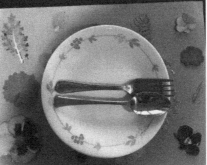

PRESSED FLOWER BOOKMARKS   PRESSED FLOWER PLACEMAT
Photo credits: Amy Wagenfeld

This multi-purpose nature-based activity can invite a conversation about memories, engage fine motor skills, and be facilitated in a group setting or one-on-one.

Materials you will need

- Flat flowers such as pansies, violas, bleeding hearts, chamomile flowers, herbs, and leaves

- Waxed paper
- Large, thick books, such as phone books
- Clear contact paper
- Colored card stock paper and blank note cards and envelopes
- Scissors to cut out bookmark strips
- Glue
- Large zip-top bags or clear plastic containers
- Silicon packets (often included in shoe boxes or bottles of vitamins)

Steps to pressing flowers and leaves

1. Carefully remove the flowers and herb leaves from their stems. Make certain the flowers, herbs, and leaves are dry. Moisture will lead to a moldy mess.
2. Tear off about 18 inches of waxed paper from the roll for each set of flowers or herbs being pressed.
3. Fold the piece of waxed paper in half so that it fits inside the pages of a thick book, such as a phonebook.
4. Open the folded piece of wax paper and open the book about 20 pages from the end.
5. Place the waxed paper inside the open pages of the book.
6. Carefully arrange flowers, herbs, and leaves on one side of the waxed paper, making sure no flowers or leaves touch each other.
7. Fold the waxed paper in half.
8. Carefully close the book.
9. Repeat the process, leaving about 15 book pages between the sheets of pressed flowers.
10. Stack additional books on top of the pressed flower book to weigh it down. The flowers and leaves will be pressed and dry in about two weeks.
11. Carefully remove the sheets of dried flowers and leaves from the book.
12. Store the flowers flat in their wax paper sheets in zip-top bags or plastic containers in a cool, dry place. Inserting several silicon packets into the zip-top bags or containers helps to absorb any residual moisture.
13. The flowers and leaves can be used for many craft projects, such as making bookmarks and stationery. The pressed flowers and leaves will be fragile, so handle them with care.
14. If making bookmarks with the pressed flowers, cover the bookmarks with clear contact paper.

How to make the activity less challenging

- Use smaller sheets of waxed paper and place fewer flowers in each sheet of waxed paper.
- Provide hand-over-hand assistance to help clients select and place dried flowers and leaves on their notecards or bookmarks.
- Precut clear contact paper and provide assistance with applying it to both sides of the bookmark.

How to make the activity more challenging

- Organize the plant materials on the waxed paper by color, size, or shape.
- Plan and prepare a flower and leaf theme or pattern for the bookmark or note card.
- Use tweezers to remove the flowers and leaves from the waxed paper and place them onto the note cards or bookmark strips.

Most recently, during the COVID-19 pandemic, a study based on older adults' self-reports found that time spent in nature was associated with improved perceptions of health. The older adult participants who reported spending more time in their garden, as compared to before the COVID-19 pandemic, also reported better physical health, emotional and mental health, and sleep quality (Corley *et al.* 2021). One of the most exciting results of Corley and colleagues' 2021 survey study is that the improved health benefits were found in older adults who reported actively gardening and also in older adults who used their garden space to simply sit and relax. As a practitioner, this may indicate that in order to harness some of the benefits of nature, the activities we provide need not be directly related to moving dirt or growing plants but can be simply provided out of doors. We are encouraged by these findings, but also hope to encourage you to be curious and look for ways to provide active interventions (Yeo *et al.* 2020).

NUGGETS OF NATURE: SEED TAPES

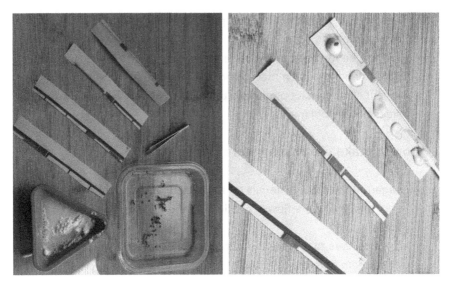

ALL SET UP TO MAKE PARSLEY SEED TAPES   FIRST SEED ADDED TO THE TAPE
Photo credits: Shannon Marder

Making seed tapes is a gardening activity that can be done in any season outdoors or indoors. Seed tapes not only make seed placement simple, but also make planting teeny-tiny seeds a bit more manageable. They are also a cool gift!

Materials you will need

- Newspaper or fairly rigid paper towels
- Scissors
- Mixing bowl(s)
- ¼ cup of flour
- ¼ cup of water
- Ruler
- Paintbrush or cotton swab
- Tweezers
- Pen (marker)
- Plant seeds
- Plastic zip-top bags or plastic containers

Steps to make seed tapes

1. Cut the newspaper (or paper towel) into one inch strips.

2. Make seed-glue by mixing equal parts flour and water in a bowl to make a paste. The consistency will be like ketchup.

3. Apply the seed-glue to the newspaper strips at the appropriate spacing distance using a ruler to measure and a paintbrush or cotton swab for application. Appropriate seed spacing is typically listed on the back of the seed packet or can be found by looking on the internet or contacting a local garden center.

4. Press a seed into each dab of seed-glue, using your fingers or tweezers.

5. Let the seed-glue dry and label the seed tapes with what seeds are glued on the newspaper strips.

6. When done, store the seed tapes in a dry plastic bag or container. The tapes can be folded or rolled.

7. When you are ready to plant them, simply lay them in your growing space on the soil, cover them with the recommended amount of soil (based on seed planting directions), and then water the soil.

How to make the activity less challenging

- Use large seeds such as peas or beans of one variety for each seed tape.
- To reduce the requirements of tool use, apply the seed-glue with fingers.

How to make the activity more challenging

- Choose tiny seeds and use tweezers to pick up the seeds.
- Encourage gardeners to design seed tapes with a variety of seeds, thinking about each plant's colors and heights in mind—being very specific with the patterns they create on the tapes.

Further adaptation

Small seeds can be glued to 1" x 1" newspaper squares to make planting individual seeds easier. This is an easy way to reduce the challenges of planting herb seeds in containers.

Evidence Beyond the Garden

We are well aware that older adults can benefit from nature-based therapy outside of a garden. Therefore, we provide a highlight of the research specific to programming for older adults and a bit of inspirational research as well. There is a very large body of evidence supporting the importance of accessible outdoor spaces and nature-based building designs for older adults, but we do not present that information here (Chang 2020; Cranney *et al.* 2016; Gharaveis 2020; Lee, Lee, and

Rodiek 2020; Xie and Yuan 2022; Yeo *et al.* 2020). Interested readers are encouraged to seek this information by researching literature on therapeutic design.

While not diving into landscape or community design (those are for another book another time), we do want to highlight the importance of access to nature. As previously mentioned, older adults may have more leisure time, which highlights the importance of easily accessible green spaces or nature-based activities (Freeman *et al.* 2019). Though not intervention based, evidence gathered during the COVID-19 pandemic demonstrated that access to and contact with nature was associated with reduced symptoms of depression and anxiety (Pouso *et al.* 2021), and that older adults found benefits, not in large, landscaped parks or grand national parks, but in local and domestic spaces, such as their own yards or within their neighborhoods (Bustamante *et al.* 2022). These findings support previous studies' findings that "as adults age, and as health and other related factors impact, the neighborhood and domestic environments become places where greater amounts of time are spent," and benefits are derived from access to nearby nature that is easily walked to and/ or able to be seen from their home, along with interaction with nature such as caring for plants (Freeman *et al.* 2019, p.25; Gilroy 2008). Interestingly, some older adult participants expressed new-found appreciation for nature, demonstrating that perhaps later in life nature-based experiences can inspire a new and positive relationship with nature (Bustamante *et al.* 2022).

CASE NARRATIVE: Hooves 4 Healing

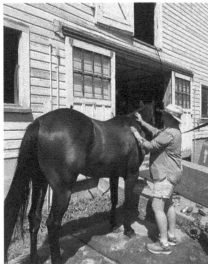
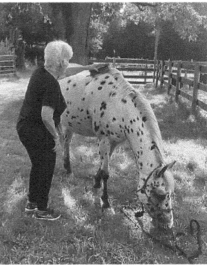

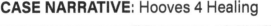

Caring for the horse and the client   Forging connections
Photo credits: Laura Ryan

Thank you to Laura Ryan, OTD, OTR/L, Founder and Lead Clinician of Hooves 4 Healing, for her help to prepare this case narrative.

With its mission of "Providing engaging and evidence-based rehabilitation for individuals with breast cancer using the therapeutic use of the horse and nature," Hooves 4 Healing represents the best of how therapy outside is an effective, meaningful, and motivating alternative to traditional rehabilitation. Located on a private family farm in Holliston, Massachusetts, Hooves 4 Healing is a holistic, wrap-around intervention incorporating the therapeutic use of horses and nature as the rehabilitative vehicles to address physical, cognitive, and psychological vulnerabilities in individuals who currently have breast cancer or had it in the past. Engaging in activities with the horse in an inherently restorative environment creates a cohesive approach to the end goal of the program, which is to return the client to their meaningful occupations.

A lifelong equestrian who has long provided hippotherapy programming for children, Dr. Ryan's motivation for Hooves 4 Healing was fortuitous. She attended a therapeutic horsemanship conference in 2019 and went to a breakout session outlining the latest research on breast cancer rehabilitation that advocated for meaningful activity, versus exercise, as the best approach for rehabilitation. The lecturers presenting the breakout session speculated on the role of the horse in this endeavor. This inspired Dr. Ryan to develop a working outline of a program using horses in meeting the physical, psychological, and cognitive needs of persons with breast cancer. Accordingly, the outcomes and goals for clients in the Hooves 4 Healing program focus on physical and mental health, cognition, and education. Hooves 4 Healing welcomed its first clients in September 2020.

The clients are adults and older adults who either currently have breast cancer or have had breast cancer. All the clients experience, in some capacity, reduced ability to perform meaningful life occupations due to diminished strength, range of motion and/or coordination of the impacted upper extremity, reduced cognition including executive functioning and/or attention, and reduced quality of life due to pain and/or fatigue. Offered as a cohort model for up to four clients at a time, the program runs twice a week for an hour for four weeks (for a total of eight sessions.) Hooves 4 Healing interventions are provided outside on five verdant acres of Dr. Ryan's family farm as well as in the horse barn. The site is maintained by the farm and barn owner where the program is situated. Because of the outdoor component of the program, it is offered ten months a year, with January and February off due to extreme cold, common in New England.

The entire Hooves 4 Healing staff is an interdisciplinary team consisting of an occupational therapist (Dr. Ryan), a physical therapist, a licensed mental health counselor who is trained in the EAGALA (Equine Assisted Growth and Learning Association) method, and a program ambassador (a volunteer role) who is a person who has had breast cancer. All licensed providers and the program ambassador who are involved in this program have experience with horses and all participated in a formal horsemanship program at the beginning of their involvement with Hooves 4 Healing. Clients are referred via physicians, social workers or psychologists, alternative health practitioners, and via word of mouth.

One component of the program involves grooming horses. This portion focuses on physical rehabilitation (increasing range of motion, strength, endurance, and coordination), and can be graded with the type of grooming brush that is used and the size of the horse. For example, a larger horse can be used to facilitate increased range of motion, and a certain brush can be used to facilitate increased strength. This grooming segment also addresses cognition through the sequencing of the specific grooming routine. Using a checklist and providing a grooming bucket that has all the necessary tools are examples of how this activity can be graded either to be more challenging or less so. The checklist can be ticked off by the client or dictated to the physical or occupational therapist. The brushes can be labeled or not, depending on the client's cognitive status. The psychosocial portion of the program involves quiet, self-guided interactions with horses using EGALA principles. The client chooses how long they would like to interact with the horse and how much they would like to process the characteristics of the interactions with the licensed mental health counselor.

The materials needed to run Hooves 4 Healing are, first and foremost, horses obtained through fee for service paid to the horse owner, and barn space, which is included in the horse fee. Other materials include grooming brushes that are acquired by the horse owner and/or the existing barn collection and energy conservation materials developed by Dr. Ryan. The purchase of formal testing materials including the QuickDASH, MMSE-2 and FACIT-F, and the Role Checklist v3 are other examples of materials needed to run the program. The cost for the program is $320 for the horse fee and $1280 for staffing, for a total of $1600. Funding is via fee for service with some costs defrayed through grant funding.

The Hooves 4 Healing program is much loved. Dr. Ryan shared some feedback from three women who participated in the program. One client commented on how relaxed and content she was after grooming a horse. She liked how she could move at her own pace; when she paused because she was tired, she could still interact with the horse, which made her feel that the quiet times during the program were still therapeutic. Another client commented on how refreshing it was to be outside (instead of in) a clinic. This woman liked feeling the breeze and the quietness of the environment. One client was too weak to hold a grooming brush and started just by patting the horse. She felt that the warmth of horses was therapeutic to her and that patting the horse gave her motivation to continue using her arm, thereby making it stronger! Nature is a powerful healer.

There are, of course, challenges associated with running a program like Hooves 4 Healing, but the benefits far outweigh any challenges. As Dr. Ryan noted above, providing your therapy in an outside setting provides added, greater benefits to enhanced cognition and mental wellbeing than providing that same therapy indoors. As you now know from the research that has been shared throughout the book, nature heals. Dr. Ryan took a great deal of inspiration from an experimental research study (Cimprich and Ronis 2003) whose results showed that just 20 minutes of interaction with nature had a significant impact on the clients' capacity to attend and focus. Therefore, providing a therapeutic intervention out of doors versus indoors can be inherently more impactful without having to alter the length of a session or an increase in the cost of providing a lengthy intervention. Dr. Ryan goes on to share that, in New England, a challenge to providing therapy outside is the unpredictability of the weather and the long and sometimes harsh winters. However, applying the principles of attention restoration theory, which we discussed in Chapter 3, inclement and colder weather have therapeutic properties as well. Being outside in the cold can be invigorating and can provide stronger proprioceptive input to the joints due to the contraction of muscles. However, another challenge could be the unpredictability of the outdoor environment. For example, for someone with reduced balance, navigating uneven ground or a tree branch in their path may be too much of a challenge. There is much to think about and much to be positive about when therapy is provided outdoors.

Dr. Ryan has some sage advice. She told us:

Take your practice outside whenever you can! Nature is an incredible healing medium. Practicing outside does not add to the cost of therapy and it is readily accessible. Even short interactions with nature and the outdoors have big impacts on cognition and mood so your interventions do not need to be long and/or robust.

We agree—just go outside!

Reference

Cimprich, B. and Ronis, D.L. (2003) 'An environmental intervention to restore attention in women with newly diagnosed breast cancer.' *Cancer Nursing 26*, 4, 284–292.

The evidence we share here is meant to inspire you to provide an active nature-based intervention with older adults. Some of our favorite examples of active nature-based interventions, outside of gardens and farming activities, include nature-based art projects (Sia *et al.* 2020), listening to birds (Lee *et al.* 2022), and walking (Salbach *et al.* 2019). Sia and colleagues (2020), as part of a larger 24-week study, provided 12 nature-based art projects; they found that after the intervention, the older adult participants experienced improved wellbeing and reduced anxiety. In addition to longer-term results, measured after the six-month intervention, each week the participants reported feeling happier after the session. Although we likely cannot bill for improved happiness on its own, we can feel a little happier ourselves knowing that nature can add a bit of happiness to our world.

When we think of active interventions, we imagine physical movement and modifying our physical environment, but there is also a need to provide older adults with opportunities to be mentally and socially active. K. Lee and colleagues' (2022) study, "Bird Tales," demonstrated a novel, informal approach to helping older adults in residential care find meaning in their lives. The study was conducted through a participatory action research framework at an assisted living facility. Please see the case narrative below to learn more about the Bird Tales program. With a small sample size, they found promising qualitative results; the older adult participants reported that the intervention was "cognitively stimulating," promoted positive social interactions, helped them feel connected to their past, and promoted "positive perceptions of birds and nature" (p.7). Lee and colleagues concluded the article with inspiring insight from their focus groups: although not all older adults like birds, there is strong support that they appreciate nature and that the changes observed were well supported by the biophilia hypothesis.

CASE NARRATIVE: Bird Tales

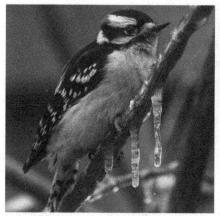

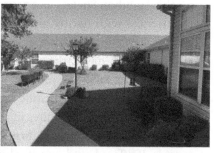

A VIEW OF BIRDS AND GARDENS FROM
INSIDE AND OUTSIDE INCREASES THE
NATURE QUOTIENT FOR OLDER ADULTS
Photo credit: Kathy Lee

A DOWNY WOODPECKER
Photo credit: Joshua Cotton via Unsplash

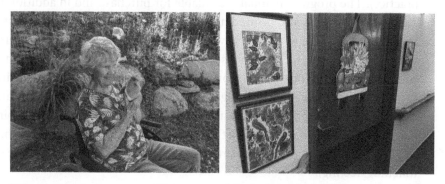

SPIRITED CONVERSATIONS INSPIRED
BY BIRD TALES
Photo credit: Shannon Marder

BIRD THEMES CAN EXTEND
BEYOND INTERVENTION
Photo credit: Kathy Lee

Thank you to Kathy Lee, PhD, LMSW, Assistant Professor at the University of Texas at Arlington School of Social Work, and Jessica Cassidy, LWSW, PhD student at the University of Texas at Arlington School of Social Work, for their help in preparing this case narrative.

Many older adults living in long-term care facilities tend to be inactive, which further contributes to adverse health outcomes, such as depression and anxiety (Schölzel-Dorenbos, Meeuwsen, and Olde Rikkert 2010). In addition, older adults, particularly those residing in long-term care facilities, are likely to be disconnected from nature and can benefit from the multisensory experiences offered through nature (Yeo *et al.* 2020). Bird Tales was developed for the Audubon Society as a program to offer opportunities for meaningful experiences with nature and to facilitate social engagement among older adults with dementia (Bryce 2013; Griffin and Elkins 2013). Designed for older adults at adult day-care centers or living in long-term care facilities (e.g., assisted living facilities and nursing homes), Bird Tales is an indoor group-based activity, though it could easily be implemented outdoors if needed/desired. The program requires minimal space, just enough for the participants to sit in a circle. Because of its flexibility, it can be run year-round, inside or outside. If offered outdoors, it is highly recommended that the outdoor space has a roof or other shade structures and comfortable seating areas, and is wheelchair accessible.

The information in the Bird Tales manual is adaptable to provide a varying number of activities, but, depending on the availability of staffing, time, and resources, it can be provided on a weekly or monthly basis for 40–50 minutes per session (the session's duration is dependent on the facility's general practice). The program manual is available for purchase and in addition to activity instructions and printed materials, includes recommendations for how to attract birds to a facility (www.healthpropress.com/product/bird-tales). Programming focuses on discussions around a specific bird, and each session includes educational information, trivia, and fun facts regarding the selected bird. Participants engage throughout each session by sharing memories and songs, and discussing their perceptions related to the bird concerned. When an ornithologist facilitates or assists with the program, a live bird can be brought to the participants for additional experiences (e.g., touching, feeling).

Dr. Lee and Ms. Cassidy facilitated Bird Tales as part of a 2019 research study in North Texas close to the University of Texas at Arlington's campus. The goals and outcomes of the research were to improve mental health, sensory regulation, and engagement in activity, and to provide an engaging and meaningful way for older adults to reminisce and socialize. Recognizing that as a meaningful, nature-based activity, Bird Tales could improve the health and wellbeing of older adults in long-term care facilities, Dr. Lee and Ms. Cassidy adapted the program and examined its impact on older adults with mild cognitive impairment living in residential care. They also focused on replicating the program from non-conservation experts' perspectives.

Dr. Lee and Ms. Cassidy delivered the six-week program, covering six different birds, in an 8 x 16-foot sunroom. The residents had an opportunity to look, listen, feel, and learn more about each bird. The typical Bird Tales session included:

- a warm-up story, indicating features of the bird's eyes, feathers, the respective bird song
- identification of the bird of the week through use of printed activity cards
- learning about the feathers and eggs of the bird of the week
- watching a video of the featured bird
- doing an activity, e.g., bird feeders and food (filling the bird feeder).

For Dr. Lee and Ms. Cassidy's research project, they initially recruited 14 of the 35 residents in the assisted living facility. However, the participants had to pass Callahan's Six-Item Screener (Callahan *et al.* 2002), which helps identify the presence of moderate or severe cognitive impairment. This was important because residents provided consent for participating in the study and were queried about depression, stress, positive and negative affect, and life satisfaction as part of the research process. As a result of the screening, 12 people were eligible for the study and completed the program. Participants were divided into two equal groups of six members. The group who did not participate in the Bird Tales program received services at the facility as usual. The research team's small-group model aligned with the Bird Tales programming model. In line with typical program scheduling at assisted living facilities, each Bird Tales research session met once weekly for approximately 40 minutes for six weeks.

Programming can be custom-tailored, and typical activities include touching bird models, listening to birds through video or audio, learning about birds using activity cards, and talking about birds in a group setting. The materials used in the research study included:

- eggs
- feathers
- plush birds (stuffed animals) that when squeezed make the particular bird song (can be purchased in discount stores and online)
- bird houses
- bird seed
- laptop and large screen, for viewing livestream footage of birds
- speakers to play songs (e.g., "Rockin' Robin" by Bobby Day released 1958, "Blackbird" by the Beatles released in 1968, "Mockingbird" by Dusty Springfield released in 1964).

All these materials can easily be stored in a small space.

While the Bird Tales program can be provided by one person, for the purposes of this research project, a trained gerontological social work intern facilitated the program under the Principal Investigator's (Dr. Lee) supervision and with assistance from Ms. Cassidy. Prior to beginning their study, the research team met virtually with one of the creators of Bird Tales (Mr. Ken Elkins) to discuss the research and made a site visit to an assisted living facility that was delivering Bird Tales once a month. Interestingly, this program was being facilitated by an ornithologist. As a future project, partnering with a local chapter of the Audubon Society and involving ornithologists, if available or desired, might be considered.

In terms of site selection for the research, initially Dr. Lee and Ms. Cassidy reached out to the marketing team of a large U.S. senior living corporation and explained the purpose and goals of the Bird Tales program and their research project. From this meeting, the marketing team directed the researchers to a local assisted living facility near the university and facilitated introductions, meetings, and scheduling arrangements. The startup costs for the research program were salary for the student interns paid through University of Texas at Arlington funds ($4500) and program materials ($500). Startup program materials included the Bird Tales program manual, eggs, feathers, plush bird toys, bird feeders, and bird food. After the research project concluded, the plush birds were gifted to the residents. Note that these can be sanitized and reused with other residents.

On an exciting note, the outcomes of the study have been published in the journal *Clinical Gerontologist*. The citation can be found in the references list below. To explore the participants' overall experiences with the program, they conducted individual, semi-structured interviews. Each interview was about 30 minutes long, audio-recorded, and transcribed by a professional company. Some of the findings showed that the participants perceived Bird Tales as a cognitively stimulating activity, enjoyed interacting with other residents in a group, were able to connect themselves to past experiences, and enjoyed this program because of their positive perceptions of birds and nature. Below are some of the comments that participants shared during the post-program interviews. One participant said, "I've enjoyed it. It got my mind off other things. Well...pleasant, informative, and getting your mind off of yourself [and] onto something else." Another told the researcher, "I love the way he [another participant] brings up something; he has such a good memory and brings up things in the past and everything. Mhmm. And I like to hear about other people's experiences with birds and I love birds." One woman said, "Well, just because for some reason I don't think about it [the past] much, I guess, since my husband's gone and... [the program] more connected to my past." And finally:

> Well, living in the city, there are not too many of those around. Maybe just a little backyard bird would become a part of your life and care about what's in his domain. That is a golden point right there, so we must be aware of it.

Extensive quotes, including those above, can be found in the published article.

Programming of any sort goes much more smoothly when there are well-prepared materials, content, and questions. The research team created a lesson plan for each session and made sure to have an abundance of content prepared in the event some information was not interesting to the participants. One of the lesson plans is included at the end of this case study. In an effort to emphasize spiritual connections to birds, the research team searched for stories and folklore. This is one way not only to honor the history of the outdoors where a current nature-based program takes place, but also to exemplify concepts of diversity, equity, justice, and inclusion as discussed in Chapter 3. Birds were often referenced in relation to the participants' previous life experiences; therefore, effort was made to include biographical and cultural references to songs or books that included the bird of the week. The facilitator also shared short clips of videos, such as an excerpt from a Woody Woodpecker cartoon, and sang or played a song each week that was related to the topic bird.

The facilitator supplemented the programming with a live stream of birds feeding, which played throughout the duration of the activity. This live stream is available at no cost through Cornell [University] Lab of Ornithology (www.allaboutbirds.org/cams). This adaptation was helpful in two ways. The program was delivered indoors and, in doing so, mitigated the participants' cognitive limitations related to difficulty paying attention to materials or following lengthy discussions. In keeping with the intention of this program, it was also important for the research team to consider and promote the multisensory nature of the materials—encouraging touching the plush birds, listening to sounds, looking at the eggs, stroking bird feathers, and watching the live feed, to name just a few.

The research team shared that the key benefits of the Bird Tales program included the ease with which the program was delivered and the amount of interest and enthusiasm many participants demonstrated almost immediately. Be prepared to laugh and learn information about birds you never knew! Dr. Lee and Ms. Cassidy's participants had a lot of information to share, including songs their research team had never heard before. The challenges of this program can be related to ensuring everyone has an opportunity to participate as some older adults may be bird enthusiasts and contribute more to discussions than those with less experience. Activity facilitators can reduce this challenge by directing questions and comments directly to participants who may not otherwise voluntarily contribute to the discussion.

And, as a last bit of advice, from Dr. Lee and Ms. Cassidy's experience, carefully consider the space to be used for the program as many older adults may have mobility and visual-perceptual challenges. Think about the layout of the space. For example, arrange chairs in a way that allows participants using wheelchairs to easily have access to joining, participating in, and exiting the group. The research team achieved this by arranging chairs in a half-moon shape and leaving spaces for wheelchairs.

Bird Tales is an excellent example of an accessible, easy-to-facilitate nature-based program that does not require a large or elaborate indoor or outdoor space, but still provides the health benefits of nature in its implementation. It exemplifies how nature can be the focus of an intervention without our having to be in it. Bird Tales shows us how programs can "sing" even when we are inside, reaping the benefits of nature.

Research article

Lee, K., Cassidy, J., Tang, W., and Kusek, V. (2022) 'Older adults' responses to a meaningful activity using indoor-based nature experiences: Bird Tales.' *Clinical Gerontologist 45*, 2, 301–311.

References

Bryce, E. (2013) 'Happy memories: The healing power of birds.' National Audubon Society May–June. Accessed on 2/12/22 at www.audubon.org/magazine/may-june-2013/the-healing-power-birds

Callahan, C.M., Unverzagt, F.W., Hui, S.L., Perkins, A.J., and Hendrie, H.C. (2002) 'Six-item screener to identify cognitive impairment among potential subjects for clinical research.' *Medical Care 40*, 9, 771–781.

Griffin, R. and Elkins, K. (2013) *Bird Tales*. Towson, MD: Health Professions Press. www.healthpropress.com/product/bird-tales

Schölzel-Dorenbos, C.J., Meeuwsen, E.J., and Olde Rikkert, M.G. (2010) 'Integrating unmet needs into dementia health-related quality of life research and care: Introduction of the Hierarchy Model of Needs in Dementia.' *Aging and Mental Health 14*, 1, 113–119.

Yeo, N.L., Elliott, L.R., Bethel, A., White, M.P., Dean, S.G., and Garside, R. (2020) 'Indoor nature interventions for health and wellbeing of older adults in residential settings: A systematic review.' *The Gerontologist 60*, 3, e184–e199.

Intended Curriculum and Lesson Plan
Feathered Friends—Lesson Plan: Downy Woodpecker

[*Italicized font text* is provided as a potential script for the facilitator.]

Materials

- Plush woodpeckers (3)

- Plush animals from previous weeks (e.g., cardinal, blue jay, robin, mockingbird)
- Woodpecker eggs
- Woodpecker ID card
- Egg ID card
- Laptop for video, connected to a large screen for easy viewing
- Speaker for sound

Time: 40 minutes

Welcome!

Greet all participants by name and remind participants of your name.

Before the bird of the week is introduced say: *This week we will be learning all about the downy woodpecker. But before we start talking about our new feathered friend, let's not forget our friends from the past few weeks...*

Spend the next few minutes reviewing previous weeks' birds and passing around respective plush birds. As each bird is being passed around, ask participants questions regarding that bird from the past lessons.

A warm-up story

Now let's learn about our bird of the week, the downy woodpecker.

Pass around the plush downy woodpecker bird.

Look: Invite participants to look at the color patterns.

Let's look at the downy woodpecker. The tail, wings, and back of the downy woodpecker have a black hue intermingled with white spots. A black cap adorns each, below which there is a white stripe. A small scarlet patch appears on the lower-back of the head. Another black stripe is below this. The downies have barred outer tail feathers not found on other birds. The tail feathers help them anchor to a tree.

Listen: *Let's listen to the downy woodpecker. As you're holding it, you may squeeze it to hear its song.* Squeeze a plush bird and have participants listen to the birds as they are passed around. *This bird uses an instrument to make noises! His drumming sound is not always looking for food: it's a way of communicating.*

> Q1: *Have you heard this sound before? Was it a woodpecker or maybe a hammer? How would you know the difference?*

After the discussion of the woodpecker's sounds, you could consider playing a short soundtrack on video to show other sounds besides drumming (www.allaboutbirds.org/guide/Downy_Woodpecker/sounds). And you could play a YouTube video of the downy woodpecker (e.g., www.youtube.com/watch?v=vuAOc6l9jhA).

Continue with further discussion by asking participants about their experience with woodpeckers, if any:

Q1: *Did you see woodpeckers growing up?*
Q2: *When was the last time you saw a woodpecker?*
Q3: *Do you like them? Why? Why not?*
Q4: *Can you think of any memories you have had with woodpeckers?*
Q5: *Have you seen any woodpeckers near where we are now? When we put the suet feeders out, they might come visit.*

Identification of the bird of the week through use of printed activity cards

Spend time exploring the woodpecker and explaining more details (see program fact sheet). Woodpeckers are known for banging on things. But they are also known as carpenters, creating apartment buildings for other forest animals!

Q1: *Do you know of anyone who reminds you of a woodpecker?*
Q2: *Have you ever worked as a carpenter? Do you know anyone who did?*
Q3: *What other types of jobs would a woodpecker do?*

Trivia: Alright, let's dive into some trivia!

Q1: *Why do woodpeckers have a different tail from other birds?*
A: They use their feathers to support them as they lean on the tree and climb it.

Q2: *Woodpeckers have extremely large . . . . ?*
A: Tongues they use to forage for insects in the tree.

Q3: *What are the three reasons woodpeckers peck on trees?*
A: To get food, to make cavities, and to claim their territories.

Q4: *What is the number-one reason woodpeckers peck?*
A: They peck for communication and even have their own language.

Q5: *Can you guess what woodpeckers are known for with the Native Americans in the U.S.?*
A: Life and spiritual energy. Woodpeckers drumming is associated with the "heartbeat" of nature itself. For Native Americans, this incredible

bird embodies the concept of life, connection with Mother Earth, and an everlasting energy that flows through all living things. The woodpecker's characteristic noise is identified with the pulse of the Earth.

Q6: *Do you know any famous woodpeckers?*

A: Woody Woodpecker. Woody was created in 1940 by Walter Lantz and storyboard artist Ben "Bugs" Hardaway, who had previously laid the groundwork for two other screwball characters, Bugs Bunny and Daffy Duck, at the Warner Bros. cartoon studio in the late 1930s. The inspiration for the character came during the producer's honeymoon with his wife, in June Lake, California. A noisy acorn woodpecker outside their cabin kept the couple awake at night, and when a heavy rain started, they learned that the bird had bored holes in their cabin's roof. As both Walter and Gracie said during a visit, Walter wanted to shoot the bird, but Gracie suggested that her husband make a cartoon about it, and thus Woody was born. Share the Woody the Woodpecker video (www.youtube.com/watch?v=RnpZpAPaLew).

Questions to prompt further discussion

Q1: *Woody Woodpecker came out in the 1940s. Do you remember what you were doing at that time?*

Q2: *What can you share about your experiences during the 1940s?*

Q3: *Do you remember hearing/watching this show? What did you think of it when you were a child?*

Continue to share information from bird fact cards and any additional information about the downy woodpecker relevant to your group.

Let's learn more about the downy woodpecker and look at these bird fact cards.

- *The downy woodpecker eats foods that larger woodpeckers cannot reach, such as insects living on or in the stems of weeds.*
- *Male and female downy woodpeckers divide up where they look for food in winter. Males feed more on small branches and weed stems, and the females feed on larger branches and trunks.*
- *Downy woodpeckers eat mainly insects, including beetle larvae that live inside wood or tree bark, as well as ants and caterpillars.*

Learning about the feathers and eggs of the bird of the week—Study bird eggs

Now let's study the downy woodpecker's eggs. Pass around the eggs and show a bird egg diagram and explain the different parts. Other facts about bird eggs:

- *All bird eggs are amniotic, which means they include a hard shell, a porous internal membrane for the exchange of oxygen and carbon dioxide, and a rich yolk that nourishes the developing chick. The yolk is made of fat and protein, and the yolk color varies depending on the quality of the laying female's diet.*
- *Eggs come in many different shapes. Budgerigars and many owls lay round or spherical eggs, but oval-shaped eggs are the most common.*
- *The colors of wild bird eggs range from plain white to a rainbow of hues such as blue, green, ivory, tan, beige, gray, red, and orange.*
- *The thickness of eggshells varies but must be thick and strong enough to support a brooding adult and the growth of the developing chick. The shell cannot be so thick, however, that the hatching chick cannot peck its way out.*
- *Because eggs are so rich in protein, fat, and nutrients, they are highly coveted sources of food for many predators. Squirrels, rats, reptiles, cats, snakes, raccoons, and many other predators will eat eggs.*

If there is time, watch this video on eggs: www.youtube.com/watch?v=-Ah-gTohTto.

Q1: *What do you think of when you see how an egg is made?*
Q2: *Did you grow up in a place where you experienced fresh eggs?*
Q3: *What have you cooked with eggs?*
Q4: *Have you ever seen a baby bird? Do they remind you of baby humans? What is it that is the same? What is the difference?*

Doing an activity—Fill bird feeder

Before we end our meeting today, let's fill the bird feeder. Give residents a chance to look at and touch the seed. If a resident is interested in filling the feeder, allow them the opportunity, otherwise designate a facilitator or volunteer to fill the feeder and hang it outside.

"Dismiss class" and remind residents to look for birds outside at the feeder!

Although no results have been published yet, we wanted to share information about a program designed for older adults living in urban areas who have difficulty walking outdoors. The task-oriented group is focused on outdoor walking training and consists of a one-day educational workshop followed by ten weekly sessions. The program is designed to increase the older adults' outdoor walking activity as well as improve their self-reports of physical activity, "emotional health, balance, leg strength, walking self-efficacy, walking speed, walking endurance, heart rate (HR) and blood pressure (BP)" (Salbach *et al.* 2019, p.2). The article clearly lays out what the education session covers and the weekly session plans, as well as a process evaluation plan to ensure the program is delivered correctly. If you are looking for a blueprint to lead an outdoor walking program, Salbach and colleagues' protocol is very helpful.

We would be remiss if we did not address a piece of literature related to nature-based interventions for older adults with dementia. There is a growing body of evidence related to addressing health needs via nature-based interventions with older adults living with dementia, and we encourage you to dig deeper if that is your field of work. Here, we provide a summary of what we consider one of the most useful studies regarding what older adults with dementia find meaningful in nature-based interventions.

Hendriks and colleagues (2016) found—through semi-structured interviews with older adults living with dementia, healthcare professionals, and volunteers who work with older adults living with dementia—that the most meaningful aspects of nature-based interventions are "pleasure, relaxation, feeling fit, enjoying the beauty of nature, feeling free, the social aspect of nature, feeling useful, and [connecting the experience to] memories" (p.1458). From those themes, they developed a client-centered questionnaire, with eight questions, which they used to guide follow-on interviews and activity designs (p.1460). The follow-up interviews, using the questionnaire, found that participants appreciated a wide variety of activities—active, passive, social, outside, and inside—"like walking, cycling, swimming...sitting outside, watching, and talking about nature...drinking coffee outside with family and friends...gardening, and inside nature activities, like watching a film about nature or handicraft with flowers" (pp.1458–1459). As an initial result, Hendriks and colleagues designed three activities: a walking group, a gardening group, and a sensory stimulation activity.

After further interviewing healthcare professionals regarding feasibility and then implementing the walking and gardening groups at various sites, they found the most important aspects of program implementation to be "preparation, guidance, location, weather, material, duration, group conditions, and cultural aspects of the organization" (Hendriks *et al.* 2016, p.1462). Facilitator preparation was the most important aspect and affected everything else. See Table 8.2 for examples of facilitator's preparation.

NUGGET OF NATURE: LEARN MORE ABOUT ANTI-AGEIST PRACTICES

Please see the Appendix for a guide to setting up your outdoor practice. A few steps specific to programming for older adults include learning about ageism before the program is designed, and delivered and incorporating actions throughout programming that will minimize ageist practices. Consider looking into free resources online, like the Old School Anti-Ageism Clearinghouse, which has a treasure trove of anti-ageism education materials (Applewhite *et al.* 2018).

Table 8.2 Examples of facilitator preparation, based on recommendations from Hendriks and colleagues (2016)

What facilitators should consider	Examples of the considerations
Meeting with stakeholders prior to the start of programming	Meeting with facility/organizational leadership to confirm programming location delivery and establish a backup location
	Meet with facility/organizational leadership to ensure sufficient personnel/staff support
	Meet with facility's maintenance team to promote communication
Study to have sufficient nature-based knowledge	Names of flowers, plants, and native birds
	Names of trees on a walk
	Gardening techniques
Knowledge of space: choose an ideal location	Names of places
	Appropriately sunny spot for gardening
	Sufficient shade to rest
Backup plans	In the event of inclement weather
	Different or fewer staff than anticipated
	Knowledge of emergency plans
	In the event participant reacts adversely
Client-centered materials, plans, and practices	Appropriately sized seeds for planting
	Adapted tools as needed
	Plan activities for an appropriate duration based on participant's needs and preferences
	Changing the activity as needed in the moment to meet the client where they are

CASE NARRATIVE: Mountain States Hand and Physical Therapy

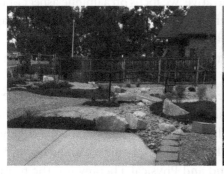

STRENGTH AND STABILITY TERRAIN
PARK AND BALANCE CENTER

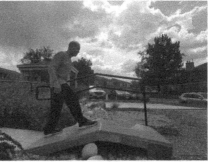

TAKING ON A BALANCE CHALLENGE
IN THE "REAL WORLD"

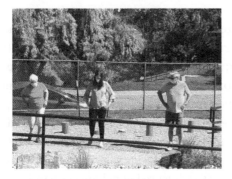

A PHYSICAL THERAPIST–LED
SMALL-GROUP BALANCE CLASS
Photo credits: Mountain States Therapy

Thank you to Pam Bohling, PT, OCS, MHS, Clinic Manager and Part-Owner, for her help preparing this case narrative.

Mountain States Hand and Physical Therapy is a clinical practice where physical, speech, and occupational therapy are provided in an environment of compassion and respect for individualized goals and lifestyles. It has a highly trained staff, many of whom have specialty certifications in orthopedic clinical specialization and hand therapy, vestibular rehabilitation, and the Lee Silverman Voice Treatment—LSVT BIG (motor focus) and LSVT LOUD (speech and language focus). Having therapists with this range of specialty certification offers an integrative approach with all three services to streamline treatment and communication between providers. Specialized and effective treatment supports each patient to meet functional goals and return to living. One of Mountain State Therapy's specialized services is the balance center, which focuses on patients at risk for falls due to injury, balance, and/ or vestibular issues. In this case narrative, we focus on a unique aspect of the balance center program that began in 2020: the Mountain States Therapy Strength and Stability Terrain Park and Balance Center ("terrain park"). As you will read, the terrain park exemplifies how a therapy clinic can expand and blend its services, outside.

Why is "taking it outside" for therapy important to consider when addressing balance and vestibular concerns? Real life. The terrain park allows patients to practice mobility in real-life conditions and on terrains such as sand, gravel, grass, mulch, river rocks, steep inclines/declines, boulders, and a log bridge. The staff at Mountain States Hand and Physical Therapy use the terrain park for balance training and fall prevention as well as for sport-specific rehabilitation such as hiking, gardening, golfing, soccer, and other leisure and recreational activities.

The motivation to start the terrain park program was multifold and included the sobering statistics that one in four people in the U.S. over the age of 65 experience falls each year; furthermore, falls are the leading cause of injury among older adults (CDC 2020). The staff saw a need in their community to address these issues, and their program idea was unique. It is unique because the terrain park helps patients navigate obstacles they would find in real life that cannot fully be simulated in the clinic. Beyond built obstacles, there are other things that cannot be simulated inside such as bright sunshine (and the demand it places on our eyes to adjust to light changes), wind gusts, an insect annoying you while you walk, a loud truck driving by, and other such realities of life outside. Installing the 4000-square-foot terrain park has allowed for a more thorough rehabilitation process. Patients are returning to and achieving outdoor goals with more success because simulating activities inside did not translate to confidence outside.

Located in a residential neighborhood in beautiful Arvada, Colorado, the clinic building and property are owned by Mountain States Hand and Physical Therapy and are privately maintained. Previously, the building was a preschool. As Ms. Bohling shared, "We turned the playground into a therapy playground!" Here is how. The design process began with clinicians making a list of all the outdoor challenges that they wanted to incorporate into the space. They submitted the list to a local landscape architect, who designed the terrain park to incorporate the features the clinicians identified, and then it was built. In the terrain park, there is an area with a ramp and steps that meet ADA code, but the great outdoors does not follow code and so the rest was designed as such. The layout progresses from the ADA compliant area with handrails to a space without rails, to steeper inclines, steps up/down from different surfaces, and a log bridge, to name a few. As with all their therapy services, intervention in the terrain park is developed to meet the individual where they are and where they hope to go.

Mountain States Hand and Physical Therapy supported the community by using all local small businesses for the materials, plants, and labor. They received a grant to help cover costs, but the total cost was roughly $80,000 for landscape design and installation. The maintenance costs for the terrain park are for lawn and plant care, as well as ongoing landscaping upkeep.

A team of physical therapists researched and developed the eight-week balance rehabilitation class in the terrain park based upon existing fall prevention programs and evidence-based balance tests including Timed Up and Go test (TUG), Single Leg Stance test (SLS), tandem stand, and the Dynamic Gait Index (DGI). The course is structured around various indoor and outdoor circuit training, including strengthening, cardio exercises, static and dynamic balance exercises, and functional activities. The indoor circuits are designed to fatigue the participants, while the follow-on outdoor circuits address functional skills. Each session includes exercises on stairs, sand, ramps, and gravel.

The class is run by staff physical therapists. Typically, the one-hour classes are provided one to one or in small groups depending on the patients' established fall risk and determination if they are appropriate for the group program. Balance skills are re-evaluated at the end of the eight-week class. Payment for the balance class is via cash, and individual sessions are billed to insurance when appropriate. The program is marketed via the Mountain States Hand and Physical Therapy website and to local physicians with a particular emphasis on ear, nose, and throat (ENT) physicians and neurologists.

Providing the terrain park program is weather dependent, as Colorado weather can be unpredictable and extreme, but all efforts are made to facilitate it outside whenever possible, and if not outside, the participants practice some of the prerequisite balance skills inside the clinic. Although the inception for the balance program was originally inspired by older adults, patients in the terrain park span all ages. Patients may have neurological diagnoses such as concussion, traumatic brain injury, Parkinson's disease, multiple sclerosis, or stroke. Patients seen for orthopedic treatment may or may not be athletes whose diagnoses include any lower-body injury. For those receiving balance treatment, their diagnoses may include Meniere's disease, benign paroxysmal positional vertigo (BPPV), other vestibular impairments, or general deconditioning.

The terrain park was completed in May 2020, at the beginning of the COVID-19 pandemic. During the COVID-19 pandemic, there was tremendous need in the community for exercise classes and safe socialization spaces since all the local recreation centers were closed. To answer the need, the staff offered group balance classes, which have since concluded. For existing patients, they provided telehealth and used a family member to spot (assist) the patients for balance challenges.

Mountain States Hand and Physical Therapy has received media attention. They were featured on the Denver Channel 7 News and in the local paper as a unique way to provide safe care during the COVID-19 pandemic and for the unique setting in which therapy is provided. The link to the story is: https://www.denver7.com/rebound/physical-therapy-clinic-says-the-future-is-outside-especially-during-covid-19-era.

As for a testimonial for the merits of the terrain park program, Ms. Bohling told us that they had a patient with a double lower-extremity amputation using the terrain park who said she was participating in the program because "I would look at something like a step or a curb and just avoid it and walk around it. I don't want to walk around it anymore." She successfully completed the program and was able to navigate sand, gravel, steep incline/declines, and curbs. For Ms. Bohling, this is what keeps a healthcare provider going, and it was definitely a bright spot in an otherwise difficult pandemic.

Here is some advice that Ms. Bohling offers to practitioners who want to take their clinic outside. She said:

> It's unpredictable, so be prepared. You must monitor patient temperatures in the heat, and be aware of bees and other insects, and anything else that might not be encountered inside. And it goes without saying that obviously use a gait belt and understand a patient's ability before taking them into a balance challenge outside (or inside).

In Ms. Bohling's mind, the benefits of taking it outside outweigh the challenges. We start with what she sees as the biggest challenges. Financially, there are maintenance costs involved with keeping the terrain park in good working order, and it is imperative that it not be accessed by the public due to liability issues related to injuries. On the positive side, the terrain park helps patients navigate real-life obstacles and challenges that they cannot encounter in the clinic. Simulating an activity inside does not translate to confidence outside. Using the terrain park as a therapeutic modality allows therapists to be more thorough in the rehabilitation of a patient whose goals include return to outdoor activities. As for the clinicians themselves, taking it outside and working in the terrain park is a change of environment and a way to get outdoors during the workday. The staff use the terrain park for their personal breaks and lunch breaks, and find that accessing the space has improved their own mental health. They also love taking patients outdoors into the beautiful Colorado weather. And we imagine the patients love being outside! Please visit Mountain States Hand and Physical Therapy's website at https://mountainstatestherapy.com/balance-center.

References
Centers for Disease Control and Prevention (2020) 'Older adult falls: A growing problem that can be prevented' [fact sheet]. Accessed on 2/12/22 at www.cdc.gov/steadi/pdf/steadi_clinicianfactsheet-a.pdf.

Wrapping It Up

In this chapter, we looked at the benefits of nature-based interventions for older adults, discussed common chronic conditions and potential accommodations, and took a closer look at a few programs. In this stage, when older adults are managing chronic conditions and potentially spending more time in leisure, nature can both provide a welcome respite and be an engaging environment. Nature is restorative across the life course and can add benefit to a treatment session with an older adult.

NUGGET OF NATURE: WARM-UP AND COOL-DOWN STRETCHING EXERCISE IDEAS FOR THE GARDENER

Devoting time to a series of warm-up and stretching exercises may reduce injuries, help clients spend more quality time in the garden, and, above all, help them feel better. These exercises are also applicable for any outdoor activity.

General thoughts and preparation tips

The following exercises can be done from a sitting or standing position. If you stand while stretching, be sure to do so within immediate reach of a wall, grab bar, or other stable and upright surface to hold on to for additional support, as needed.

Getting ready to warm up and stretch

- Stand or sit up straight!
- Visualize a length of gardening twine running up from the base of your spine, going up along the spine and through your back, neck, and head, and

coming out of the top of your skull. This twine is taut and helps you stand upright or sit up straight.

The stretches

1. Slowly and gently, bend head and neck towards chest. Slowly and gently, return head and neck to upright position.
2. Bend head and neck towards right shoulder. Slowly and gently, return head and neck to upright position.
3. Bend head and neck towards left shoulder. Slowly and gently, return head and neck to upright position.
4. Slowly and gently, rotate head and neck towards right side. Return head and neck to forward-facing position.
5. Slowly and gently, rotate head and neck towards left side. Return head and neck to forward-facing position.
6. Roll right shoulder back and then lower it down to a position of comfort.
7. Roll left shoulder back and then lower it down to a position of comfort.
8. Slowly and gently, rotate trunk, neck, and head towards right side. Return trunk, neck, and head to forward-facing position.
9. Rotate trunk, neck, and head towards left side. Return trunk, neck, and head to forward-facing position.
10. Bend body forward. Slowly and gently, return body to upright position.
11. Bend hip and knee and raise right leg, as if marching. Slowly and gently, return leg to ground.
12. Bend hip and knee and raise left leg, as if marching. Slowly and gently, return leg to ground.
13. Bring right leg out to the side. Slowly and gently, return leg to ground.
14. Bring left leg out to the side. Slowly and gently, return leg to ground.
15. Rotate right ankle from side to side. Slowly and gently, return leg to ground.
16. Rotate left ankle from side to side. Slowly and gently, return leg to ground.
17. Slowly and gently, wiggle toes on right foot.
18. Slowly and gently, wiggle toes on left foot.
19. Slowly and gently, place right arm close to body and raise arm straight up towards the sky. Return arm to side.
20. Slowly and gently, place left arm close to body and raise arm straight up towards the sky. Return arm to side.
21. Slowly and gently, place right arm close to body and raise arm out to the right side. Return arm to side.
22. Slowly and gently, place left arm close to body and raise arm out to the left side. Return arm to side.

23. Slowly and gently, place right arm close to body and reach behind. Return arm to side.
24. Slowly and gently, place left arm close to body and reach behind. Return arm to side.
25. Slowly and gently, bend and straighten right arm. Return arm to side.
26. Slowly and gently, bend and straighten left arm. Return arm to side.
27. Keeping arm tucked in close to body, rotate right forearm palm up and then down.
28. Keeping arm tucked in close to body, rotate left forearm palm up and then down.
29. Keeping arm tucked in close to body, bend right wrist up and then down.
30. Keeping arm tucked in close to body, bend left wrist up and then down.
31. Keeping arm tucked in close to body, bend right wrist to right and then left side.
32. Keeping arm tucked in close to body, bend left wrist to right and then left side.
33. Slowly and gently, spread fingers and thumb apart and then together on right hand.
34. Slowly and gently, spread fingers and thumb apart and then together on left hand.
35. Slowly and gently, open and close fingers on right hand.
36. Slowly and gently, open and close fingers on left hand.

Happy gardening!

Disclaimer: The materials presented here are for informational purposes and should only be used as a guide.

CHAPTER 9

Program Evaluation

Introduction

The reality is that innovative and out-of-the-box programs often must prove their viability quickly and demonstrate their worth and value to continue to be supported. By now, we think you will agree that "taking therapy outside" is one example of a novel therapy-delivery model worth perpetuating. Measuring the effectiveness of an outdoor therapy program for clients and for the staff can help you better understand how the program impacts everyone involved. And sharing the data from measuring outcomes of your program with funders and other decision makers lends further support for them to understand why it is necessary and should continue to be funded.

There are many reasons and ways to evaluate an outdoor therapy program's effectiveness. The first is that you believe in it because you love being outside. This reason alone is a key motivator for providing therapy outside and doing all you can to keep the program running. We are passionate about providing therapy outside, and our reason for writing this book has been to help you see its worth and value, and to inspire you to "take it outside" wherever it is you work or to create your own model of an outside therapy program. We want as many people as possible to experience the benefits of being in nature while healing. Hence, we want you to have an outdoor therapy program and to evaluate your program so others can know that it matters and makes a positive difference in your clients' lives.

As mentioned above, one of the reasons for evaluating your program could include seeking funding and grants. Having data to demonstrate the effectiveness of your program will increase your chances of obtaining funding to continue and/or expand the program's capacity. In other words, can you provide the data to verify that your program is meeting its intended key performance indicators so that funders will take notice and provide funding? This is important.

Another reason for evaluating your outside therapy program may be to do research and publish and present on findings that demonstrate if/how/why providing therapy outside improves client function and goal attainment. Or you may want to measure therapist satisfaction with outdoor therapy programs. Regarding diversity, equity, inclusion, and justice, here is a further reason that program evaluation is important. According to the National Institute of Health (2017), since a primary aim of research is to provide scientific evidence leading to a change in health policy or standard of care, it is imperative to determine whether the intervention or therapy being studied affects women or men or members of minority groups and their subpopulations differently (para. 1).

We hope you are now inspired not only to take it outside but also to measure its impact on your clients. Gathering baseline information is foundational for a research platform. Research drives innovation, and the reality is that there have been very few published studies that validate why therapy outdoors provided by licensed healthcare professions (such as music therapy, occupational therapy, physical therapy, recreational therapy, and speech and language therapy) is important. There is good reason to facilitate this research, and we hope you will consider it! The bulk of the research looking at therapy outdoors has come out of the mental health professions such as counseling, psychology, and social work. Keep it coming, as we need more of it. The more that good research gets published and presented at professional conferences, the more likely it is that taking therapy outside will become standard practice rather than the current out-of-the-box practice model that it is. Another day at the office can become another day in the forest, park, garden, mountain, or body of water. Does that sound wonderful to you?

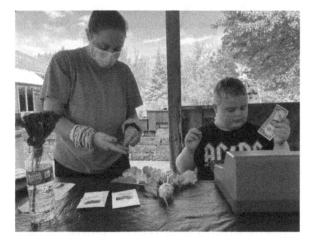

PRACTICAL ASSESSMENT OF MONEY MANAGEMENT
Photo credit: Monarch School of New England

How you choose to evaluate your program is a decision that is based on many factors and best discussed with staff and administration at your facility. If you are in solo practice, spend some time brainstorming about it. If you feel intimidated at the thought of doing research, first take a deep, nature-filled breath and know that every time you evaluate a client you are doing research. As part of practice, you do many initial and final evaluations to measure client progress and goal achievement. You may do home evaluations to assess whether it is safe for a client to return after an accident or illness. And you constantly evaluate yourself and your practice to ensure that you are providing the best intervention possible. With that said, partnering with a college or university who will work with you to develop and carry out a research study that pertains to your outside therapy program is a wonderful option and builds great connections.

Your program evaluation and research may be designed as a qualitative study that tells a "story." Qualitative research includes interviews, survey questions that ask you to elaborate on responses, observations, and focus groups, to name just a few. Findings from qualitative research are determined by identifying words and themes. Quantitative research includes administering assessments such as surveys, questionnaires, standardized assessment tools, obtaining physiological data, doing observations (used in both qualitative and quantitative research), and analyzing/measuring the "numbers." Both methods involve collecting and analyzing data, just differently. Many studies include both quantitative and qualitative methods. Thanks to technology, qualitative and quantitative data are often analyzed through computer programs. It is the rare researcher who does hand calculations for quantitative data, although many qualitative researchers still prefer to analyze their data by hand, despite the availability of qualitative data analysis software.

Evaluation Tools

In this chapter, we present a series of tables containing information about suggested standardized assessment tools used in quantitative research that can be used to support the evaluation tools that you currently use to assess client progress. The assessment tools that we include can also, should your program be intended as such, be useful for research purposes. The list of assessment tools is not intended to be exhaustive but will get you started with gathering evidence to demonstrate the worth and purpose of outside therapy programs. For easier readability, we organized this chapter by standardized measures of physical/physiological, social-emotional, sensory, cognitive function, and other for assessment tools that are useful for multiple areas of function, such as quality of life and visual analogue scales that measure a single item such as pain level (see p.297). We begin with physical and physiological measures of function.

Physical and Physiological Measures of Function

The assessments in Table 9.1 are examples of standardized tools to measure strength, endurance, range of motion, fatigue, balance, heart rate variability, blood pressure, and cortisol levels.

Table 9.1 Physical and physiological measures of function

Tool	Access	What it measures
Goniometer	Medical supply companies	Range of motion
Pinch meter	Medical supply companies	Pinch strength
Dynamometer	Medical supply companies	Grip strength
Cortisol testing—various methods such as hair and saliva	Medical laboratory supply companies	Cortisol hormone level
Chest-strap heart rate monitor	Medical supply companies	Heart rate variability
Blood pressure cuff	Medical supply companies	Blood pressure
Pulse oximeter	Medical supply companies	Oxygen saturation level
Timed Up and Go (TUG) test	www.cdc.gov/steadi/pdf/TUG_test-print.pdf	Balance, gait, mobility
2 Minute Walk Test (2MWT)	www.sralab.org/rehabilitation-measures/2-minute-walk-test	Gait, aerobic capacity, mobility
Nine Hole Peg Test	www.sralab.org/sites/default/files/2017-07/Nine Hole Peg Test Instructions.pdf	Fine motor skills and dexterity
Functional Assessment of Chronic Illness Therapy—Fatigue	www.facit.org/measures/FACIT-F	Self-reported levels of fatigue and its impact on daily activities
Quick Disabilities of the Arm, Shoulder, and Hand questionnaire (QuickDASH)	www.physio-pedia.com/DASH_Outcome_Measure	Ability to engage in upper-extremity activities
Senior Fitness Test	Rikli, R.E. and C.J. Jones (2013) *Senior Fitness Test Manual*. Champaign, IL: Human Kinetics.	Physical functional ability in older adults
Waist circumference and waist–hip ratio	Use a fabric tape measurer to measure a client's waist circumference and hip circumference	Both measurements are important indicators of the risks of cardiovascular disease and abdominal obesity (Huxley et al. 2010)

Social-Emotional Measures of Function

The assessments in Table 9.2 are examples of standardized tools to measure mood, emotions, sense of coherence, resilience, hope, stress, and social connectivity.

Table 9.2 Social-emotional measures of function

Tool	Access	What it measures
UCLA Loneliness Scale	https://fetzer.org/sites/default/files/images/ stories/pdf/selfmeasures/Self_Measures_for_ Loneliness_and_Interpersonal_Problems_ UCLA_LONELINESS_REVISED.pdf	Social isolation
De Jong Gierveld Scale (6 item)	Gierveld, J.D.J. and Tilburg, T.V. (2006) 'A 6-item scale for overall, emotional, and social loneliness: Confirmatory tests on survey data.' *Research on Aging 28*, 5, 582–598.	Social isolation
Lubben Social Network Scale	Lubben, J., Blozik, E., Gillmann, G., Iliffe, S. *et al.* (2006) 'Performance of an abbreviated version of the Lubben Social Network Scale among three European community-dwelling older adult populations.' *The Gerontologist 46*, 4, 503–513. Other versions are available.	Social isolation
Friendship Scale	Hawthorne, D.G. and Griffith, P. (2000) 'The Friendship Scale: Development and Properties' (Working Paper No. 114). Centre for Health Program Evaluation. Accessed on 2/12/22 at https://core.ac.uk/download/ pdf/36962344.pdf	Social isolation
Brief Hypervigilance Scale	https://dynamic.uoregon.edu/jjf/ hypervigilance/index.html	Level of hypervigilance
Life Events Checklist	www.ptsd.va.gov/professional/assessment/ te-measures/life_events_checklist.asp Weathers, F.W., Blake, D.D., Schnurr, P.P., Kaloupek, D.G., Marx, B.P., and Keane, T.M. (2013) *The Life Events Checklist for DSM-5 (LEC-5).* White River Junction, VT: National Center for PTSD.	Traumatic events in a lifetime
The Child and Youth Resilience Measure (CYRM-28)	Resilience Research Centre (2009) *The Child and Youth Resilience Measure-28: User Manual.* Halifax: Dalhousie University Resilience Research Centre.	Screening tool to explore resources available to adolescents and young adults to foster resilience

cont.

Tool	Access	What it measures
Four Mood Introspection Scale	Mayer, J.D., Allen, J., and Beauregard, K. (1995) 'Mood inductions for four specific moods: Procedure employing guided imagery vignettes with music.' *Journal of Mental Imagery 19*, 133–150.	Four moods: happiness, anger, fear, and sadness
Brief Mood Introspection Scale	Mayer, J.D. and Gaschke, Y.N. (1988) 'The experience and meta-experience of mood.' *Journal of Personality and Social Psychology 55*, 102–111.	Eight mood states
Agitated Behavior Scale	www.sralab.org/rehabilitation-measures/ agitated-behavior-scale	Behavioral observation
Observed Emotion Rating Scale	This scale was first published as the Philadelphia Geriatric Center Rating Scale. Lawton, M.P., Van Haitsma, K.S., and Klapper, J.A. (1996) 'Observed affect in nursing home residents.' *Journals of Gerontology B 51*, 1, 3–15.	Observation of emotions in older adults
Positive and Negative Affect Schedule (PANAS)	Watson, D., Clark, L.A., and Tellegan, A. (1988) 'Development and validation of brief measures of positive and negative affect: The PANAS scales.' *Journal of Personality and Social Psychology 54*, 6, 1063–1070.	Emotional state
Profile of Mood States (POMS)	McNair, D., Lorr, M., and Droppleman, L. (1992) *Profile of Mood States Manual* (rev. ed.). Princeton, NJ: Educational and Industrial Testing Service.	Variety of mood states
Patient Health Questionnaire-9 (PHQ-9)	Kroenke, K., Spitzer, R.L., and Williams, J.B. (2001) 'The PHQ-9: Validity of a brief depression severity measure.' *Journal of General Internal Medicine 16*, 9, 606–613.	Depression
Beck Depression Inventory (BDI-II)	www.ismanet.org/doctoryourspirit/pdfs/ Beck-Depression-Inventory-BDI.pdf	Depression
Resiliency Scales for Children and Adolescents	Prince-Embury, S. (2006) *Resiliency Scales for Children and Adolescents: Profiles of Personal Strengths.* San Antonio, TX: Harcourt Assessments. Prince-Embury, S. (2008) 'The Resiliency Scales for Children and Adolescents, psychological symptoms, and clinical status in adolescents.' *Canadian Journal of School Psychology 23*, 1, 41–56.	Resilience

Strengths and Difficulties Questionnaire (SDQ)	Goodman, R. (1997) 'The Strengths and Difficulties Questionnaire: A research note.' *Journal of Child Psychology and Psychiatry 38*, 581–586.	Resilience
Emotional and Behavioral Development Scale (EBDS)	Riding, R., Rayner, S., Morris, S., Grimley, M., and Adams, D. (2002) *Emotional and Behavioral Development Scales*. Birmingham, UK: Assessment Research Unit, School of Education, University of Birmingham.	Emotions and behavior responses
The Warwick-Edinburgh Mental Wellbeing Scale (WEMWBS)	https://warwick.ac.uk/fac/sci/med/ research/platform/wemwbs/using/register/ resources?isRenderPage=true	Mental (health) wellbeing
Sense of Coherence Scale	Antonovsky, A. (1993) 'The structure and properties of the Sense of Coherence Scale.' *Social Science & Medicine 36*, 6, 725–733.	Construct of sense of coherence; a belief that life is manageable, comprehensible, and has meaning
Hope Scale (adult and child)	Snyder, C.R., Harris, C., Anderson, J.R., Holleran, S.A. *et al.* (1991) 'The will and the ways: Development and validation of an individual-differences measure of hope.' *Journal of Personality and Social Psychology 60*, 570–585. Snyder, C.R., Hoza, B., Pelham, W.E., Rapoff, M. et al. (1997) 'The development and validation of the Children's Hope Scale.' *Journal of Pediatric Psychology 22*, 3, 399–421.	Hopefulness and sense that goals can be met
Perceived Restorativeness for Activities Scale (PRAS)	Norling, J., Sibthorp, J., and Ruddell, E. (2008) 'Perceived Restorativeness for Activities Scale (PRAS): Development and validation.' *Journal of Physical Activity & Health 5*, 1, 184–195.	Impact of attentional restoration on physical activity

Cognitive Measures of Function

The assessments in Table 9.3 are examples of standardized tools to measure attention, memory, processing, and concentration.

Table 9.3 Cognitive measures of function

Tool	Access	What it measures
Mini-Mental State Examination (MMSE)	https://cgatoolkit.ca/Uploads/ ContentDocuments/MMSE.pdf	Cognitive function in older adults

cont.

Tool	Access	What it measures
Montreal Cognitive Assessment test (MoCA)	www.mocatest.org/the-moca-test	Attention, short-term memory, visuospatial function, concentration, language, orientation to time and place
WPPSI-IV and WISC-V	www.pearsonassessments.com/professional-assessments/featured-topics/cognitive-concerns/cognitive-development.html	Cognitive skills in preschoolers to 6 years (WPPSI-IV) and children 6–16 years
Weschler Memory Scale	Wechsler, D. (2009) *WMS-IV: Wechsler Memory Scale: Administration and Scoring Manual.* New York, NY: Pearson.	Memory
Stroop Test	Scarpina, F. and Tagini, S. (2017) 'The Stroop Color and Word Test.' *Frontiers in Psychology 8*, 557.	Ability to inhibit cognitive interference

Other Measures of Function

The assessments in Table 9.4 are examples of standardized and non-standardized tools to measure constructs such as quality of life, pain, and sensation.

Table 9.4 Other measures of function

Tool	Access	What it measures
WHO Quality of Life-BREF (WHOQOL-BREF)	World Health Organization—www.who.int/toolkits/whoqol	Self-perceived quality of life
Pediatric Evaluation of Disability Inventory (PEDI)	www.pearsonassessments.com/store/usassessments/en/Store/Professional-Assessments/Developmental-Early-Childhood/Pediatric-Evaluation-of-Disability-Inventory/p/100000505.html	Children's functional capabilities and performance
Canadian Occupational Performance Measure	www.thecopm.ca	Self-perception in performance of daily activities
Life Satisfaction Questionnaire 9 and 11 (LISAT-9 and LISAT-11)	https://scireproject.com/outcome/life-satisfaction-questionnaire-lisat9-lisat11	Occupational performance, social relationships, social support

Global Rating of Change scale (GRC)	Kamper, S.J., Maher, C.G., and Mackay, G. (2009) 'Global Rating of Change scales: A review of strengths and weaknesses and considerations for design.' *Journal of Manual & Manipulative Therapy 17*, 3, 163–170.	Self-rating of improvement of health conditions
Goal Attainment Scaling (GAS)	Kiresuk, T.J. and Sherman, M.R.E. (1968) 'Goal attainment scaling: A general method for evaluating comprehensive community mental health programs.' *Community Mental Health Journal 4*, 6, 443–453.	Physical and mental health goals and outcomes
Role Checklist	www.sralab.org/rehabilitation-measures/role-checklist-version-3 Oakley, F., Kielhofner, G., Barris, R., and Reichler, R.K. (1986) 'The Role Checklist: Development and empirical assessment of reliability.' *Occupational Therapy Journal of Research 6*, 3, 157–170.	Participation, satisfaction with participation, or reasons for non-participation
Brief Pain Inventory (BPI)	www.mdanderson.org/documents/Departments-and-Divisions/Symptom-Research/BPI_UserGuide.pdf	Pain levels
McGill Pain Questionnaire	https://onlinelibrary.wiley.com/doi/10.1002/art.11440	Pain levels
Wong–Baker FACES Pain Rating Scale	Wong, D.L., Hockenberry-Eaton, M., Wilson, D. and Winkelstein, M.L. (2001) *Wong's Essentials of Pediatric Nursing* (6th ed.). Maryland Heights, MO: Mosby.	Visual analog scale that uses range of negative to positive emoticons to identify pain level
Sensory Processing Measure (SPM-2)	www.wpspublish.com/spm-2	Sensory integration and processing

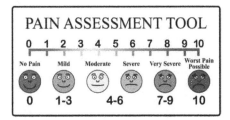

VISUAL ANALOG PAIN SCALE

Wrapping It Up

Before closing, we would like to remind you not to limit yourself to using only standardized assessment tools. Your program's efficacy can also be measured and demonstrated with a tool you create. Consider what change you are trying to effect, and then write questions to measure that construct or idea. It is possible to show change with a simple questionnaire that you develop. Program evaluation can take on many forms and be conducted for various reasons, including funding and research. Evaluation is a reflective process. It offers an opportunity to step back and think about the impact that the program is making on the lives of those we serve and those we work with. Consider all that can be learned and shared when you engage in an evaluative process. In the words of the philosopher Friedrich Nietzsche, "Evaluation is creation: hear it, you creators! Evaluating is itself the most valuable treasure of all that we value. It is only through evaluation that value exists and without evaluation the nut of existence would be hollow" (AZ Quotes n.d.).

Afterword

As we wrap up the book, we thought it would be a timely ending to share our own "This Much I Know" stories because they each truly represent the seed and inspiration for writing *Nature-Based Allied Health Practice: Creative and Evidence-Based Strategies*.

Out of Amy's profound "Aha!" moment came the realization that nature matters and everyone who wants to experience what it has to offer deserves the right to do so—for recreation, adventure, leisure, exercise, social connection, learning, respite, reflection, restoration, joy, or for therapy. Here is **Amy's story**.

Twenty-two years ago, on a balmy mid-spring afternoon in Boston, there we were, my then 13-year-old son and I, each perched in front of our respective computers, doing our homework. At that time, I was writing my dissertation, editing my first textbook, teaching at a local college, maintaining a small private pediatrics practice, and, oh yes, planning David's Bar Mitzvah. I am not quite sure what happened, but something triggered my inner thermo-nuclear button, and I unleashed a torrent of profanities and complaints, pretty out of character for me. David, obviously surprised and, yes, amused as any 13-year-old would be to witness Mom "having a moment," calmly stopped typing, gazed over at his out-of-control mother, and quietly offered, "Hey, Mom, why don't you go outside in your garden for a while?" I paused, looked at him, and responded somewhat sheepishly, "Okayyyyyyyy."

So off I went, still dressed for work, high heels and all, into my backyard sanctuary. For the next 20 minutes, I stroked and smelled my herbs, poked around, did some weeding, gazed at the vibrant palette of colors in the garden, looked at the sky, felt the light breeze on my shoulders, and just breathed. All the angst I was feeling simply melted away. I was transformed and I was restored. I went back inside and was fully attentive, calm, and focused. Little did I know then that there is a name for what I had experienced. Environmental psychologists Stephen and Rachel Kaplan developed the attention restoration theory, which in its simplest iteration means that the most efficacious way to recover from mental fatigue, which arguably we all deal with daily, is through interaction with nature. For some, it is a walk in the mountains, a stroll along the shores of a sandy beach, the opportunity to look out of a window at a verdant green expanse, or, for many, to be in a garden.

This was a pivotal moment for me. All my life I have loved being in nature and gardening. Growing up in a very busy household, tending the vegetable garden was not a chore; it was solace and comfort for me. But at that time, 20-plus years ago, during my moment of complete transformation, I thought that if I experienced restoration in nature, perhaps it happens for others as well. Being the curious occupational therapist that I am, I wondered, even more globally, if being in and engaging with nature through gardening and other types of green interactions could be healthful therapeutic interventions for our clients.

I wanted to know if my ideas were sheer folly or if there really was a connection with occupational therapy. I hoped that looking at the roots of my profession could give me some answers. I learned that occupational therapy has a long-standing history of using gardening as intervention. Early in the evolution of occupational therapy as a profession, practitioners used gardening as therapy, particularly with veterans and those with mental health diagnoses. While there was no evidence available to support the value of nature as therapy at that time, there was expert opinion, including a prescient statement by occupational therapist Elizabeth Clarke who shared in "Gardening as a Therapeutic Experience," published in a 1950 issue of the *American Journal of Occupational Therapy*, "There are many types of activities in which patients may become interested; perhaps one of the most profitable, yet relaxing and enjoyable to all those requiring physical exercise, is that of gardening. The values derived from gardening, whether the participation is passive or very strenuous, are far reaching and give each person a chance to re-create and express themself" (p.110).

Knowing that, historically, occupational therapists used gardening as intervention led me to want to know if it is being used in contemporary practice. Survey research on the use of gardening as an intervention that myself and Dr. Ben Atchison, PhD, OTR/L, FAOTA, Professor and Occupational Therapy Department Chair Emeritus at Western Michigan University, published in the *Open Journal of Occupational Therapy* ("Putting the Occupation Back in Occupational Therapy" (Wagenfeld and Atchison 2014)) showed that many occupational therapy practitioners are engaging in gardening as occupations-centered intervention in varied practice settings, such as skilled nursing, home health, schools, clinics, hospitals, and even at some universities. This was incredible to learn and made me want to be a passionate voice to encourage licensed healthcare practitioners to either initiate or continue to take therapy outside and to measure its effectiveness and promote its value. It is my humble hope that I have done and will continue to do my job.

For Shannon, her connection with nature stems in large part from the wisdom, passion, and love of being outside she learned from her grandma. There was no "Aha!" moment for Shannon, but a series of "Oh, okay then" reflections that have culminated into the opinion that nature-based therapies are not just possible but a mandatory option every client should be offered. Here is **Shannon's story**.

My originating connection to nature-based experiences is not an actual memory, but one based on photos and stories. From birth through childhood, I spent the majority of my summers outdoors as my grandma Ellen—who is an enthusiastic and creative gardener—cared for me. By preschool, I had my first garden plot because she carved out a space for me in our front yard. And some of my first memories are of all the imaginative fun we had in the woods near her farmette. As I reflect now, I think that my grandma has been an inspiration for some of the biggest decisions in my life.

I became an occupational therapist based on seeing the care she received after her first hip replacement. I became curious about garden therapy programming, and pursued it as my doctoral capstone focus, due to the benefits I saw my grandma derive from her active gardening hobby as she has lived with Parkinson's disease for almost 20 years. And, most recently, I have become a fiercer advocate for outdoor therapy, based on the care my grandma received after a subsequent hip injury. I was in the middle of working on this book when my grandma broke her hip a third time. After leaving the rehabilitation hospital, she received home healthcare from multiple therapy disciplines. Depending on the season, my grandma typically spends between seven and fifty hours a week outside in her garden or on the porch. Being outside is important and meaningful to her. I was saddened and angry when I learned that none of the therapists asked her about gardening, or how she planned to get onto the porch, or even what mattered to her. I hope this book inspires at least one healthcare provider to consider what matters to their clients and thinks to ask about going outside.

And now, from both of us, one final thought we would like to leave you with is: please, for the health and wellbeing of your clients and patients, and for yourselves, "Take it outside!"

Appendix

Program Readiness Guide 1: Unmodifiable Public Site

This guide is for you to edit, add, delete, and use to help you plan an outdoor therapy program on *a public site that you cannot permanently modify*.

Program name . . . .

Client population . . . .

Program Intention
Start with addressing your program's intention. Check all that apply in each category.

General Health
☐ Reduce pain

☐ Reduce fatigue

☐ Improve planning and organizational skills

☐ Increase response to external stimuli

☐ Promote communication

☐ Improve memory and attentional skills

☐ Increase language skills

☐ Improve social skills

Physical Health

- ☐ Increase or maintain strength and endurance
- ☐ Improve or maintain range of motion
- ☐ Address weight issues
- ☐ Reduce pain
- ☐ Encourage use of weak or affected extremities
- ☐ Improve balance and coordination
- ☐ Increase mobility skills

Mental Health

- ☐ Reduce isolation
- ☐ Address autonomy
- ☐ Increase attention span
- ☐ Decrease anxiety
- ☐ Reduce depression
- ☐ Reduce stress
- ☐ Reduce rumination
- ☐ Decrease impact of trauma
- ☐ Improve mood
- ☐ Increase resilience
- ☐ Encourage relaxation
- ☐ Spark memory
- ☐ Encourage creativity and self-expression
- ☐ Enhance self-esteem and confidence
- ☐ Improve self-efficacy
- ☐ Provide a purpose—caring and nurturing for a living thing
- ☐ Improve social skills

Cognition

- ☐ Promote communication
- ☐ Improve memory and attentional skills

☐ Increase language skills

☐ Improve planning and organizational skills

☐ Improve decision-making skills

☐ Increase problem-solving skills

Sensory Integration

☐ Address sensory challenges

☐ Increase response to external stimuli

☐ Address self-regulation

Vocational Skills

☐ Address pre-vocational skills

☐ Explore career options

☐ Simulated outdoor work experience

Other

☐ Other . . . .

Business Model

☐ New business model within an existing organization

    ☐ Sole proprietorship

    ☐ Limited Liability Corporation

    ☐ Corporation

    ☐ Non-profit

☐ Updating an existing business model within existing organization

Note: In the U.S., SCORE (www.score.org) provides free business mentoring.

Operating Costs

This section of the readiness guide helps you to plan for funding needs.

★

Staffing needs

Therapy. . . . .

    # . . . .

    Salaries . . . .

Administrative. . . . .

    # . . . .

    Salaries . . . .

Maintenance. . . . .

    # . . . .

    Salaries . . . .

Volunteer . . . .

    # . . . .

Other . . . .

    # . . . .

    Salaries . . . .

Maintenance

Startup cost . . . .

Ongoing costs . . . .

Supplies

Startup cost . . . .

Ongoing costs . . . .

Supplies list . . . .

. . . .

. . . .

. . . .

Storage

Type of storage . . . .

Startup cost . . . .

Ongoing costs . . . .

Insurance and Permitting

Startup . . . .

Annual . . . .

Total Budgeting

Startup budget . . . .

Annual budget. . . . .

Revenue Sources for Program

Now that you've done the work of planning, it's time to pitch your program to funding sources.

☐ Fee for service

☐ Insurance

☐ Grants

☐ Other . . . .

Grant sources . . . .

. . . .

Fundraising options . . . .

. . . .

Stakeholders necessary to meet with for "take it outside" funding

. . . .

. . . .

☐ Prepare a 10–15-minute program overview to present to relevant funders

☐ Prepare a few "elevator speeches"; each should be about 30 seconds to 2 minutes long and crafted with a specific stakeholder in mind

★

Marketing

The checklist below is a start—continue to brainstorm to find ways that serve your concept best.

☐ Social media

☐ Website

☐ Mass mailing

☐ Magazine advertisements

☐ Media appearances

☐ Craft articles for local news outlets

☐ Email blasts

☐ Posters

☐ Word of mouth

☐ Networking through professional communities of practice

☐ Other . . . .

Proposed Program Location and Existing Conditions

Site location . . . .

Distance from nearest accessible restroom . . . .

Does the restroom have a child-sized changing table?

☐ Yes

☐ No

Does the restroom have an adult-sized changing table?

☐ Yes

☐ No

Number of accessible parking spaces . . . .

Distance from parking lot to therapy site . . . .

Distance to closest public transit station . . . .

★

Assessment of Existing Site Conditions

Average hours of sunlight . . . .

Orientation (east, west, north, south) . . . .

Existing shade

☐ Trees

☐ Shelter

☐ Shade sails

☐ Other . . . .

Existing terrain

☐ Flat

☐ Hilly

☐ Combination

Existing paving

Type/s . . . .

Existing fencing

☐ Yes

☐ No

Type of fencing . . . .

Height of fencing . . . .

Existing water source

☐ Yes

☐ No

Existing surveillance

☐ None

☐ Cameras

☐ Security staff

☐ Site visibility (describe). . . . .

Furnishings: Existing seating

☐ Benches with arm rests

☐ Benches without arm rests

☐ Moveable chairs with arm rests

☐ Moveable chairs without arm rests

☐ Hammocks

☐ Gliders/rocking

☐ Swings

☐ Stools

☐ Seating walls

☐ Tree stumps

☐ Boulders

☐ Other . . . .

Furnishings: Existing tables

☐ Moveable

☐ Fixed in place

☐ Adjustable height

☐ Wheelchair accessible

Existing access to drinkable water

☐ One level

☐ Multi-level

☐ Water bottle filling station

Existing storage

☐ Wheeled carts for transporting supplies

☐ Storage unit

Program Readiness Guide 2: Modifiable Site

This guide is for you to edit, add, delete, and use to plan a program on *a site that you can permanently modify.*

Program name . . . .

Client population . . . .

Program Intention
Start with addressing your program's intention. Check all that apply in each category.

General Health

☐ Reduce pain

☐ Reduce fatigue

☐ Address sensory challenges

☐ Improve planning and organizational skills

☐ Increase response to external stimuli

☐ Promote communication

☐ Improve memory and attentional skills

☐ Increase language skills

☐ Improve social skills

Physical Health

☐ Increase strength and endurance

☐ Improve range of motion

☐ Address weight issues

★

- ☐ Reduce pain
- ☐ Encourage use of weak or affected extremities
- ☐ Improve balance and coordination
- ☐ Increase mobility skills

Mental Health

- ☐ Reduce isolation
- ☐ Address autonomy
- ☐ Increase attention span
- ☐ Decrease anxiety
- ☐ Reduce depression
- ☐ Reduce stress
- ☐ Reduce rumination
- ☐ Decrease impact of trauma
- ☐ Improve mood
- ☐ Increase resilience
- ☐ Encourage relaxation
- ☐ Spark memory
- ☐ Encourage creativity and self-expression
- ☐ Enhance self-esteem and confidence
- ☐ Improve self-efficacy
- ☐ Provide a purpose—caring and nurturing for a living thing
- ☐ Improve social skills

Cognition

- ☐ Promote communication
- ☐ Improve memory and attentional skills
- ☐ Increase language skills
- ☐ Improve planning and organizational skills
- ☐ Improve decision-making skills
- ☐ Increase problem-solving skills

Sensory Integration

☐ Address sensory challenges

☐ Increase response to external stimuli

☐ Address self-regulation

Vocational Skills

☐ Address pre-vocational skills

☐ Explore career options

☐ Simulated outdoor work experience

Other

☐ Other . . . .

Business Model

☐ New business model within an existing organization

    ☐ Sole proprietorship

    ☐ Limited Liability Corporation

    ☐ Corporation

    ☐ Non-profit

☐ Updating an existing business model within existing organization

Note: In the U.S., SCORE (www.score.org) provides free business mentoring.

Operating Costs

This section of the readiness guide helps you to plan for funding needs.

Staffing needs

Therapy . . . .

    # . . . .

    Salaries . . . .

Administrative. . . . .

    #. . . . .

    Salaries . . . .

Maintenance. . . . .

    #. . . . .

    Salaries . . . .

Volunteer. . . . .

    #. . . . .

Other . . . .

    #. . . . .

    Salaries . . . .

Maintenance

Startup cost . . . .

Ongoing costs . . . .

Supplies

Startup cost . . . .

Ongoing costs . . . .

Supplies list . . . .

. . . .

. . . .

. . . .

Total Budgeting

Startup budget . . . .

Annual budget . . . .

Propose Your Program

Now that you've done the work of planning, it's time to pitch your program.

Stakeholders necessary to meet with for "take it outside" buy-in:

. . . .

. . . .

☐ Prepare a 10–15-minute program overview to present to relevant administrators and funders

☐ Prepare a few "elevator speeches"; each should be about 30 seconds to 2 minutes long and crafted with a specific stakeholder in mind

☐ Set meeting date with stakeholders

☐ Permission obtained to "take it outside"

☐ Identify and meet with the maintenance or facilities manager to establish a working relationship (this cannot be emphasized enough—as a practitioner taking it outside, you need the support of the maintenance and facilities team)

Revenue Sources for Program

☐ Fee for service

☐ Insurance

☐ Grants

☐ Donations

☐ Other . . . .

Grant sources . . . .

. . . .

Fundraising options. . . . .

. . . .

Marketing

The checklist below is a start—continue to brainstorm to find ways that serve your community best.

★

☐ Social media

☐ Website

☐ Mass mailing

☐ Magazine advertisements

☐ Media appearances

☐ Craft articles for local news outlets

☐ Email blasts

☐ Posters

☐ Word of mouth

☐ Networking through professional communities of practice

☐ Other . . . .

Onsite Design and Installation

This section is about who will help you design your site if you plan on modifying the space.

☐ Landscape architect or designer

☐ Facilities and maintenance staff

☐ Therapy staff

☐ Volunteer

☐ Other . . . .

Proposed Program Location and Existing Conditions

Site location . . . .

Distance from indoor therapy space . . . .

Is there a direct door from therapy space to outdoor space?

☐ Yes

☐ No

Does the door from the indoor therapy space to outdoor space have an electronic opener?

☐ Yes

☐ No

Distance from nearest accessible restroom . . . .

Does the restroom have a child-sized changing table?

☐ Yes

☐ No

Does the restroom have an adult-sized changing table?

☐ Yes

☐ No

Site Access

☐ Public will have access to the space during therapy sessions

☐ Public is not allowed access to space

☐ Public is not allowed access to space during therapy hours

Number of accessible parking spaces . . . .

Distance from parking lot to therapy site . . . .

Distance to closest public transit station . . . .

Assessment of Existing Site Conditions

Average hours of sunlight . . . .

Orientation (east, west, north, south) . . . .

Existing shade

☐ Trees

☐ Shelter

☐ Shade sails

☐ Other . . . .

Desired type/s of shade . . . .

★

Existing terrain

☐ Flat

☐ Hilly

☐ Combination

Desired type/s of terrain . . . .

Existing paving

Type/s . . . .

Desired type/s of paving . . . .

Existing fencing

☐ Yes

☐ No

Type of fencing . . . .

Height of fencing . . . .

Desired type/s of fencing . . . .

Existing water source

☐ No

☐ Yes

    ☐ Hose

    ☐ Irrigation

    ☐ Both

Desired type/s of water sources . . . .

Existing electrical outlets

☐ Yes

☐ No

Desired type/s of electrical outlets or lighting . . . .

★

Existing surveillance

☐ None

☐ Cameras

☐ Security staff

☐ Site visibility (describe) . . . .

Desired type/s of security . . . .

Furnishings

This is a tool to help you assess what your space currently has.

Existing planters for gardening programs

☐ Raised planting beds

☐ Wheelchair roll under planting beds

☐ Ground-level planting beds

☐ Potted plants

☐ Hanging planters

☐ Vertical gardens

☐ Greenhouse

☐ Planting trays and grow lights

Desired type/s of planters . . . .

Existing seating

☐ Benches with arm rests

☐ Benches without arm rests

☐ Moveable chairs with arm rests

☐ Moveable chairs without arm rests

☐ Hammocks

☐ Gliders/rocking

☐ Swings

☐ Stools

☐ Seating walls

★

☐ Tree stumps

☐ Boulders

☐ Other . . . .

Desired type/s of seating . . . .

Existing tables

☐ Moveable

☐ Fixed in place

☐ Adjustable height

☐ Wheelchair accessible

Desired type/s of tables . . . .

Existing access to drinkable water

☐ One level

☐ Multi-level

☐ Water bottle filling station

Desired type of drinking fountain . . . .

Existing storage

☐ Shed

☐ Bins

☐ Inside storage

☐ Locking storage

☐ Non-locking storage

Desired type/s of storage . . . .

Site Maintenance Plan

☐ Develop in collaboration with facilities manager

☐ Plan in place

☐ Administration approved

★

References

Abrego, L.J. (2019) 'Relational legal consciousness of U.S. citizenship: Privilege, responsibility, guilt, and love in Latino mixed status families.' *Law & Society Review 53*, 3, 641–670.

Adams, D. and Beauchamp, G. (2018) 'Portals between worlds: A study of the experiences of children aged 7–11 years from primary schools in Wales making music outdoors.' *Research Studies in Music Education 40*, 1, 50–66.

Adams, M. and Morgan, J. (2018) 'Mental health recovery and nature: How social and personal dynamics are important.' *Ecopsychology 10*, 1, 44–52.

Administration on Aging (2021) '*2020 Profile of Older Americans.*' Department of Health and Human Services, Administration for Community Living. Accessed on 12/8/22 at https://acl.gov/sites/default/files/Aging and Disability in America/2020ProfileOlderAmericans.Final_.pdf

AgrAbility (n.d.) 'The Toolbox.' AgrAbislity. Accessed on 2/12/22 at www.agrability.org/toolbox

Ainsworth, M.D. (1979) 'Attachment as Related to Mother-Infant Interaction.' In J.S. Rosenblatt, R.A. Hinde, C. Beer, and M.-C. Busnel (eds) *Advances in the Study of Behavior* (vol. 9). Cambridge, MA: Academic Press.

Allen, B.A. and Waterman, H. (2019) 'Stages of Adolescence.' American Academy of Pediatrics. Accessed on 2/12/22 at www.healthychildren.org/English/ages-stages/teen/Pages/Stages-of-Adolescence.aspx

Amarya, S., Singh, K., and Sabharwal, M. (2018) 'Ageing Process and Physiological Changes.' In G. D'Onofrio, A. Greco, and D. Sancarlo (eds) *Gerontology*. London: IntechOpen.

American Academy of Pediatrics (2007) 'Active Healthy Living: Prevention of Childhood Obesity through Increased Physical Activity.' Policy Statement. Accessed on 30/11/22 at https://pediatrics.aappublications.org/content/117/5/1834.full.pdf

American Occupational Therapy Association (AOTA) (2017) 'Productive Aging for Community Dwelling Older Adults.' AOTA Critically Appraised Topics and Papers Series. Accessed on 3/11/22 at www.aota.org/Practice/Productive-Aging/Evidence-based/CAT-PA-Social.aspx (member only access).

American Occupational Therapy Association (2020) 'AOTA occupational therapy code of ethics.' *American Journal of Occupational Therapy 74*, Suppl 3, 7413410005p1–p13.

American Optometric Association (n.d.) 'Adult vision: 41–60 years of age.' Accessed on 2/12/22 at www.aoa.org/healthy-eyes/eye-health-for-life/adult-vision-41-to-60-years-of-age?

Anderson, K.A. (2019) 'The virtual care farm: A preliminary evaluation of an innovative approach to addressing loneliness and building community through nature and technology.' *Activities, Adaptation & Aging 43*, 4, 334–344.

Anderson, L., Campbell-Sills, L., Ursano, R.J., Kessler, R.C. *et al.* (2019) 'Prospective associations of perceived unit cohesion with postdeployment mental health outcomes.' *Depression and Anxiety 36*, 6, 511–521.

Anil, M.A. and Bhat, J.S. (2020) 'Transitional changes in cognitive-communicative abilities in adolescents: A literature review.' *Journal of Natural Science, Biology and Medicine 11*, 85–92.

Anti-Defamation League (2017) 'Understanding and challenging ageism' [lesson plan]. Accessed on 12/6/22 at https://www.adl.org/education/educator-resources/lesson-plans/understanding-and-challenging-ageism

Antonovsky, A. (1993) 'The structure and properties of the Sense of Coherence Scale.' *Social Science & Medicine 36*, 6, 725–733.

Appleton, J. (1996) *The Experience of Landscape* (rev. ed.). Hoboken, NJ: Wiley. (Original work published 1975.)

Applewhite, A., Backer, R., and Carpenter, K. (2018) 'What is Old School?' Old School: Anti-Ageism Clearinghouse. Accessed on 2/12/22 at https://oldschool.info

Arnett, J.J. (2000) 'Emerging adulthood: A theory of development from the late teens through the twenties.' *American Psychologist 55*, 469–480.

Arnett, J.J. and Jensen, L.A. (2019) *Human Development: A Cultural Approach* (3rd ed.). New York, NY: Pearson.

Ashton-Shaeffer, C. and Constant, A. (2006) 'Why do older adults garden?' *Activities, Adaptation & Aging 30*, 2, 1–18.

Askew, R. and Walls, M.A. (2019) 'Diversity in the great outdoors: Is everyone welcome in America's parks and public lands?' *Resources Magazine*, May 24. Accessed on 30/11/22 at www.resourcesmag.org/common-resources/diversity-in-the-great-outdoors-is-everyone-welcome-in-americas-parks-and-public-lands

Attwell, C., Jöhr, J., Pincherle, A., Pignat, J.M. *et al.* (2019) 'Neurosensory stimulation outdoors enhances cognition recovery in cognitive motor dissociation: A prospective crossover study.' *NeuroRehabilitation 44*, 4, 545–554.

AZ Quotes (n.d.) 'Friedrich Nietzsche Quotes About Creation.' Accessed on 27/2/2023 at www.azquotes.com/author/10823-Friedrich_Nietzsche/tag/creation

Bailey, A.W., Allen, G., Herndon, J., and Demastus, C. (2018) 'Cognitive benefits of walking in natural versus built environments.' *World Leisure Journal 60*, 4, 293–305.

Baker, P. (2018) 'Identifying the connection between Roman conceptions of "Pure Air" and physical and mental health in Pompeian gardens (c.150BC–AD79): A multi-sensory approach to ancient medicine.' *World Archaeology 50*, 3, 404–417.

Barfield, P.A., Ridder, K., Hughes, J., and Rice-McNeil, K. (2021) 'Get outside! Promoting adolescent health through outdoor after-school activity.' *International Journal of Environmental Research and Public Health 18*, 14, 7223.

Barrett, D.E. (1996) 'The three stages of adolescence.' *High School Journal 79*, 4, 333–339.

Barton, J. and Pretty, J. (2010) 'What is the best dose of nature and green exercise for improving mental health? A multi-study analysis.' *Environmental Science & Technology 44*, 10, 3947–3955.

Bates, C. (2020) 'Rewilding education? Exploring an imagined and experienced outdoor learning space.' *Children's Geographies 18*, 3, 364–374.

Beauchamp, T.L. and Childress, J.F. (2019) *Principles of Biomedical Ethics* (8th ed.). Oxford: Oxford University Press.

Beery, T. and Jørgensen, K.A. (2018) 'Children in nature: Sensory engagement and the experience of biodiversity.' *Environmental Education Research 24*, 1, 13–25.

Behrendt, H.F., Scharke, W., Herpertz-Dahlman, B., Konrad, K., and Firk, C. (2019) 'Like mother, like child? Maternal determinants of children's early social-emotional development.' *Infant Mental Health Journal 40*, 2, 234–247.

Beil, K. (2021) 'Nature therapy: Part one: Evidence for the healing power of contact with nature.' *Journal of Restorative Medicine 11*, 1.

Bélanger, M., Gallant, F., Doré, I., O'Loughlin, J.L. *et al.* (2019) 'Physical activity mediates the relationship between outdoor time and mental health.' *Preventive Medicine Reports 16*, 101006.

Best, O. and Ban, S. (2021) 'Adolescence: Physical changes and neurological development.' *British Journal of Nursing 30*, 5, 272–275.

Beyer, K.M., Szabo, A., Hoormann, K., and Stolley, M. (2018) 'Time spent outdoors, activity levels, and chronic disease among American adults.' *Journal of Behavioral Medicine 41*, 4, 494–503.

Birch, J., Rishbeth, C., and Payne, S.R. (2020) 'Nature doesn't judge you: How urban nature supports young people's mental health and wellbeing in a diverse UK city.' *Health & Place 62*, 102296.

Blakemore, S.J., Burnett, S., and Dahl, R.E. (2010) 'The role of puberty in the developing adolescent brain.' *Human Brain Mapping 31*, 6, 926–933.

Blanchard-Fields, F. (2007) 'Everyday problem solving and emotion: An adult developmental perspective.' *Current Directions in Psychological Science 16*, 1, 26–31.

Bowers, E.P., Larson, L.R., and Parry, B.J. (2021) 'Nature as an ecological asset for positive youth development: Empirical evidence from rural communities.' *Frontiers in Psychology 12*, 688574.

Bowlby, J. (2008) *A Secure Base*. New York, NY: Basic Books. (Original work published 1988.)

Bratman, G.N., Hamilton, J.P., and Daily, G.C. (2012) 'The impacts of nature experience on human cognitive function and mental health: Nature experience, cognitive function, and mental health.' *Annals of the New York Academy of Sciences 1249*, 1, 118–136.

Bratman, G.N., Daily, G.C., Levy, B.J., and Gross, J.J. (2015) 'The benefits of nature experience: Improved affect and cognition.' *Landscape and Urban Planning 138*, 41–50.

Bratman, G.N., Anderson, C.B., Berman, M.G., Cochran, B. *et al.* (2019) 'Nature and mental health: An ecosystem service perspective.' *Science Advances 5*, 7, eaax0903.

Brook, G., Wagenfeld, A., and Thompson, C. (2016) *Fingergym Fine Motor Skills School Readiness Program*. Brisbane: Australian Academic Press.

Broom, C. (2017) 'Exploring the relations between childhood experiences in nature and young adults' environmental attitudes and behaviours.' *Australian Journal of Environmental Education 33*, 1, 34–47.

Brown, V.M., Allen, A.C., Dwozan, M., Mercer, I., and Warren, K. (2004) 'Indoor gardening and older adults: Effects on socialization, activities of daily living, and loneliness.' *Journal of Gerontological Nursing 30*, 10, 34–42.

Browning, M.H., Mimnaugh, K.J., Van Riper, C.J., Laurent, H.K., and LaValle, S.M. (2020) 'Can simulated nature support mental health? Comparing short, single-doses of 360-degree nature videos in virtual reality with the outdoors.' *Frontiers in Psychology 10*, 2667.

Bryce, E. (2013) 'Happy memories: The healing power of birds.' National Audubon Society May–June. Accessed on 2/12/22 at www.audubon.org/magazine/may-june-2013/the-healing-power-birds

Bustamante, G., Guzman, V., Kobayashi, L.C., and Finlay, J. (2022). 'Mental health and wellbeing in times of COVID-19: A mixed-methods study of the role of neighborhood parks, outdoor spaces, and nature among US older adults.' *Health & Place 76*, 102813.

Callahan, C.M., Unverzagt, F.W., Hui, S.L., Perkins, A.J., and Hendrie, H.C. (2002) 'Six-Item Screener to identify cognitive impairment among potential subjects for clinical research.' *Medical Care 40*, 9, 771–781.

Calogiuri, G., Litleskare, S., Fagerheim, K.A., Rydgren, T.L., Brambilla, E., and Thurston, M. (2018) 'Experiencing nature through immersive virtual environments: Environmental perceptions, physical engagement, and affective responses during a simulated nature walk.' *Frontiers in Psychology 8*, 2321.

Cameron-Faulkner, T., Melville, J., and Gattis, M. (2018) 'Responding to nature: Natural environments improve parent-child communication.' *Journal of Environmental Psychology 59*, 9–15.

Cartwright, T., Mason, H., Porter, A., and Pilkington, K. (2020) 'Yoga practice in the UK: A cross-sectional survey of motivation, health benefits and behaviours.' *BMJ Open 10*, 1, e031848.

Centers for Disease Control and Prevention (CDC) (2020) 'Older adult falls: A growing problem that can be prevented' [fact sheet]. Accessed on 2/12/22 at www.cdc.gov/steadi/pdf/steadi_clinicianfactsheet-a.pdf

Centers for Disease Control and Prevention (2022a) 'How much physical activity do children need?' Accessed on 2/12/22 at www.cdc.gov/physicalactivity/basics/children/index.htm#:~:text=Children ages 3 through 5, the recommended physical activity levels

Centers for Disease Control and Prevention (2022b) 'CDC's developmental milestones.' Accessed on 30/11/22 at www.cdc.gov/ncbddd/actearly/milestones/index.html.

Chang, M. and Netzer, D. (2019) 'Exploring natural materials: Creative stress-reduction for urban working adults.' *Journal of Creativity in Mental Health 14*, 2, 152–168.

Chang, P.-J. (2020) 'Effects of the built and social features of urban greenways on the outdoor activity of older adults.' *Landscape and Urban Planning 204*, 103929.

Chang, T.H., Tucker, A., Norton, C., Gass, M., and Javorski, S. (2016) 'Cultural issues in adventure programming: Applying Hofstede's five dimensions to assessment and practice.' *Journal of Adventure Education and Outdoor Learning 17*, 4, 307–320.

Chang, Y. (2021) 'Engaging in autonomous learning in the outdoors: Final expedition and youth autonomy.' *Journal of Outdoor and Environmental Education 24*, 2, 191–214.

Chaudhary, G. and Sehgal, A. (2019) 'Teratogens.' *International Journal of Emerging Technologies and Innovative Research 6*, 1, 305–308.

Chawla, L. (2015) 'Benefits of nature contact for children.' *Journal of Planning Literature 30*, 4, 433–452.

Chawla, L., Keena, K., Pevec, I., and Stanley, E. (2014) 'Green schoolyards as havens from stress and resources for resilience in childhood and adolescence.' *Health & Place 28*, 1–13.

Chen, Y.-M. and Ji, J.-Y. (2015) 'Effects of horticultural therapy on psychosocial health in older nursing home residents: A preliminary study.' *Journal of Nursing Research 23*, 3, 167–171.

Chiumento, A., Mukherjee, I., Chandna, J., Dutton, C., Rahman, A. and Bristow, K. (2018) 'A haven of green space: Learning from a pilot pre-post evaluation of a school-based social and therapeutic horticulture intervention with children.' *BMC Public Health 18*, 1, 836.

Choe, E.Y., Jorgensen, A., and Sheffield, D. (2020) 'Does a natural environment enhance the effectiveness of Mindfulness-Based Stress Reduction (MBSR)? Examining the mental health and wellbeing, and nature connectedness benefits.' *Landscape and Urban Planning 202*, 103886.

Christiana, R.W., Besenyi, G.M., Gustat, J., Horton, T.H., Penbrooke, T.L., and Schultz, C.L. (2021) 'A scoping review of the health benefits of nature-based physical activity.' *Journal of Healthy Eating and Active Living 1*, 3, 142–160.

Cimprich, B. and Ronis, D.L. (2003) 'An environmental intervention to restore attention in women with newly diagnosed breast cancer.' *Cancer Nursing 26*, 4, 284–292.

Clarke, E. (1950) 'Gardening as a therapeutic experience.' *American Journal of Occupational Therapy 4*, 3, 109–110, 116.

Clemson, L., Stark, S., Pighills, A.C., Torgerson, D.J., Sherrington, C. and Lamb, S.E. (2019) 'Environmental interventions for preventing falls in older people living in the community.' *Cochrane Database of Systematic Reviews 2019*, 2, CD013258.

Cook, R., Catmur, C., Press, C. and Heyes, C. (2014) 'Mirror neurons: From origin to function.' *Behavioral and Brain Sciences 37*, 2, 177–192.

Corazon, S.S., Sidenius, U., Poulsen, D.V., Gramkow, M.C., and Stigsdotter, U.K. (2019) 'Psycho-physiological stress recovery in outdoor nature-based interventions: A systematic review of the past eight years of research.' *International Journal of Environmental Research and Public Health 16*, 10, 1711.

Cordoza, M., Ulrich, R.S., Manulik, B.J., Gardiner, S.K. *et al.* (2018) 'Impact of nurses taking daily work breaks in a hospital garden on burnout.' *American Journal of Critical Care 27*, 6, 508–512.

Corley, J., Okely, J.A., Taylor, A.M., Page, D. *et al.* (2021) 'Home garden use during COVID-19: Associations with physical and mental wellbeing in older adults.' *Journal of Environmental Psychology 73*, 101545.

Council on School Health, Murray, R., Ramstetter, C., Devore, C. *et al.* (2013) 'The crucial role of recess in school.' *Pediatrics 131*, 1, 183–188.

Course Hero (2023) 'Early and middle adulthood.' Accessed on 13/3/22 at www.coursehero.com/study-guides/boundless-psychology/early-and-middle-adulthood

Courtin, E. and Knapp, M. (2017) 'Social isolation, loneliness and health in old age: A scoping review.' *Health & Social Care in the Community 25*, 3, 799–812.

Coventry, P.A., Brown, J.E., Pervin, J., Brabyn, S. *et al.* (2021) 'Nature-based outdoor activities for mental and physical health: Systematic review and meta-analysis.' *SSM-Population Health 16*, 100934.

Cranney, L., Phongsavan, P., Kariuki, M., Stride, V. *et al.* (2016) 'Impact of an outdoor gym on park users' physical activity: A natural experiment.' *Health & Place 37*, 26–34.

Crocetti, E., Moscatelli, S., Kaniušonytė, G., Meeus, W., Žukauskienė, R., and Rubini, M. (2019) 'Developing morality, competence, and sociability in adolescence: A longitudinal study of gender differences.' *Journal of Youth and Adolescence 48*, 5, 1009–1021.

Cronin, A. and Mandich, M.B. (2016) *Human Development and Performance throughout the Life Span*. Boston, MA: Cengage Learning.

D'Agostino, E.M., Frazier, S.L., Hansen, E., Patel, H.H. *et al.* (2019) 'Two-year changes in neighborhood juvenile arrests after implementation of an afterschool park-based mental health promotion program in Miami-Dade County, Florida, 2015-2017.' *American Journal of Public Health 109*, S214–S220.

D'Andrea, S.J., Batavia, M., and Sasson, N.J. (2008) 'Effect of horticultural therapy on preventing the decline of mental abilities of patients with Alzheimer's type dementia.' *Journal of Therapeutic Horticulture 18*, 9–13.

Dean, J.H., Shanahan, D.F., Bush, R., Gaston, K.J. *et al.* (2018) 'Is nature relatedness associated with better mental and physical health?' *International Journal of Environmental Research and Public Health 15*, 7, 1–18.

Demark-Wahnefried, W., Cases, M.G., Cantor, A.B., Frugé, A.D. *et al.* (2018) 'Pilot randomized controlled trial of a home vegetable gardening intervention among older cancer survivors shows feasibility, satisfaction, and promise in improving vegetable and fruit consumption, reassurance of worth, and the trajectory of central adiposity.' *Journal of the Academy of Nutrition and Dietetics 118*, 4, 689–704.

Determan, J., Akers, M.A., Albright, T., Browning, B. *et al.* (2019) 'The impact of biophilic learning spaces on student success.' Craig Goulding Davis. Accessed on 2/12/22 at https://cgdarch.com/biophilic-learning-space-study

Dettweiler, U., Becker, C., Auestad, B.H., Simon, P. and Kirsch, P. (2017) 'Stress in school: Some empirical hints on the circadian cortisol rhythm of children in outdoor and indoor classes.' *International Journal of Research and Public Health 14*, 475.

Detweiler, M.B., Sharma, T., Detweiler, J.G., Murphy, P.F. *et al.* (2012) 'What is the evidence to support the use of therapeutic gardens for the elderly?' *Psychiatry Investigation 9*, 2, 100–110.

Dodson, M.J. (2004) 'Vestibular stimulation in mania: A case report.' *Journal of Neurology, Neurosurgery & Psychiatry 75*, 168–169.

Dong, J., Zhang, S., Xia, L., Yu, Y. *et al.* (2018) 'Physical activity, a critical exposure factor of environmental pollution in children and adolescents' health risk assessment.' *International Journal of Environmental Research and Public Health 15*, 2, 176.

Dosen, A.S. and Ostwald, M.J. (2016) 'Evidence for prospect-refuge theory: A meta-analysis of the findings of environmental preference research.' *City, Territory, and Architecture 3*, 4, 1–14.

Dzhambov, A.M., Dimitrova, D.D., and Dimitrakova, E.D. (2014) 'Association between residential greenness and birth weight.' *Urban Forestry and Urban Greening 13*, 4, 621–629.

Eiland, L. and Romeo, R.D. (2013) 'Stress and the developing adolescent brain.' *Neuroscience 249*, 162–171.

encyclopedia.com (n.d.) 'Ethics, History of.' Encyclopedia of Philosophy. Accessed on 30/11/22 at www.encyclopedia.com/humanities/encyclopedias-almanacs-transcripts-and-maps/ethics-history

Fang, B.B., Lu, F., Gill, D.L., Liu, S.H., Chyi, T. and Chen, B. (2021) 'A systematic review and meta-analysis of the effects of outdoor education programs on adolescents' self-efficacy.' *Perceptual and Motor Skills 128*, 5, 1932–1958.

Fieldhouse, J. (2003) 'The impact of an allotment group on mental health clients' health, wellbeing and social networking.' *British Journal of Occupational Therapy 66*, 7, 286–296.

Figueroa, L.P. (2020) 'Nature-based occupational therapy for children with developmental disabilities.' *AOTA Special Interest Section Quarterly Practice Connections 5*, 3, 2–5.

Fjortoft, I. (2001) 'The natural environment as a playground for children.' *Early Childhood Education Journal 29*, 2, 111–117.

Flannigan, C. and Dietze, B. (2017) 'Children, outdoor play, and loose parts.' *Journal of Childhood Studies*, 53–60.

Fletcher, J.M. and Kim, J. (2019) 'Learning hope and optimism: Classmate experiences and adolescent development.' *Applied Economics Letters 26*, 5, 409–412.

Flowers, L., Houser, A., Noel-Miller, C., Shaw, J. *et al.* (2017) 'Medicare spends more on socially isolated older adults.' AARP Public Policy Institute. Accessed on 30/11/22 at www.aarp.org/ppi/info-2017/medicare-spends-more-on-socially-isolated-older-adults.html

Foster, S. and Powell, J. (1992) 'Making gardening easier: Gardening strategies for people with heart and lung problems.' Oregon State University Extension Catalog, EM8501, 1–2. Accessed on 2/12/22 at https://catalog.extension.oregonstate.edu/em8501

Foster, S., Duvall, C., and Powell, J. (1992) 'Making Gardening Easier: Adaptive Gardening Techniques for the Visually Impaired.' Oregon State University Extension Catalog, EM8498, 1–4. Accessed on 2/12/22 at https://catalog.extension.oregonstate.edu/em8498

Foxx, C.L., Heinze, J.D., González, A., Fernando, V. *et al.* (2021) 'Effects of immunization with the soil-derived bacterium *Mycobacterium vaccae* on stress coping behaviors and cognitive performance in a "two hit" stressor model.' *Frontiers in Physiology 11*, 524833.

Frank, M.G., Fonken, L.K., Dolzani, S.D., Annis, J.L. *et al.* (2018) 'Immunization with *Mycobacterium vaccae* induces an anti-inflammatory milieu in the CNS: Attenuation of stress-induced microglial priming, alarmins and anxiety-like behavior.' *Brain, Behavior, and Immunity 73*, 352–363.

Freeman, C., Waters, D.L., Buttery, Y., and van Heezik, Y. 2019. 'The impacts of ageing on connection to nature: The varied responses of older adults.' *Health & Place 56*, 24–33.

Frömel, K., Šafář, M., Jakubec, L., Groffik, D., and Žatka, R. (2020) 'Academic stress and physical activity in adolescents.' *BioMed Research International 2020*, 4696592.

Fry, R. (2021) 'Amid the pandemic, a rising share of older U.S. adults are now retired.' Pew Research Center. Accessed on 2/12/22 at www.pewresearch.org/fact-tank/2021/11/04/amid-the-pandemic-a-rising-share-of-older-u-s-adults-are-now-retired

Gaillard, R., Wright, J., and Jaddoe, V. (2019) 'Lifestyle intervention strategies in early life to improve pregnancy outcomes and long-term health of offspring: A narrative review.' *Journal of Developmental Origins of Health and Disease 10*, 3, 314–321.

Galambos, N.L. and Martínez, M.L. (2007) 'Poised for emerging adulthood in Latin America: A pleasure for the privileged.' *Child Development Perspectives 1*, 2, 109–114.

Garst, B.A. and Whittington, A. (2020) 'Defining moments of summer camp experiences: An exploratory study with youth in early adolescence.' *Journal of Outdoor Recreation, Education, and Leadership 12*, 3, 306–321.

Gelman, R. (1978) 'Cognitive development.' *Annual Review of Psychology 29*, 1, 297–332.

Gharaveis, A. (2020) 'A systematic framework for understanding environmental design influences on physical activity in the elderly population: A review of literature.' *Facilities 38*, 9/10, 625–649.

Gierveld, J.D.J. and Tilburg, T.V. (2006) 'A 6-item scale for overall, emotional, and social loneliness: Confirmatory tests on survey data.' *Research on Aging 28*, 5, 582–598.

Giles, G.M. (2017) 'Occupational Therapy's Role with Adult Cognitive Disorder' [fact sheet]. AOTA. Accessed on 2/12/22 at www.aota.org/-/media/Corporate/Files/AboutOT/Professionals/WhatIsOT/PA/Facts/Cognition fact sheet.pdf

Gill, E., Goldenberg, M., Starnes, H., and Phelan, S. (2016) 'Outdoor adventure therapy to increase physical activity in young adult cancer survivors.' *Journal of Psychosocial Oncology 34*, 3, 184–199.

Gilroy, R. (2008) 'Places that support human flourishing: Lessons from later life.' *Planning, Theory & Practice 9*, 2, 145–163.

Ginsburg, K.R., Committee on Communications, and Committee on Psychosocial Aspects of Child and Family Health (2007) 'The importance of play in promoting healthy child development and maintaining strong parent-child bonds.' *Pediatrics 119*, 1, 182–191.

Glover, R.J. (2000) 'Developmental tasks of adulthood: Implications for counseling community college students.' *Community College Journal of Research and Practice 24*, 6, 505–514.

Goodman, R. (1997) 'The Strengths and Difficulties Questionnaire: A research note.' *Journal of Child Psychology and Psychiatry 38*, 581–586.

Gorman, M. (2015) *Our Enduring Values, Revisited: Librarianship in an Ever-Changing World.* Chicago: ALA Editions.

Grabherr, L., Macauda, G., and Lenggenhager, B. (2015) 'The moving history of vestibular stimulation as a therapeutic intervention.' *Multisensory Research 28*, 5–6, 653–687.

Graf, A.S., Long, D.M., and Patrick, J.H. (2017) 'Successful aging across adulthood: Hassles, uplifts, and self-assessed health in daily context.' *Journal of Adult Development 24*, 3, 216–225.

Griffin, R. and Elkins, K. (2013) *Bird Tales.* Towson, MD: Health Professions Press.

Gunderman, R.B. (2020) 'Medical valor in plague time: Dr. Benjamin Rush.' *Perspective 27*, 6, 889–891.

Hall, C.R., and Knuth, M.J. (2019) 'An update of the literature supporting the well-being benefits of plants: Part 3-Social benefits.' *Journal of Environmental Horticulture 37*, 4, 136–142.

Halle, T.G. and Darling-Churchill, K.E. (2016) 'Review of measures of social and emotional development.' *Journal of Applied Developmental Psychology 45*, 8–18.

Han, K.T. and Wang, P.C. (2018) 'Empirical examinations of effects of three-level green exercise on engagement with nature and physical activity.' *International Journal of Environmental Research and Public Health 15*, 2, 375.

Hanscom, A.J. (2016) *Balanced and Barefoot: How Unrestricted Play Makes for Strong, Confident, and Capable Children.* Oakland, CA: New Harbinger Publications.

Hansen, M.M., Jones, R., and Tocchini, K. (2017) 'Shinrin-yoku (forest bathing) and nature therapy: A state-of-the-art review.' *International Journal of Environmental Research and Public Health 14*, 8, 851.

Harada, K., Lee, S., Park, H., Shimada, H. *et al.* (2016) 'Going outdoors and cognitive function among community-dwelling older adults: Moderating role of physical function.' *Geriatrics & Gerontology International 16*, 1, 65–73.

Harris, K.I. (2016) 'Let's play at the park! Family pathways promoting spiritual resources to inspire nature, pretend play, storytelling, intergenerational play and celebrations.' *International Journal of Children's Spirituality 21*, 2, 90–103.

Havighurst, R.J. (1952) *Developmental Tasks and Education.* Philadelphia: David McKay.

Havighurst, R. (1972) *Developmental Tasks and Education* (3rd ed.). Philadelphia: McKay.

Hawkins, J.E., Mercer, J., Thirlaway, K.J., and Clayton, D.A. (2013) '"Doing" gardening and "being" at the allotment site: Exploring the benefits of allotment gardening for stress reduction and healthy aging.' *Ecopsychology 5*, 2, 110–125.

Hawthorne, D.G. and Griffith, P. (2000) 'The Friendship Scale: Development and Properties' (Working Paper 114). Centre for Health Program Evaluation. Accessed on 2/12/22 at https://core.ac.uk/download/pdf/36962344.pdf

Healthy Aging Team (2021) 'The top 10 most common chronic diseases for older adults.' National Council on Aging, April 23. Accessed on 2/12/22 at www.ncoa.org/article/the-top-10-most-common-chronic-conditions-in-older-adults

Hendriks, I.H., van Vliet, D., Gerritsen, D.L., and Dröes, R.-M. (2016) 'Nature and dementia: Development of a person-centered approach.' *International Psychogeriatrics 28*, 9, 1455–1470.

Hertzog, C., Kramer, A.F., Wilson, R.S., and Lindenberger, U. (2008) 'Enrichment effects on adult cognitive development: Can the functional capacity of older adults be preserved and enhanced?' *Psychological Science in the Public Interest 9*, 1, 1–65.

Heyerdahl, C. (n.d.) 'Mother Nature is the great equalizer.' quotefancy.com. Accessed on 30/11/22 at https://quotefancy.com/quote/1688758/Christopher-Heyerdahl-Mother-Nature-is-the-great-equalizer-You-can-t-get-away-from-it

Hickman-Dunne, J. (2019) 'Experiencing the outdoors: Embodied encounters in the Outward Bound Trust.' *Geographical Journal 185*, 3, 279–291.

History of Medicine Division (2012) 'Greek Medicine: The Hippocratic Oath' (M. North, trans.). U.S. National Library of Medicine, National Institutes of Health. Accessed on 30/11/22 at www.nlm.nih.gov/hmd/greek/greek_oath.html

Hobbs, L.K. (2015) 'Play-based science learning activities: Engaging adults and children with informal science learning for preschoolers.' *Science and Communication 37*, 3, 405–414.

Hochberg, Z. and Konner, M. (2020) 'Emerging adulthood: a pre-adult life-history stage.' *Frontiers in Endocrinology 10*, 918.

Holt-Lunstad, J. (2017) 'The potential public health relevance of social isolation and loneliness: Prevalence, epidemiology, and risk factors.' *Public Policy & Aging Report 27*, 4, 127–130.

Honig, A.S. (2019) 'Outdoors in nature: Special spaces for young children's learning.' *Early Child Development and Care 189*, 4, 659–669.

Hornor, G. (2019) 'Attachment disorders.' *Journal of Pediatric Health Care 33*, 5, 612–622.

Howarth, M., Brettle, A., Hardman M., and Maden, M. (2020) 'What is the evidence for the impact of gardens and gardening on health and well-being? A scoping review and evidence-based logic model to guide healthcare strategy decision making on the use of gardening approaches as a social prescription.' *BMJ Open 10*, e036923.

Hunter, S.B., Barber, B.K., and Stolz, H.E. (2015) 'Extending knowledge of parents' role in adolescent development: The mediating effect of self-esteem.' *Journal of Child and Family Studies 24*, 8, 2474–2484.

Huxley, R., Mendis, S., Zheleznyakov, E., Reddy, S., and Chan, J. (2010) 'Body mass index, waist circumference and waist:hip ratio as predictors of cardiovascular risk: A review of the literature.' *European Journal of Clinical Nutrition 64*, 1, 16–22.

Ibes, D.C., Rakow, D.A., and Kim, C.H. (2021) 'Barriers to nature engagement for youth of color.' *Children, Youth and Environments 31*, 3, 49–73.

Ireland, A.V., Finnegan-John, J., Hubbard, G., Scanlon, K., and Kyle, R.G. (2019) 'Walking groups for women with breast cancer: Mobilising therapeutic assemblages of walk, talk and place.' *Social Science & Medicine 231*, 38–46.

Irvine, K., Fisher, D., Currie, M., Marselle, M., and Warber, S. (2021) 'Social isolation of older adults: A qualitative study of the effects of group outdoor health walks on social wellbeing.' *Global Advances in Health and Medicine 10*, 57.

Ismail, K.H., Rahman, A., Badayai, A., and Rubini, K. (2017) 'Children's development and well-being: A review of environmental stressors in children's physical environments.' *Journal of Social Sciences and Humanities 3*, 1–10.

Iwasaki, S. and Yamasoba, T. (2014) 'Dizziness and imbalance in the elderly: Age-related decline in the vestibular system.' *Aging and Disease 6*, 1, 38–47.

Izenstark, D. and Ebata, A.T. (2016) 'Theorizing family-based nature activities and family functioning: The integration of attention restoration theory with a family routines and rituals perspective.' *Journal of Family Theory & Review 8*, 2, 137–153.

Izenstark, D. and Ebata, A.T. (2019) 'Why families go outside: An exploration of mothers' and daughters' family-based nature activities.' *Leisure Sciences 44*, 5, 559–577.

Izenstark, D. and Middaugh, E. (2022) 'Patterns of family-based nature activities across the early life course and their association with adulthood outdoor participation and preference.' *Journal of Leisure Research 53*, 1, 4–26.

Jackson, S.B., Stevenson, K.T., Larson, L.R., Peterson, M.N., and Seekamp, E. (2021a) 'Connection to nature boosts adolescents' mental well-being during the COVID-19 pandemic.' *Sustainability 13*, 21, 12297.

Jackson, S.B., Stevenson, K.T., Larson, L.R., Peterson, M.N., and Seekamp, E. (2021b) 'Outdoor activity participation improves adolescents' mental health and well-being during the COVID-19 pandemic.' *International Journal of Environmental Research and Public Health 18*, 5, 2506.

Jennings, V. and Bamkole, O. (2019) 'The relationship between social cohesion and urban green space: An avenue for health promotion.' *International Journal of Environmental Research and Public Health 16*, 3, 452.

Jennings, V., Baptiste, A.K., Osborne Jelks, N.T., and Skeete, R. (2017) 'Urban green space and the pursuit of health equity in parts of the United States.' *International Journal of Environmental Research and Public Health 14*, 11, 1432.

Johnstone, A., McCrorie, P., Cordovil, R., Fjørtoft, I. *et al.* (2022) 'Nature-based early childhood education and children's physical activity, sedentary behavior, motor competence, and other physical health outcomes: A mixed-methods systematic review.' *Journal of Physical Activity and Health 19*, 6, 456–472.

Kamper, S.J., Maher, C.G. and Mackay, G. (2009) 'Global rating of change scales: A review of strengths and weaknesses and considerations for design.' *Journal of Manual & Manipulative Therapy 17*, 3, 163–170.

Kaplan, R. and Kaplan, S. (1989) *The Experience of Nature: A Psychological Perspective.* Cambridge: Cambridge University Press.

Kaplan, S. (1995) 'The restorative benefits of nature: Toward an integrative framework.' *Journal of Environmental Psychology 15*, 3, 169–182.

Kellert, S.R., Case, D.J., Escher, D., Witter, D.J., Mikels-Carrasco, J., and Seng, P.T. (2017) 'The Nature of Americans: Disconnection and Recommendation for Reconnection.' National Report. https://conservationtools.org/library_items/1574/files/1716

Keniger, L.E., Gaston, K.J., Irvine, K.N., and Fuller, R.A. (2013) 'What are the benefits of interacting with nature?' *International Journal of Environmental Research and Public Health 10*, 913–935.

Kepper, M.M., Staiano, A.E., Katzmarzyk, P.T., Reis, R.S. *et al.* (2020) 'Using mixed methods to understand women's parenting practices related to their child's outdoor play and physical activity among families living in diverse neighborhood environments.' *Health & Place 62*, 102292.

Kiresuk, T.J. and Sherman, M.R.E. (1968) 'Goal attainment scaling: A general method for evaluating comprehensive community mental health programs.' *Community Mental Health Journal 4*, 6, 443–453.

Kirk, G. and Jay, J. (2018) 'Supporting kindergarten children's social and emotional development: Examining the synergetic role of environments, play, and relationships.' *Journal of Research in Childhood Education 32*, 4, 472–485.

Kleisiaris, C.F., Sfakianakis, C., and Papathanasiou, I.V. (2014) 'Health care practices in ancient Greece: The Hippocratic ideal.' *Journal of Medical Ethics and History of Medicine 7*, 6.

Klotz, A., McClean, S.T., and Yim, J. (2020) 'When does a daily dose of nature matter? Linking extra-work contact with nature to employee behavior.' *Academy of Management Proceedings* 20, 1, 14337.

Kobaş, M., Kizildere, E., Doğan, I., Aktan-Erciyes, A. *et al.* (2022) 'Motor skills, language development, and visual processing in preterm and full-term infants.' *Current Psychology.* https://doi.org/10.1007/s12144-021-02658-8

Koh, C., Kondo, M.C., Rollins, H., and Bilal, U. (2022) 'Socioeconomic disparities in hypertension by levels of green space availability: A cross-sectional study in Philadelphia, PA.' *International Journal of Environmental Research and Public Health* 19, 4, 2037.

Korpela, K.M. and Ratcliffe, E. (2021) 'Which is primary: Preference or perceived instoration?' *Journal of Environmental Psychology* 75, 101617.

Kroenke, K., Spitzer, R.L., and Williams, J.B. (2001) 'The PHQ-9: Validity of a brief depression severity measure.' *Journal of General Internal Medicine* 16, 9, 606–613.

Kuo, F.E. and Faber-Taylor, A. (2004) 'A potential natural treatment for attention-deficit/hyperactivity disorder: Evidence from a national study.' *American Journal of Public Health* 94, 1580–1586.

Kuo, M., Browning, M.H.E.M., and Penner, M.L. (2018) 'Do lessons in nature boost subsequent Classroom engagement? Refueling students in flight.' *Frontiers in Psychology* 8, 2253.

Kuo, M., Barnes, M., and Jordan, C. (2019) 'Do experiences with nature promote learning? Converging evidence of a cause-and-effect relationship.' *Frontiers in Psychology* 10, 305.

Lambert, A., Vlaar, J., Herrington, S., and Brussoni, M. (2019) 'What is the relationship between the neighbourhood built environment and time spent in outdoor play? A systematic review.' *International Journal of Environmental Research and Public Health* 16, 20, 3840.

Landeiro, F., Barrows, P., Musson, E.N., Gray, A.M., and Leal, J. (2017) 'Reducing social isolation and loneliness in older people: A systematic review protocol.' *BMJ Open* 7, 5, 1–5.

Langa, K.M. and Levine, D.A. (2014) 'The diagnosis and management of mild cognitive impairment: A clinical review.' *Journal of the American Medical Association* 312, 23, 2551–2561.

Larouche, R., Garriguet, D., and Tremblay, M.S. (2016) 'Outdoor time, physical activity and sedentary time among young children: The 2012–2013 Canadian Health Measures Survey.' *Canadian Journal of Public Health*, 10, 6, e500–e506.

Larsen, B. and Luna, B. (2018) 'Adolescence as a neurobiological critical period for the development of higher-order cognition.' *Neuroscience & Biobehavioral Reviews* 94, 179–195.

Larson, L.R., Cooper, C.B., Stedman, R.C., Decker, D.J. and Gagnon, R.J. (2018) 'Place-based pathways to proenvironmental behavior: Empirical evidence for a conservation–recreation model.' *Society & Natural Resources* 31, 871–891.

Larson, L.R., Zhang, Z., Oh, J.I., Beam, W. *et al.* (2021) 'Urban park use during the COVID-19 pandemic: Are socially vulnerable communities disproportionately impacted?' *Frontiers in Sustainable Cities* 3, 710243.

Lawton, M.P., Van Haitsma, K.S. and Klapper, J.A. (1996) 'Observed affect in nursing home residents.' *Journals of Gerontology B* 51, 1, 3–15.

Leavell, M.A., Leiferman, J.A., Gascon, M., Braddick, F., Conzalez, J.C. and Litt, J.S. (2019) 'Nature-based social prescribing in urban settings to improve social connectedness and mental well-being: A review.' *Current Environmental Health Reports* 6, 297–308.

Lee, H.S., Song, J.G., and Lee, J.Y. (2022) 'Influences of dog attachment and dog walking on reducing loneliness during the COVID-19 pandemic in Korea.' *Animals* 12, 4, 483.

Lee, K., Cassidy, J., Tang, W., and Kusek, V. (2022) 'Older adults' responses to a meaningful activity using indoor-based nature experiences: Bird Tales.' *Clinical Gerontologist* 45, 2, 301–311.

Lee, S., Lee, C., and Rodiek, S. (2020) 'Outdoor exposure and perceived outdoor environments correlated to fear of outdoor falling among assisted living residents.' *Aging & Mental Health* 24, 12, 1968–1976.

Leimert, K. and Olson, D.M. (2020). 'Racial disparities in pregnancy outcomes: Genetics, epigenetics, and allostatic load.' *Current Opinion in Physiology 13*, 155–165.

Levinger, P., Sales, M., Polman, R., Haines, T. *et al.* (2018) 'Outdoor physical activity for older people—The senior exercise park: Current research, challenges and future directions.' *Health Promotion Journal of Australia 29*, 3, 353–359.

Lewis, M. and Feiring, C. (1989) 'Infant, mother, and mother–infant interaction behavior and subsequent attachment.' *Child Development 60*, 4, 831–837.

Li, D. and Sullivan, W.C. (2016) 'Impact of views to school landscapes on recovery from stress and mental fatigue.' *Landscape and Urban Planning 148*, 149–158.

Lingham, G., Yazar, S., Lucas, R.M., Milne, E. *et al.* (2021) 'Time spent outdoors in childhood is associated with reduced risk of myopia as an adult.' *Scientific Reports 11*, 1, 6337.

Littman, A.J., Bratman, G.N., Lehavot, K., Engel, C.C. *et al.* (2021) 'Nature versus urban hiking for veterans with post-traumatic stress disorder: A pilot randomised trial conducted in the Pacific Northwest USA.' *BMJ Open 11*, e051885.

Lottrup, L., Grahn, P., and Stigsdotter, U.K. (2013) 'Workplace greenery and perceived level of stress: Benefits of access to a green outdoor environment at the workplace.' *Landscape and Urban Planning 110*, 5–11.

Louv, R. (2010) *Last Child in the Woods: Saving our Children from Nature-Deficit Disorder.* London: Atlantic Books.

Loveland, J. (2017) 'Hands down: Upper extremity challenges that can occur in individuals with diabetes.' *OT Practice 22*, 8, 8–13.

Lovelock, B., Walters, T., Jellum, C., and Thompson-Carr, A. (2016) 'The participation of children, adolescents, and young adults in nature-based recreation.' *Leisure Sciences 38*, 5, 441–460.

Lubben, J., Blozik, E., Gillmann, G., Iliffe, S. *et al.* (2006) 'Performance of an abbreviated version of the Lubben Social Network Scale among three European community-dwelling older adult populations.' *The Gerontologist 46*, 4, 503–513.

Lumen Learning (2022) 'Adulthood.' Accessed on 2/12/22 at https://courses.lumenlearning.com/waymaker-psychology/chapter/reading-adulthood

MacKerron, G. and Mourato, S. (2013) 'Happiness is greater in natural environments.' *Global Environmental Change 23*, 5, 992–1000.

MacNaughton, P., Eitland, E., Kloog, I., Schwartz, J., and Allen, J. (2017) 'Impact of particulate matter exposure and surrounding "greenness" on chronic absenteeism in Massachusetts public schools.' *International Journal of Research and Public Health 14*, 2, 207.

Mahler, K. (2018) *The Interoception Curriculum: A Step-by-Step Guide to Developing Mindful Self-regulation.* Shawnee, KS: AAPC Publishing.

Malani, P., Kullgren, J., Solway, E., Ober-Allen, J., Singer, D., and Kirch, M. (2020) 'Everyday Ageism and Health.' National Poll on Healthy Aging. Accessed on 19/06/23 at https://www.healthyagingpoll.org/reports-more/report/everyday-ageism-and-health

Malcolm, M., Frost, H., and Cowie, J. (2019) 'Loneliness and social isolation causal association with health-related lifestyle risk in older adults: A systematic review and meta-analysis protocol.' *Systematic Reviews 8*, 1, 48.

Maresca, G., Portaro, S., Naro, A., Crisafulli, R. *et al.* (2020) 'Hippotherapy in neurodevelopmental disorders: A narrative review focusing on cognitive and behavioral outcomes.' *Applied Neuropsychology: Child 11*, 3, 553–560.

Marselle, M.R., Warber, S.L., and Irvine, K.N. (2019) 'Growing resilience through interaction with nature: Can group walks in nature buffer the effects of stressful life events on mental health?' *International Journal of Environmental Research and Public Health 16*, 6, 986.

Marshall, J., Ferrier, B., Ward, P.B., and Martindale, R. (2020) '"When I was surfing with those guys I was surfing with family": A grounded exploration of program theory within the Jimmy Miller Memorial.' *Global Journal of Community Psychology Practice 11*, 2, 1–19.

Mather, M. and Kilduff, L. (2020) 'The U.S. population is growing older, and the gender gap in life expectancy is narrowing.' Population Reference Bureau, February 19. Accessed on 2/13/23 at www.prb.org/resources/u-s-population-is-growing-older

Matthews, D.M. and Jenks, S.M. (2013) 'Ingestion of *Mycobacterium vaccae* decreases anxiety-related behavior and improves learning in mice.' *Behavioural Processes 96*, 27–35. https://doi.org/10.1016/j.beproc.2013.02.007

Mayer, F.S., Frantz, C.M., Bruehlman-Senecal, E., and Dolliver, K. (2009) 'Why is nature beneficial? The role of connectedness to nature.' *Environment and Behavior 41*, 5, 617–643.

Mayer, J.D. and Gaschke, Y.N. (1988) 'The experience and meta-experience of mood.' *Journal of Personality and Social Psychology 55*, 102–111.

Mayer, J.D., Allen, J., and Beauregard, K. (1995) 'Mood inductions for four specific moods: Procedure employing guided imagery vignettes with music.' *Journal of Mental Imagery 19*, 133–150.

McAllister, E., Bhullar, N., and Schutte, N.S. (2017) 'Into the woods or a stroll in the park: How virtual contact with nature impacts positive and negative affect.' *International Journal of Environmental Research and Public Health 14*, 7, 786.

McNair, D., Lorr, M., and Droppleman, L. (1992) *Revised Manual for the Profile of Mood States*. Princeton, NJ: Educational and Industrial Testing Service.

Merriam, S. and Mullins, L. (1981) 'Havighurst's adult developmental tasks: A study of their importance relative to income, age and sex.' *Adult Education 31*, 3, 123–141.

Mitchell, R. (2013) 'What is equigenesis and how might it help narrow health inequalities? Centre for Research of Environment, Society and Health. Accessed on 30/11/22 at https://cresh.org.uk/2013/11/08/what-is-equigenesis-and-how-might-it-help-narrow-health-inequalities/

Mitchell, R.J., Richardson, E.A., Shortt, N.K., and Pearce, J.R. (2015) 'Neighborhood environments and socioeconomic inequalities in mental well-being.' *American Journal of Preventive Medicine 49*, 1, 8–84.

Miyazaki, Y. (2018) *Shinrin Yoku: The Japanese Art of Forest Bathing*. Portland, OR: Timber Press.

Miyazaki, Y., Song, C., and Ikei, H. (2015) 'Preventive medical effects of nature therapy and their individual differences.' *Japanese Journal of Physiological Anthropology 20*, 1, 19–32.

Moore, D., Morrissey, A.-M., and Robertson, N. (2021) '"I feel like I'm getting sad there": Early childhood outdoor play spaces as places for children's wellbeing.' *Early Child Development and Care 191*, 6, 933–951.

Moss, S. (2012) 'Natural Childhood.' National Trust. Accessed on 30/11/22 at www.lotc.org.uk/wp-content/uploads/2012/04/National-Trust-natural_childhood.pdf

Mulholland, R. and Williams, A. (1998) 'Exploring together outdoors: A family therapy approach based in the outdoors for troubled mother/daughter relationships.' *Journal of Outdoor and Environmental Education 3*, 21–31.

Mulry, C., Gardner, J., Hardaway, H., Zissler-Syers, K. *et al.* (2017) 'Preemptive home modifications for fall prevention and facilitating participation in older adults in PACE program.' *SIS Quarterly Practice Connections 2*, 2, 21–23.

Murphy, D., Kahn-D'Angelo, L., and Gleason, J. (2008) 'The effect of hippotherapy on functional outcomes for children with disabilities: A pilot study.' *Pediatric Physical Therapy 20*, 3, 264–270.

Murray-Browne, S. (2022) 'Courses.' Kindred Wellness. Accessed on 2/12/22 at www.shawnamurraybrowne.com/courses

Murry, V.M. and Lippold, M.A. (2018) 'Parenting practices in diverse family structures: Examination of adolescents' development and adjustment.' *Journal of Research on Adolescence 28*, 3, 650–664.

Mutz, M. and Müller, J. (2016) 'Mental health benefits of outdoor adventures: Results from two pilot studies.' *Journal of Adolescence 49*, 1, 105–114.

Mygind, L., Stevenson, M.P., Liebst, L.S., Konvalinka, I., and Bentsen, P. (2018) 'Stress response and cognitive performance modulation in classroom versus natural environments: A quasi-experimental pilot study with children.' *International Journal of Environmental Research and Public Health 15*, 6, 1098.

Mygind, L., Kjeldsted, E., Hartmeyer, R., Mygind, E., Bølling, M., and Bentsen, P. (2019) 'Mental, physical and social health benefits of immersive nature-experience for children and adolescents: A systematic review and quality assessment of the evidence.' *Health & Place 58*, 102136.

Nanthakumar, C. (2018) 'The benefits of yoga in children.' *Journal of Integrative Medicine 16*, 1, 14–19.

National Institute of Health (2017) 'NIH policy and guidelines on the inclusion of women and minorities as subjects in clinical research.' Accessed on 2/12/22 at https://grants.nih.gov/policy/inclusion/women-and-minorities/guidelines.htm

Naval Postgraduate School (n.d.) 'Operational risk management.' Accessed on 30/11/22 at https://nps.edu/web/safety/orm

North Carolina State University (2019 [1997]) 'Universal design principles.' Center for Universal Design. Accessed on 3/11/22 at www.udinstitute.org/principles

Nedovic, S. and Morrissey, A.-M. (2013) 'Calm, active and focused: Children's responses to an organic outdoor learning environment.' *Learning Environments Research 16*, 2, 281–295.

Ng, K.S.T., Sia, A., Ng, M.K.W., Tan, C.T.Y. *et al.* (2018) 'Effects of horticultural therapy on Asian older adults: A randomized controlled trial.' *International Journal of Environmental Research and Public Health 15*, 8.

Nicholas, S.O., Giang, A.T., and Yap, P.L.K. (2019) 'The effectiveness of horticultural therapy on older adults: A systematic review.' *Journal of the American Medical Directors Association 20*, 10, 1351.e1–1351.e11.

Nigg, C., Niessner, C., Nigg, C.R., Oriwol, D., Schmidt, S.C.E., and Woll, A. (2021) 'Relating outdoor play to sedentary behavior and physical activity in youth: Results from a cohort study.' *BMC Public Health 21*, 1, 1716.

Noar, L. and Mayseless, O. (2020) 'The therapeutic value of experiencing spirituality in nature.' *Spirituality in Clinical Practice 7*, 2, 114–133.

Norling, J., Sibthorp, J., and Ruddell, E. (2008) 'Perceived Restorativeness for Activities Scale (PRAS): Development and validation.' *Journal of Physical Activity & Health 5*, 1, 184–195.

Norling, M., Sandberg, A., and Almqvist, L. (2015) 'Engagement and emergent literacy practices in Swedish preschools.' *European Early Childhood Education Research Journal 23*, 5, 619–634.

Norwood, M.F., Lakhani, A., Fullagar, S., Maujean, A. *et al.* (2019) 'A narrative and systematic review of the behavioural, cognitive and emotional effects of passive nature exposure on young people: Evidence for prescribing change.' *Landscape and Urban Planning 189*, 71–79.

Oakley, F., Kielhofner, G., Barris, R., and Reichler, R K. (1986) 'The Role Checklist: Development and empirical assessment of reliability.' *Occupational Therapy Journal of Research 6*, 3, 157–170.

Oliveros, M.J., Serón, P., Lanas, F., and Bangdiwala, S.I. (2021) 'Impact of outdoor gyms on adults' participation in physical activity: A natural experiment in Chile.' *Journal of Physical Activity and Health 18*, 11, 1412–1418.

Opper, B., Maree, J.G., Fletcher, L., and Sommerville, J. (2014) 'Efficacy of outdoor adventure education in developing emotional intelligence during adolescence.' *Journal of Psychology in Africa 24*, 2, 193–196.

Orben, A., Tomova, L., and Blakemore, S.J. (2020) 'The effects of social deprivation on adolescent development and mental health.' *The Lancet: Child & Adolescent Health 4*, 8, 634–640.

Outward Bound (2021) 'Our Mission.' Accessed on 2/12/22 at www.outwardbound.org/our-difference/mission-and-vision

Owens, P.E. and McKinnon, I. (2009) 'In pursuit of nature: The role of nature in adolescents' lives.' *Journal of Developmental Processes 4*, 1, 43–58.

Özdemir, A., Utkualp, N., and Palloş, A. (2016) 'Physical and psychosocial effects of the changes in adolescence period.' *International Journal of Caring Sciences 9*, 2, 717.

Padro-Guzman, J. (2022) 'Answers to 8 FAQ about Chemotherapy-Induced Peripheral Neuropathy (CIPN).' Accessed 27/02/2023 at www.mskcc.org/news/answers-faq-about-chemotherapy-induced-peripheral-neuropathy-cipn

Pagels, P., Raustorp, A., Ponce De Leon, A., Mårtensson, F., Kylin, M. and Boldemann, C. (2014) 'A repeated measurement study investigating the impact of school outdoor environment upon physical activity across ages and seasons in Swedish second, fifth and eighth graders.' *Biomed Central Public Health 14*, 803.

Park, B.J., Tsunetsugu, Y., Kasetani, T., Kagawa, T., and Miyazaki, Y. (2010) 'The physiological effects of Shinrin-yoku (taking in the forest atmosphere or forest bathing): Evidence from field experiments in 24 forests across Japan.' *Environmental Health and Preventive Medicine 15*, 1, 18–26.

Park, S.A., Shoemaker, C.A., and Haub, M.D. (2008) 'A preliminary investigation on exercise intensities of gardening tasks in older adults.' *Perceptual and Motor Skills 107*, 3, 974–980.

Park, S.A., Lee, A.Y., Son, K.C., Lee, W.L., and Kim, D.S. (2016) 'Gardening intervention for physical and psychological health benefits in elderly women at community centers.' *HortTechnology 26*, 4, 474–483.

Pearson, D.G. and Craig, T. (2014) 'The great outdoors? Exploring the mental health benefits of natural environments.' *Frontiers in Psychology 5*, 1178.

Penn Medicine (n.d.) 'Dr. Benjamin Rush.' University of Pennsylvania. Accessed on 30/11/22 at www.uphs.upenn.edu/paharc/features/brush.html

Petencin, K., Diaz, K., and Kirchen, T. (2016) 'Harvesting memories with older adults using therapeutic gardening.' *OT Practice 21*, 12, 23–25.

Pfeifer, E., Fiedler, H., and Wittmann, M. (2019) 'Increased relaxation and present orientation after a period of silence in a natural surrounding.' *Nordic Journal of Music Therapy 29*, 1, 75–92.

Piccininni, C., Michaelson, V., Janssen, I., and Pickett, W. (2018) 'Outdoor play and nature connectedness as potential correlates of internalized mental health symptoms among Canadian adolescents.' *Preventive Medicine 112*, 168–175.

Pouso, S., Borja, Á., Fleming, L.E., Gómez-Baggethun, E., White, M.P., and Uyarra, M.C. (2021) 'Contact with blue-green spaces during the COVID-19 pandemic lockdown beneficial for mental health.' *Science of the Total Environment 756*, 143984.

Pretty, J. (2004) 'How nature contributes to mental and physical health.' *Spirituality and Health International 5*, 2, 68–78.

Pretty, J., Bragg, R., and Barton, J. (2006) 'Green exercise: The benefits of activities in green places.' *Biologist 53*, 143–148.

Price, M.J. and Trbovich, M. (2018) 'Thermoregulation Following Spinal Cord Injury.' In A. Romanovsky (ed.) *Handbook of Clinical Neurology*. Amsterdam: Elsevier.

Prince-Embury, S. (2006) *Resiliency Scales for Children and Adolescents: Profiles of Personal Strengths.* San Antonio, TX: Harcourt Assessments.

Prince-Embury, S. (2008) 'The Resiliency Scales for Children and Adolescents, psychological symptoms, and clinical status in adolescents.' *Canadian Journal of School Psychology 23*, 1, 41–56.

Puhakka, S., Pyky, R., Lankila, T., Kangas, M. *et al.* (2018) 'Physical activity, residential environment, and nature relatedness in young men: A population-based MOPO study.' *International Journal of Environmental Research and Public Health 15*, 10, 2322.

Pusch, S., Mund, M., Hagemeyer, B., and Finn, C. (2019) 'Personality development in emerging and young adulthood: A study of age differences.' *European Journal of Personality 33*, 3, 245–263.

Pynoos, J., Steinman, B.A., and Nguyen, A.Q.D. (2010) 'Environmental assessment and modification as fall-prevention strategies for older adults.' *Clinics in Geriatric Medicine 26*, 4, 633–644.

Quillen, D.A. (1999) 'Common causes of vision loss in elderly patients.' *American Family Physician 60*, 1, 99–108.

Rantala, O. and Puhakka, R. (2020) 'Engaging with nature: Nature affords well-being for families and young people in Finland.' *Children's Geographies 18*, 4, 490–503.

Rebeiro, K.L. (2001) 'Enabling occupation: The importance of an affirming environment.' *Canadian Journal of Occupational Therapy 68*, 2, 80–89.

Resilience Research Centre (2009) *The Child and Youth Resilience Measure-28: User Manual.* Halifax, NS: Dalhousie University Resilience Research Centre.

Riding, R., Rayner, S., Morris, S., Grimley, M., and Adams, D. (2002) *Emotional and Behavioral Development Scales.* Birmingham, UK: Assessment Research Unit, School of Education, University of Birmingham.

Rigolon, A. and Flohr, T.L. (2014) 'Access to parks for youth as an environmental justice issue: Access inequalities and possible solutions.' *Buildings 4*, 2, 69–94.

Rikli, R.E. and C.J. Jones (2013) *Senior Fitness Test Manual.* Champaign, IL: Human Kinetics.

Rishbeth, C. and Rogaly, B. (2018) 'Sitting outside: Conviviality, self-care and the design of benches in urban public space.' *Transactions of the Institute of British Geographers 43*, 2, 284–298.

Roberts, S.D., Stroud, D., Hoag, M.J., and Combs, K.M. (2016) 'Outdoor behavioral health care: Client and treatment characteristics effects on young adult outcomes.' *Journal of Experiential Education 39*, 3, 288–302.

Robertson, N., Yim, B., and Paatsch, L. (2020) 'Connections between children's involvement in dramatic play and the quality of early childhood environments.' *Early Child Development and Care 190*, 3, 376–389.

Rogers, C.M., Mallinson, T., and Peppers, D. (2014) 'High-intensity sports for posttraumatic stress disorder and depression: Feasibility study of ocean therapy with veterans of Operation Enduring Freedom and Operation Iraqi Freedom.' *American Journal of Occupational Therapy 68*, 4, 395–404.

Rogers, P. and Powell, J. (1992) 'Making gardening easier: Gardening with limited range of motion.' Oregon State University Extension Catalog, EM8505, 1–2. Accessed on 2/12/22 at https://catalog.extension.oregonstate.edu/em8505

Rogerson, M., Wood, C., Pretty, J., Schoenmakers, P., Bloomfield, D., and Barton, J. (2020) 'Regular doses of nature: The efficacy of green exercise interventions for mental wellbeing.' *International Journal of Environmental Research and Public Health 17*, 5, 1526.

Rose, V., Stewart, I., Jenkins, K.G., Tabbaa, L., Ang, C.S., and Matsangidou, M. (2021) 'Bringing the outside in: The feasibility of virtual reality with people with dementia in an inpatient psychiatric care setting.' *Dementia 20*, 1, 106–129.

Rosenberg, R.S., Lange, W., Zebrack, B., Moulton, S., and Kosslyn, S.M. (2014) 'An outdoor adventure program for young adults with cancer: Positive effects on body image and psychosocial functioning.' *Journal of Psychosocial Oncology 32*, 5, 622–636.

Rowland-Shea, J., Doshi, S., Edberg, S., and Fanger, R. (2020) 'The Nature Gap: Confronting racial and economic disparities in the destruction and protection of nature in America.' Center for American Progress. Accessed on 30/11/22 at www.americanprogress.org/article/the-nature-gap

Runkle, J.D., Matthews, J.L., Sparks, L., McNicholas, L., and Sugg, M.M. (2022) 'Racial and ethnic disparities in pregnancy complications and the protective role of greenspace: A retrospective birth cohort study.' *Science of the Total Environment 808*, 152145.

Saadi, D., Schnell, I., Tirosh, E., Basagaña, X., and Agay-Shay, K. (2020) 'There's no place like home? The psychological, physiological, and cognitive effects of short visits to outdoor urban environments compared to staying in the indoor home environment: A field experiment on women from two ethnic groups.' *Environmental Research 187*, 109687.

Sääkslahti, A. and Niemistö, D. (2021) 'Outdoor activities and motor development in 2–7-year-old boys and girls.' *Journal of Physical Education and Sport 21*, Suppl. 1, 463–468.

Salbach, N.M., Barclay, R., Webber, S.C., Jones, C.A. *et al.* (2019) 'A theory-based, task-oriented, outdoor walking programme for older adults with difficulty walking outdoors: Protocol for the Getting Older adults OUTdoors (GO-OUT) randomised controlled trial.' *BMJ Open 9*, 4, e029393.

Salzman, B. (2010) 'Gait and balance disorders in older adults.' *American Family Physician 82*, 1, 61–68.

Sarkisian, G.V., Curtis, C., and Rogers, C.M. (2020) 'Emerging hope: Outcomes of a one-day surf therapy program with youth at-promise.' *Global Journal of Community Psychology Practice 11*, 2, 1–16.

Sasso, D.A. (2020) 'The walking cure.' *Psychiatric Times*, August 3. Accessed on 12/3/2023 at www.psychiatrictimes.com/view/walking-cure.

Sawyer, S.M., Afifi, R.A., Bearinger, L.H., Blakemore, S.-J. *et al.* (2012) 'Adolescence: A foundation for future health.' *The Lancet 379*, 9826, 1630–1640.

Scarpina, F. and Tagini, S. (2017) 'The Stroop Color and Word Test.' *Frontiers in Psychology 8*, 557.

Scheimer, D. and Chakrabarti, M. (2020) 'Former Surgeon General Vivek Murthy: Loneliness is a Public Health Crisis' [audio podcast episode]. WBUR: On Point. Accessed on 30/11/22 at www.wbur.org/onpoint/2020/03/23/vivek-murthy-loneliness

Schmidt, S.N. (2020) 'Beekeeping as a healing intervention: Historical background, recent programs and proposed mechanisms of action.' Cascade Girl. Accessed on 2/12/22 at www.cascadegirl.org/beekeeping-for-healing-and-therapy

Schölzel-Dorenbos, C.J., Meeuwsen, E.J., and Olde Rikkert, M.G. (2010) 'Integrating unmet needs into dementia health-related quality of life research and care: Introduction of the Hierarchy Model of Needs in Dementia.' *Aging and Mental Health 14*, 1, 113–119.

Scorza, P., Araya, R., Wuermli, A.J., and Betancourt, T.S. (2015) 'Towards clarity in research on "non-cognitive" skills: Linking executive functions, self-regulation, and economic development to advance life outcomes for children, adolescents, and youth globally.' *Human Development 58*, 6, 313–317.

Seaman, J., Sharp, E.H., Tucker, C.J., Van Gundy, K., and Rebellon, C. (2019) 'Outdoor activity involvement and postsecondary status among rural adolescents: Results from a longitudinal analysis.' *Journal of Leisure Research 50*, 1, 18–27.

Shanahan, D.F., Bush, R., Gaston, K.J., Lin, B.B. *et al.* (2016) 'Health benefits from nature experiences depend on dose.' *Scientific Reports 6*, 1, 1–10.

Shanahan, D.F., Franco, L., Lin, B.B., Gaston, K.J., and Fuller, R.A. (2016) 'The benefits of natural environments for physical activity.' *Sports Medicine 46*, 989–995.

Shanahan, D.F., Astell-Burt, T., Barber, E., Brymer, E. *et al.* (2019) 'Nature-based interventions for improving health and wellbeing: The purpose, the people and the outcomes.' *Sports 7*, 6, 141.

Shankar, A., McMunn, A., Demakakos, P., Hamer, M., and Steptoe, A. (2017) 'Social isolation and loneliness: Prospective associations with functional status in older adults.' *Health Psychology 36*, 2, 179–187.

Sharma, M., Largo-Wight, E., Kanekar, A., Kusumoto, H., Hooper, S., and Nahar, V.K. (2020) 'Using the Multi-Theory Model (MTM) of health behavior change to explain intentional outdoor nature contact behavior among college students.' *International Journal of Environmental Research and Public Health 17*, 17, 6104.

Shimada, H., Ishizaki, T., Kato, M., Morimoto, A. *et al.* (2010) 'How often and how far do frail elderly people need to go outdoors to maintain functional capacity?' *Archives of Gerontology and Geriatrics 50*, 2, 140–146.

Shuda, Q., Bougoulias, M.E., and Kass, R. (2020) 'Effect of nature exposure on perceived and physiologic stress: A systematic review.' *Complementary Therapies in Medicine 53*, 102514.

Sia, A., Tam, W.W., Fogel, A., Kua, E.H., Khoo, K., and Ho, R. (2020) 'Nature-based activities improve the well-being of older adults.' *Scientific Reports 10*, 1, 1–8.

Simpson, A.R. (2018) 'Changes in young adulthood.' Massachusetts Institute of Technology. Accessed on 2/12/22 at https://hr.mit.edu/static/worklife/youngadult/changes.html

Singer, C. (2018) 'Health effects of social isolation and loneliness.' *Journal of Aging Life Care* 28, 1, 4–8.

Sjögren, K. and Stjernberg, L. (2010) 'A gender perspective on factors that influence outdoor recreational physical activity among the elderly.' *BMC Geriatrics* 10, 1, 1–9.

Smith, J.M. (2012) 'Toward a better understanding of loneliness in community-dwelling older adults.' *Journal of Psychology* 146, 3, 293–311.

Snyder, C.R., Harris, C., Anderson, J.R., Holleran, S.A. *et al.* (1991) 'The will and the ways: Development and validation of an individual-differences measure of hope.' *Journal of Personality and Social Psychology* 60, 570–585.

Snyder, C.R., Hoza, B., Pelham, W.E., Rapoff, M. *et al.* (1997) 'The development and validation of the Children's Hope Scale.' *Journal of Pediatric Psychology* 22, 3, 399–421.

Söderström, M., Boldemann, C., Sahlin, U., Mårtensson, F., Raustorp, A., and Blennow, M. (2013) 'The quality of the outdoor environment influences childrens health: A cross-sectional study of preschools.' *Acta Paediatrica* 102, 1, 83–91.

Soga, M., Gaston, K.J., and Yamaura, Y. (2017) 'Gardening is beneficial for health: A meta-analysis.' *Preventive Medical Reports* 5, 92–99.

Soga, M., Evans, M.J., Tsuchiya, K., and Fukano, Y. (2020) 'A room with a green view: The importance of nearby nature during the COVID-19 pandemic.' *Ecological Applications* 31, 2, e2248.

Souter-Brown, G., Hinckson, E., and Duncan, S. (2021) 'Effects of a sensory garden on workplace wellbeing: A randomised control trial.' *Landscape and Urban Planning* 207, 10399.

Spano, G., D'Este, M., Giannico, V., Carrus, G. *et al.* (2020) 'Are community gardening and horticultural interventions beneficial for psychosocial well-being? A meta-analysis.' *International Journal of Environmental Research and Public Health* 17, 10, 3584.

Steigen, A.M., Eriksson, B., Kogstad, R.E., Toft, H.P., and Bergh, D. (2018). 'Young adults in nature-based services in Norway: In-group and between-group variations related to mental health problems.' *Nordic Journal of Social Research* 9, 110–133.

Stigsdotter, U.K., Palsdottir, A.M., Burls, A., Chermaz, A., Ferrini, F., and Grahn, P. (2011) 'Nature-Based Therapeutic Interventions.' In K. Nilsson, M. Sangster, C. Gallis, T. Hartig *et al.* (eds) *Forests, Trees and Human Health*. Dordrecht: Springer.

Stolt, S., Lind, A., Matomäki, J., Haataja, L., Lapinleimu, H., and Lehtonen, L. (2016) 'Do the early development of gestures and receptive and expressive language predict language skills at 5;0 in prematurely born very-low-birth-weight children?' *Journal of Communication Disorders* 61, 16–28.

Strooband, K.F.B., Howard, S.J., Okely, A.D., Neilson Hewitt, C., and de Rosnay, M. (2022) 'Validity and reliability of a fine motor assessment for preschool children.' *Early Childhood Education Journal*. https://doi.org/10.1007/s10643-022-01336-z

Sugiyama, T., Carver, A., Koohsari, M.J., and Veitch, J. (2018) 'Advantages of public green spaces in enhancing population health.' *Landscape and Urban Planning* 178, 12–17.

Sugiyama, N., Hosaka, T., Takagi, E., and Numata, S. (2021) 'How do childhood nature experiences and negative emotions towards nature influence preferences for outdoor activity among young adults?' *Landscape and Urban Planning* 205, 103971.

Taylor, B. (ed.) (2010) 'Friluftsliv.' In *The Encyclopedia of Religion and Nature*. New York, NY: Continuum Press.

Terrapin Bright Green (2014) *14 Patterns of Biophilic Design: Improving Health and Well-Being in the Built Environment*. New York, NY: Terrapin Bright Green. Accessed on 30/11/22 at www.terrapinbrightgreen.com/reports/14-patterns

Tester-Jones, M., White, M.P., Elliott, L.R., Weinstein, N. *et al.* (2020) 'Results from an 18 country cross-sectional study examining experiences of nature for people with common mental health disorders.' *Scientific Reports* 10, 1, 19408.

Thorburn, M. and Marshall, A. (2014) 'Cultivating lived-body consciousness: Enhancing cognition and emotion through outdoor learning.' *Journal of Pedagogy 5*, 1, 115–132.

Tidball, K. (2018) 'Farming and veterans: Why agricultural programs resonate with returning combatants.' *Journal of Veterans Studies 3*, 1, 85–88.

Tillmann, S., Tobin, D., Avison, W., and Gilliland, J. (2018) 'Mental health benefits of interactions with nature in children and teenagers: A systematic review.' *Journal of Epidemiology and Community Health 72*, 10, 958–966.

Tse, M.M.Y. (2010) 'Therapeutic effects of an indoor gardening programme for older people living in nursing homes.' *Journal of Clinical Nursing 19*, 78, 949–958.

Ulrich, R. (1984) 'View through a window may influence recovery from surgery.' *Science 224*, 420–421.

Ulrich, R.S., Simons, R.F., Losito, B.D., Fiorito, E., Miles, M.A., and Zelson, M. (1991) 'Stress recovery during exposure to natural and urban environments.' *Journal of Environmental Psychology 11*, 201–203.

U.S. Department of Health and Human Services (2018) *Adolescent Development Explained.* Washington, DC: HHS, Office of Population Affairs. Accessed on 2/12/22 at https://opa. hhs.gov/sites/default/files/2021-03/adolescent-development-explained-download.pdf

Valevicius, A.M., Boser, A., Lavoie, E.B., Murgatroyd, G.S. *et al.* (2018) 'Characterization of normative hand movements during two functional upper limb tasks.' *PLoS One 13*, 6, e0199549.

Van Hecke, L., Ghekiere, A., Van Cauwenberg, J., Veitch, J. *et al.* (2018) 'Park characteristics preferred for adolescent park visitation and physical activity: A choice-based conjoint analysis using manipulated photographs.' *Landscape and Urban Planning 178*, 144–155.

Vella-Brodrick, D.A. and Gilowska, K. (2022) 'Effects of nature (greenspace) on cognitive functioning in school children and adolescents: A systematic review.' *Educational Psychology Review 34*, 1217–1254.

Visser-Bochane, M.I., Reijneveld, S.A., Krijnen, W.P., van der Schans, C.P., and Luinge, M.R. (2020) 'Identifying milestones in language development for young children ages 1 to 6 years.' *Academic Pediatrics 20*, 3, 421–429.

Wade, L., Lubans, D.R., Smith, J.J., and Duncan, M.J. (2020) 'The impact of exercise environments on adolescents' cognitive and psychological outcomes: A randomised controlled trial.' *Psychology of Sport and Exercise 49*, 101707.

Wagenfeld, A. and Atchison, B. (2014) '"Putting the occupation back in occupational therapy": A survey of occupational therapy practitioners' use of gardening as an intervention.' *Open Journal of Occupational Therapy 4*, 2, 4.

Wagenfeld, A., Schefkind, S., and Hock, N. (2019) 'Measuring emotional response to a planting activity for staff at an urban office setting.' *Open Journal of Occupational Therapy 7*, 2, 5.

Wales, M., Mårtensson, F., Hoff, E., and Jansson, M. (2022) 'Elevating the role of the outdoor environment for adolescent wellbeing in everyday life.' *Frontiers in Psychology 13*, 774592.

Wallner, P., Kundi, M., Arnberger, A., Eder, R. *et al.* (2018) 'Reloading pupils' batteries: Impact of green spaces on cognition and wellbeing.' *International Journal of Environmental Research and Public Health 15*, 6, 1205.

Wang, D. and MacMillan, T. (2013) 'The benefits of gardening for older adults: A systematic review of the literature.' *Activities, Adaptation & Aging 37*, 2, 153–181.

Wang, W.-C., Wu, C.-C., and Wu, C.-Y. (2013) 'Early-life outdoor experiences and involvement in outdoor recreational activities in adulthood: A case study of visitors in Da-Keng, Taiwan.' *Journal of Quality Assurance in Hospitality & Tourism 14*, 1, 66–80.

Warber, S.L., DeHudy, A.A., Bialko, M.F., Marselle, M.R., and Irvine, K.N. (2015) 'Addressing "nature-deficit disorder": A mixed methods pilot study of young adults attending a wilderness camp.' *Evidence-Based Complementary and Alternative Medicine 2015*, 651827.

Watson, D., Clark, L.A., and Tellegan, A. (1988) 'Development and validation of brief measures of positive and negative affect: The PANAS scales.' *Journal of Personality and Social Psychology 54*, 6, 1063–1070.

Weathers, F.W., Blake, D.D., Schnurr, P.P., Kaloupek, D.G., Marx, B.P., and Keane, T.M. (2013) *The Life Events Checklist for DSM-5 (LEC-5)*. White River Junction, VT: National Center for PTSD. Accessed on 2/10/23 at www.ptsd.va.gov/professional/assessment/te-measures/life_events_checklist.asp

Wechsler, D. (2009) *WMS-IV: Wechsler Memory Scale: Administration and Scoring Manual*. New York, NY: Pearson.

Wells, N.M., Myers, B.M., Todd, L.E., Barale, K. *et al.* (2015) 'The effects of school gardens on children's science knowledge: A randomized controlled trial of low-income elementary schools.' *International Journal of Science Education 37*, 2858–2878.

Wen, Y., Yan, Q., Pan, Y., Gu, X., and Liu, Y. (2019) 'Medical empirical research on forest bathing (Shinrin-yoku): A systematic review.' *Environmental Health and Preventive Medicine 24*, 1, 1–21.

White, M.P., Pahl, S., Ashbullby, K., Herbert, S., and Depledge, M.H. (2013) 'Feelings of restoration from recent nature visits.' *Journal of Environmental Psychology 35*, 40–51.

White, M.P., Alcock, I., Grellier, J., Wheeler, B.W. *et al.* (2019) 'Spending at least 120 minutes a week in nature is associated with good health and wellbeing.' *Scientific Reports 9*, 1, 1–11.

White, R. (2012) 'A sociocultural investigation of the efficacy of outdoor education to improve learning engagement.' *Emotional and Behavioural Difficulties 17*, 13–23.

Whiteford, G. (2000) 'Occupational deprivation: Global challenge in the new millennium.' *British Journal of Occupational Therapy 63*, 5, 200–204.

Widmer, M.A., Duerden, M.D., and Taniguchi, S.T. (2014) 'Increasing and generalizing self-efficacy: The effects of adventure recreation on the academic efficacy of early adolescents.' *Journal of Leisure Research 46*, 2, 165–183.

Wildlife Trusts (n.d.) 'How to Make a Seed Bomb.' Accessed on 2/12/22 at www.wildlifetrusts.org/actions/how-make-seed-bomb

Wilkie, S. and Davinson, N. (2021) 'Prevalence and effectiveness of nature-based interventions to impact adult health-related behaviours and outcomes: A scoping review.' *Landscape and Urban Planning 214*, 104166.

Williams, I.R. (2009) Depression prevention and promotion of emotional wellbeing in adolescents using a therapeutic outdoor adventure intervention: Development of a Best Practice Model (unpublished doctoral thesis). University of Melbourne.

Williams, I.R., Rose, L.M., Olsson, C.A., Patton, G.C., and Allen, N.B. (2018) 'The impact of outdoor youth programs on positive adolescent development: Study protocol for a controlled crossover trial.' *International Journal of Educational Research 87*, 22–35.

Wilson, E.O. (1984) *Biophilia*. Cambridge, MA: Harvard University Press.

Winerman, L. (2005) 'Helping men to help themselves.' *Monitor on Psychology 36*, 7, 57.

Wiseman, T. and Sadlo, G. (2015) 'Gardening: An Occupation for Recovery and Wellness.' In I. Söderback (ed.) *International Handbook of Occupational Therapy Interventions*. New York, NY: Springer International.

Wolf, I.D. and Wohlfart, T. (2014) 'Walking, hiking and running in parks: A multidisciplinary assessment of health and well-being benefits.' *Landscape and Urban Planning 130*, 89–103.

Wong, D.L., Hockenberry-Eaton, M., Wilson, D., and Winkelstein, M.L. (2001) *Wong's Essentials of Pediatric Nursing* (6th ed.). Maryland Heights, MO: Mosby.

Woodward, A. and Wild, K. (2020) 'Active Transportation, Physical Activity, and Health.' In M.J. Nieuwenhuijsen and H. Khreis (eds) *Advances in Transportation and Health*. Amsterdam: Elsevier.

World Health Organization (2020) 'Physical activity.' Accessed on 30/11/22 at www.who.int/news-room/fact-sheets/detail/physical-activity

World Health Organization (2001) *International Classification of Functioning, Disability and Health.* Geneva: World Health Organization. Accessed on 13/3/23 at www.who.int/standards/classifications/international-classification-of-functioning-disability-and-health

Woy, J. (1997) 'Make your garden accessible.' *Country Journal*, February, 21–70.

Wyver, S., Tranter, P., Naughton, G., Little, H., Sandseter, E.B.H., and Bundy, A. (2010) 'Ten ways to restrict children's freedom to play: The problem of surplus safety.' *Contemporary Issues in Early Childhood 11*, 3, 263–277.

Xie, Q. and Yuan, X. (2022) 'Functioning and environment: Exploring outdoor activity-friendly environments for older adults with disabilities in a Chinese long-term care facility.' *Building Research & Information 50*, 1–2, 43–59.

Yamasaki, T., Yamada, K., and Laukka, P. (2013) 'Viewing the world through the prism of music: Effects of music on perceptions of the environment.' *Psychology of Music 43*, 1, 61–74.

Yao, Y.-F. and Chen, K.-M. (2017) 'Effects of horticulture therapy on nursing home older adults in southern Taiwan.' *Quality of Life Research 26*, 4, 1007–1014.

Yao, Y., Xu, C., Yin, H., Shao, L. and Wang, R. (2022) 'More visible greenspace, stronger heart? Evidence from ischaemic heart disease emergency department visits by middle-aged and older adults in Hubei, China.' *Landscape and Urban Planning 224*, 104444.

Yeo, N.L., Elliott, L.R., Bethel, A., White, M.P., Dean, S.G., and Garside, R. (2020) 'Indoor nature interventions for health and wellbeing of older adults in residential settings: A systematic review.' *The Gerontologist 60*, 3, e184–e199.

Yu, J.J., Capio, C.M., Abernethy, B., and Sit, C. (2021) 'Moderate-to-vigorous physical activity and sedentary behavior in children with and without developmental coordination disorder: Associations with fundamental movement skills.' *Research in Developmental Disabilities 118*, 104070.

Zamora, A.N., Waselewski, M.E., Frank, A.J., Nawrocki, J.R., Hanson, A.R., and Chang, T. (2021) 'Exploring the beliefs and perceptions of spending time in nature among U.S. youth.' *BMC Public Health 21*, 1, 1586.

Zarr, R., Cottrell, L., and Merrill, C. (2017) 'Park prescription (DC Park Rx): A new strategy to combat chronic disease in children.' *Journal of Physical Activity and Health 14*, 1–2.

Zebrack, B., Kwak, M., and Sundstrom, L. (2017) 'First Descents, an adventure program for young adults with cancer: Who benefits?' *Supportive Care in Cancer 25*, 12, 3665–3673.

Zijlema, W.L., Triguero-Mas, M., Smith, G., Cirach, M. *et al.* (2017) 'The relationship between natural outdoor environments and cognitive functioning and its mediators.' *Environmental Research 155*, 268–275.

Zimmermann, P. and Iwanski, A. (2014) 'Emotion regulation from early adolescence to emerging adulthood and middle adulthood: Age differences, gender differences, and emotion-specific developmental variations.' *International Journal of Behavioral Development 38*, 2, 182–194.

Subject Index

Sub-headings in *italics* indicate tables.

Author Index